Aspects of Nutritional Physiology

World Review of Nutrition and Dietetics

Vol. 56

Series Editor
Geoffrey H. Bourne, St. Georges, Grenada, West Indies

KARGER

Basel · München · Paris · London · New York · New Delhi · Singapore · Tokyo · Sydney

Aspects of Nutritional Physiology

Volume Editor
Geoffrey H. Bourne
St. Georges University School of Medicine, Grenada, West Indies

44 figures and 24 tables, 1988

KARGER

Basel · München · Paris · London · New York · New Delhi · Singapore · Tokyo · Sydney

World Review of Nutrition and Dietetics

Library of Congress Cataloging-in-Publication Data
Aspects of nutritional physiology / volume editor, Geoffrey H. Bourne.
(World review of nutrition and dietetics; vol. 56)
Includes bibliographies and index.
1. Nutrition. 2. Metabolism. 3. Chronic diseases – Nutritional aspects.
I. Bourne, Geoffrey H. (Geoffrey Howard), 1909 – . II. Series.
[DNLM: 1. Nutrition. 2. Physiology. W1 WO898 v. 56 / QU 145 A8385]
[QP141.A1W59 vol. 56]
612'.3 s – dc19 [599'.013] DNLM/DLC 88-8077
ISBN 3-8055-4785-4

Bibliographic Indices

This publication is listed in bibliographic services, including Current Contents® and Index Medicus.

Drug Dosage

The authors and the publisher have exerted every effort to ensure that drug selection and dosage set forth in this text are in accord with current recommendations and practice at the time of publication. However, in view of ongoing research, changes in government regulations, and the constant flow of information relating to drug therapy and drug reactions, the reader is urged to check the package insert for each drug for any change in indications and dosage and for added warnings and precautions. This is particularly important when the recommended agent is a new and/or infrequently employed drug.

Printed in Switzerland by Thür AG, Offsetdruck, Pratteln
ISBN 3-8055-4785-4

Advisory Board

Contents

Vitamin D: Experimental Research and Its Practical Application

Nutritional and Health Properties of Yogurt

Wld Rev. Nutr. Diet., vol. 56, pp. 1–42 (Karger, Basel 1988)

Nutritional Implications of Human and Mammalian Large Intestinal Function

N.I. McNeil

Department of Medicine, Faculty of Clinical Sciences, University College London, London, UK

Contents

Introduction

The importance of the large intestine in providing nourishment has long been recognised in monogastric herbivores. The horse, for example, has a capacious caecum and colon which act as a fermentation chamber for the bacterial breakdown of plant polysaccharides in a manner very similar to the rumen of ruminant animals. Animals that are omnivorous have been more recently re-assessed and in these animals the contribution of the large intestine to nutrition is now recognised as being substantial. Even the large intestine of man, which has been considered an organ for final absorption of salt and water from faeces and as a social convenience, is now recognised as an asset with nutritional potential, well able to support the small intestine.

Carbohydrate metabolism within the colon and the subsequent absorption of the major products of fermentation is the principal source of energy arising from the large intestine. A nitrogen pool that is particularly mobile exists and proteins can be metabolised so that they are available to the mammalian host. The fate of fat in the large intestine is poorly understood. Vitamin synthesis by the microflora is well known but the ability of the colon to absorb minerals is less widely appreciated.

This review will be biased towards knowledge about and pertaining to the human large intestine, with an assessment of the considerably broader experience of mammalian colonic function.

Carbohydrate Metabolism in the Colon

Sources of Carbohydrate

Both plant and animal foods contain carbohydrates. Plants contain carbohydrates of varying complexity and of differing properties whose purposes include energy storage, cell wall construction [217] and protection. Animal foods contain some storage polysaccharide and in milk there is a considerable amount of the disaccharide lactose. Mammals have the ability to digest only some of these many carbohydrates in the stomach and small intestine [91], the remainder passing into the large intestine.

Mammalian digestion and absorption of carbohydrate goes through the processes of luminal breakdown of starch and glycogen to oligosaccharides. These are subsequently hydrolysed at the brush border to monosaccharides. Glucose and galactose share an active transport system for absorption. Fructose is absorbed by 'facilitated diffusion'. Other hexoses and pentoses are absorbed much less rapidly by passive diffusion [135].

Starch digestion and absorption in the small intestine is variable. It is likely that the source of the starch, the maturity of the plant from which it is obtained and also whether degradation, such as cooking, has occurred will influence the amount of starch digestion. In ponies 40% of available carbohydrate passed into the large intestine: this is likely to be mainly starch [104]. It has been known for at least 35 years that much of dietary starch consumed by both ruminants and non-ruminants is not digested in the stomach and small intestine [12]. Potato starch seems to be resistant to mammalian digestion: in the pig with a re-entrant ileal cannula, 56% of dietary potato starch passes into the large intestine [57]. Starch digestion also varies in man. In people with an ileostomy, McNeil et al. [154] found only 1–2 g daily on a normal diet, and about 5 g of other sugars that may represent recently hydrolysed starch within the intestinal lumen. Studies examining more specific types of starch in ileostomists have shown that 1.3–5% starch from cooked (baked) potatoes was not absorbed [40] and that up to 90% of banana starch appeared in ileostomy effluent [76].

An alternative approach to measuring starch malabsorption involves terminal ileal intubation and measurements of amounts passing this region of the intestine after meals. When meals containing 20 or 60 g of starch were consumed, 9.3 and 6%, respectively, of the starch from one meal only was not digested and absorbed in the small intestine [226]. Indirect measurements of starch malabsorption have also been made using the quantitative breath hydrogen technique. Anderson et al. [4] studied various foods and estimated that 10–20% of a meal of white bread reached the right colon. Different foods were malabsorbed to different extents, rice starch being fully absorbed [4].

Simple sugars can also fail to be absorbed by the small intestine. Lactose is the best known example. In both rats and pigs 30% of dietary lactose passed the terminal ileum [133, 134]. Lactose malabsorption is well recognised in man and has been extensively studied, because of the symptoms produced and of the importance of dairy foods in some diets [48]. Other sugars can be malabsorbed and various small intestinal defects have been recognised including sucrose-isomaltase deficiency [146, 242], trehalase deficiency and glucose/galactose malabsorption [142]. Intestinal infection will reduce brush border disaccharidases [183] and, in some parts of the world, contribute to small intestinal malabsorption of sugars.

Non-starch polysaccharides in plants comprise cellulose, hemicellulose, gums and gels. The gastrointestinal tract of mammals is unable to hydrolyse these polymers and they pass intact into the large intestine. They represent the polysaccharides present in dietary fibre. These substances are principally components of plant cell walls [217] and thus are likely to protect cellular contents from digestion, by sequestering them from mammalian digestive enzymes. The quantities consumed by man vary greatly. The British diet contains about 20 g daily with a range of 8–32 g [21], and similar intakes have been reported from Scandinavia [125] and the USA [221]. In rural Sub-Saharan Africa estimates of dietary fibre intake are 5–8 times higher [20].

Clearly in omnivorous animals and particularly herbivores, the non-starch polysaccharides are a particularly important source of carbohydrate for the animals. Their metabolism holds the key to the success of the animal in its environment.

The final source of carbohydrate entering the colon is mucus. Colonic mucus is 85% carbohydrate (dry weight) [220], but the amount produced daily is not known. A small amount of mucus enters the colon from the stomach and small intestine. This was found to be of the order of 1 g daily be Stephen et al. [226].

Breakdown of Carbohydrate within the Colon

The carbohydrates that pass into the large intestine are subsequently metabolised there, evidence collected in several ways demonstrating this. Oligosaccharides are almost completely lost in passage from ileum to anus. In the large intestine of both rat and man, Bond and Levitt [27] found rapid metabolism of instilled ^{14}C-glucose and ^{14}C-sucrose with production of labelled carbon dioxide. One sixth of the radioactivity was recovered in faeces, the rest being metabolised and lost from the intestinal lumen. Similarly, studies have been carried out in patients having a jejuno-ileal bypass, that short circuits most of the small intestine [26]. After a 50-gram sucrose drink, 30–84% was not absorbed by the jejunum and ileum. Of the sucrose (and its monosaccharides) that entered the colon 50–60% did not appear in the faeces in any form [26]. Oligosaccharides, such as lactulose, resistant to mammalian enzymes undergo degradation in the large intestine in a similar manner [214].

Starch is also broken down by the microflora of the large intestine and this applies to readily digestible starch and to 'resistant' starch which is not digestible by mammalian enzymes [78].

Non-starch polysaccharides are also broken down in the large intestine, though the extent of the breakdown varies with the polysaccharides. Soluble non-cellulose polymers are readily broken down. Pectin is almost wholly metabolised [56] and so is isphaghula [187]. Pure cellulose is broken down to a lesser extent. In young men and women about 40% is lost, and about 50% is metabolised in the elderly [130]. This may reflect the purification process for cellulose, with highly purified products being less well metabolised than cellulose present in its normal state as a part of mixed carbohydrates [51].

Bacterial Metabolism of Carbohydrate

The physical conditions in the large intestine and the presence of a large microbial flora are very like those found in the rumen. The range of pH and redox potential are similar and oxygen tensions are very low in both organs [29, 36, 123]. Microbial counts are similar at 10^{11} to 10^{12} organisms/g, with well over 95% anaerobes [103, 123]. Under these conditions anaerobic fermentation of carbohydrate proceeds. The processes involved have been particularly well established for the rumen, because of the economic importance of domesticated ruminants. Similar processes are believed to occur in the mammalian large intestine.

In the rumen, extracellular microbial enzymes break down the complex carbohydrates to simple sugars. These are subsequently absorbed by the bacteria and metabolised further [163]. The pathways involved are shown in figures 1 and 2.

Cellulose and starch are broken down to glucose [138] which is taken up by the micro-organisms of the rumen and metabolised to pyruvate by glycolysis [13]. Hemicelluloses are hydrolysed to the constituent pentose and hexose sugars [121, 166, 249]. The pentoses are converted to hexose via the pentose phosphate pathway [178, 179], after which they undergo glycolysis. Pectins are hydrolysed to pectic acid then galacturonic acid and finally pentose sugars [120]. Pyruvate is metabolised by several pathways to short chain fatty acids (SCFA), lactic acid, hydrogen, methane and carbon dioxide [138].

Individual bacterial species in the rumen have specialised metabolism such that these pathways may involve reactions occurring in more than one species, the intermediate products being released by one bacterium and taken up by the next. For example, succinate is an intermediate in propionate production but is the limit for metabolism in *Bacteroides succinogenes* and the starting point in *Veillonella gazogenes* [25]. Individual cul-

1

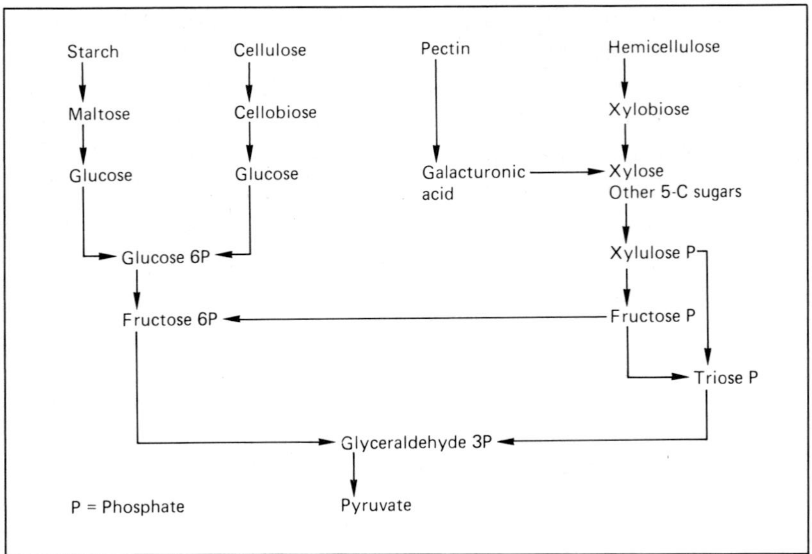

2

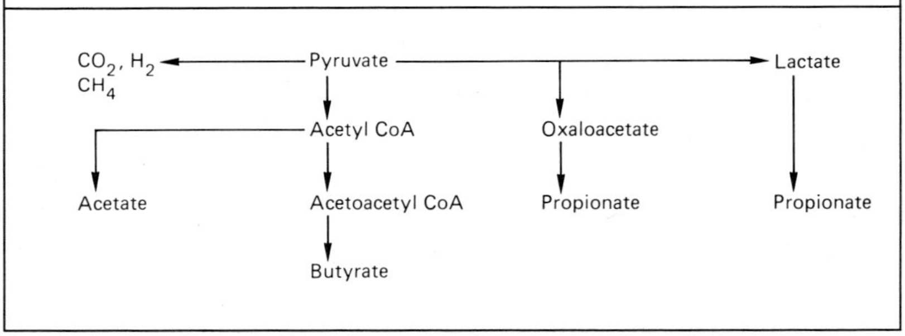

Fig. 1. Production of pyruvate from carbohydrate in the rumen.
Fig. 2. Metabolism of pyruvate to short chain fatty acids in the rumen.

ture studies show that most organisms produce acetic acid (acetate) but only one quarter each produce propionic and butyric acids [123]. This presumably accounts in part for the molar ratio of SCFA in the rumen of acetate 50: propionate 17: butyrate 8 [139, 213].

In the large intestine of man and animals a number of the resident bacterial species are able to ferment dietary residues, including pectin, hemicelluloses and cellulose [210]. Incubation systems set up to study the faecal and hence colonic microflora are able to ferment a variety of carbohydrates producing SCFA [29, 70, 252]. Finally, glycoprotein such as mucus can be degraded, indeed blood group glycoproteins are degraded by bacteria specific for the individual's blood group [109, 110].

An alternative approach to demonstrate fermentation is to measure the end products. Not only are hydrogen [140] and methane [141] produced but so are SCFA. In the human small bowel SCFA are at a low concentration, under 0.4 m*M* in the jejunum [41] rising to 3.7–7.7 m*M* in the terminal ileum [59, 169]. Faecal concentrations are much higher, up to 140 m*M* [5, 43, 54, 147] with a molar ratio similar to that found in the rumen [203, 257]. With hydrogen and methane occurring in expired air and flatus and SCFA appearing in the large intestinal contents as digesta pass, this all adds up to fermentation of carbohydrate occurring within the large intestine.

Short Chain Fatty Acid Absorption from the Large Intestine

The absorption of SCFA has been studied in at least 10 species [5, 8, 10, 73, 100, 128, 137, 155, 167, 168] and all absorb these acids. The three major acids, acetic, propionic and butyric, are all absorbed. The acids are absorbed in proportion to their concentration in the lumen [147, 205] and absorption is associated with the accumulation of bicarbonate within the lumen [10, 155, 205]. In man the absorption of SCFA in vivo exceeds sodium absorption from equimolar solutions over the whole large bowel [205] or a short length [155]. Sodium absorption appears to be stimulated by SCFA [201, 205]. Absorption rates at physiological luminal concentrations of 80–100 m*M* are remarkably constant, being 6–12 $\mu mol/cm^2/h$ for man [152, 155], 8–10 $\mu mol/cm^2/h$ in the pig [6] and 8 $\mu mol/cm^2/h$ in equine large intestine [8].

The mechanisms involved are incompletely understood and several have been put forward (fig. 3). Firstly, though the pK_a of SCFA is around 4.8 and therefore at colonic pH of 6.5–7.5 [160], the major part of the acids are going to be ionised, it is believed that both ionized and unionized acids are absorbed. Unionized acids are believed to be more rapidly absorbed as they are lipid-soluble [205]. Ionized SCFA can be absorbed in association with sodium. It is postulated that unionized acids are absorbed in relation to hydrogen ion and bicarbonate handling.

It has been put forward that a sodium-hydrogen exchange occurs when sodium is absorbed, the hydrogen ion subsequently combining with ionized SCFA prior to their absorption [7]. This will only account for that proportion of SCFA absorption that is equal to sodium absorption (fig. 3a). The excess, which matches bicarbonate 'secretion', has been

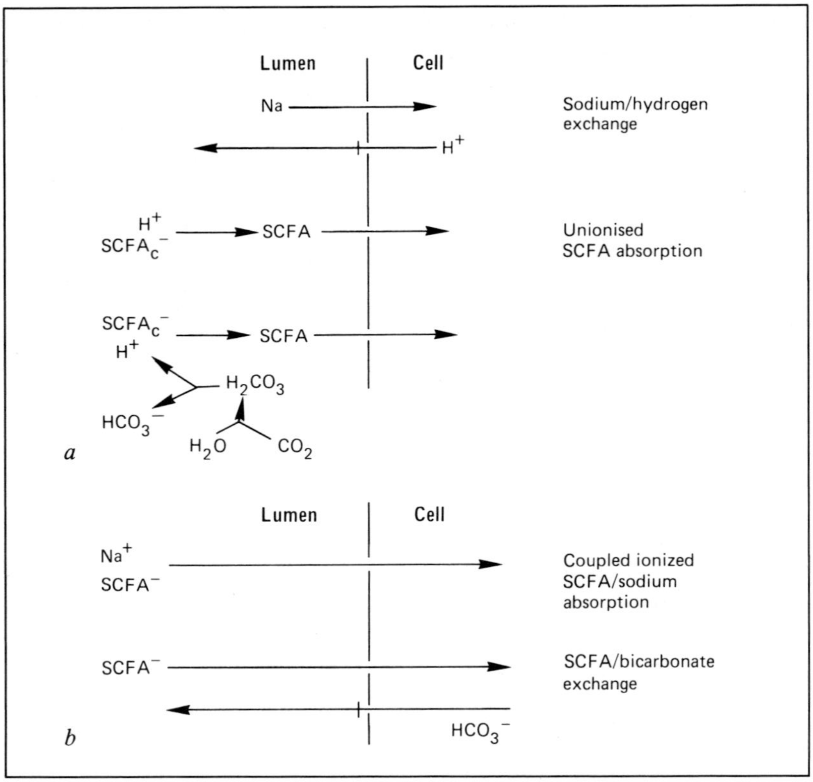

Fig. 3. Potential mechanism for absorbing short chain fatty acids.

ascribed to luminal production of bicarbonate and H^+ from carbon dioxide and water [205]. The H^+ will be utilized in SCFA absorption leaving an excess of bicarbonate in the lumen. This utilization of CO_2 for bicarbonate production will result in a fall in pCO_2 in the luminal fluid. However, this fall in pCO_2 has been reported for some species [10, 205], but not others [233]. An alternative mechanism for producing luminal bicarbonate would be a bicarbonate-SCFA exchange analogous to the bicarbonate-chloride exchange [65] (fig. 3b). Certainly the accumulation of bicarbonate is independent of chloride [156]. Arguments in support of bicarbonate-SCFA exchange include (1) similar absorption rate in the distal colon for chloride and acetate [148, 149], (2) the finding that the juxta-mucosal region of the large intestine has a pH 6.5 which is difficult to change and which will maintain the SCFA ionized at the cell surface [157], (3) no differences in absorption with respect to chain length and lipid solubility have been found as would be expected [149, 205].

The ability to present a consensus is made more difficult by suggestions that different species have different absorptive mechanisms and that different large intestinal regions may also differ in how SCFA are absorbed [73].

The fate of absorbed SCFA varies with species and with the acid. A major proportion of butyrate is metabolised in the mucosa of man [198] and guinea-pig [96] but lesser amounts in that of rat [202] and rabbit [97, 98]. Part of both the absorbed acetate and butyrate are converted to ketone bodies [97, 98], which pass to the liver. Hepatic extraction of butyrate is virtually complete [52, 184]. Propionate is variably metabolised (to lactate) by the mucosa and much passes unchanged to the liver where again extraction from portal blood is virtually complete [52, 184]. In ruminants propionate is very important for gluconeogenesis, but its importance in other animals is not properly known though recent evidence suggests a valuable place in the rat [195]. Acetate is present in arterial blood [184] and plays an important part in the aerobic metabolism of all cells. Nonetheless substantial amounts of acetate absorbed in the large intestine fail to pass the liver, where they must be presumed to enter the metabolic pool of acetate [184].

Because the breakdown of carbohydrate is undertaken in anaerobic conditions the microflora is able to obtain only a fraction of the potential energy available. For any quantity of carbohydrate in the lumen a very small fraction will be retained by bacteria for future energy supplies and for cell synthesis, the rest being metabolised for immediate energy requirements. In the rumen Hungate [123] has represented the metabolism of carbohydrate in the form:

$$58 \text{ mol hexose} \rightarrow 100 \text{ mol SCFA} + 60.5 \text{ mol } CO_2 + 33.5 \text{ mol } CH_4.$$

In the large intestine similar equations have been derived [50, 163]. The assumptions employed include hexose as the only carbohydrate source, SCFA, carbon dioxide, hydrogen and methane as the end products and that 1 mol hexose yields 4–5 mol adenosine triphosphate (ATP) by glycolysis [163]. This will tend to overestimate the energy yield slightly. The equation used is [163]:

$$34.5 \text{ mol hexose} \rightarrow 48 \text{ mol acetate} + 11 \text{ mol propionate} + 5 \text{ mol butyrate}$$
$$+ 23.75 \text{ mol } CH_4 + 34.25 \text{ mol } CO_2.$$

The amounts of SCFA yielded in some species will be considered below. Thus, SCFA, which are absorbed, will become an energy source for the animal and these calculations are used to estimate the energy produced by these metabolic and absorptive processes.

Species Differences in Carbohydrate Metabolism and the Energy Yielded

Aspects of the sequence, carbohydrate delivery to the large intestine, fermentation, SCFA absorption and the metabolic benefits obtained (fig. 4) will be discussed in this section.

Ruminants

In ruminant animals studies of the metabolic processes that occur in the rumen, their control and manipulation, have predominated. However, some attention has been accorded the large intestine too. Considerable quantities of carbohydrate are not digested in the rumen and pass to the large intestine. For example, Ulyatt and Macrae [232] found 28–31% of organic matter consumed passing the ileum. Though some passes intact through the entire gastro-intestinal tract, starch being present in reasonable quantities in ruminant faeces [243], about 10% of dietary intake is metabolised in the large intestine [232]. Both cellulose (3–30% of intake) and hemicellulose (7–34% of intake) are digested there [16]. Concentrations of SCFA are high in the rumen then fall as digesta passes along the small intestine [71, 173]. Within the caecum and large intestine SCFA concentrations rise to approximately the levels found in the rumen [31, 71, 173], though there was some variation with time after feeding [31].

Absorption of SCFA has been studied in the large intestine of sheep, goats and some inferences drawn from deer. In the sheep caecum Myers et al. [168] found that absorption varied with pH, falling as pH rose from 6.7 to 7.5. At the lower pH, chain length was also a determinant of absorption. Increasing the concentration of an acid increased its absorption and this was not inhibited by the presence of other SCFA [168]. They concluded that absorption was likely to be by passive diffusion. Rubsamen and Engelhardt [204] found that SCFA absorption was closely linked to hydrogen ion availability and that a change in the proportion of acetate and propionate in the infusate did not alter total SCFA absorption. In the goat it has been

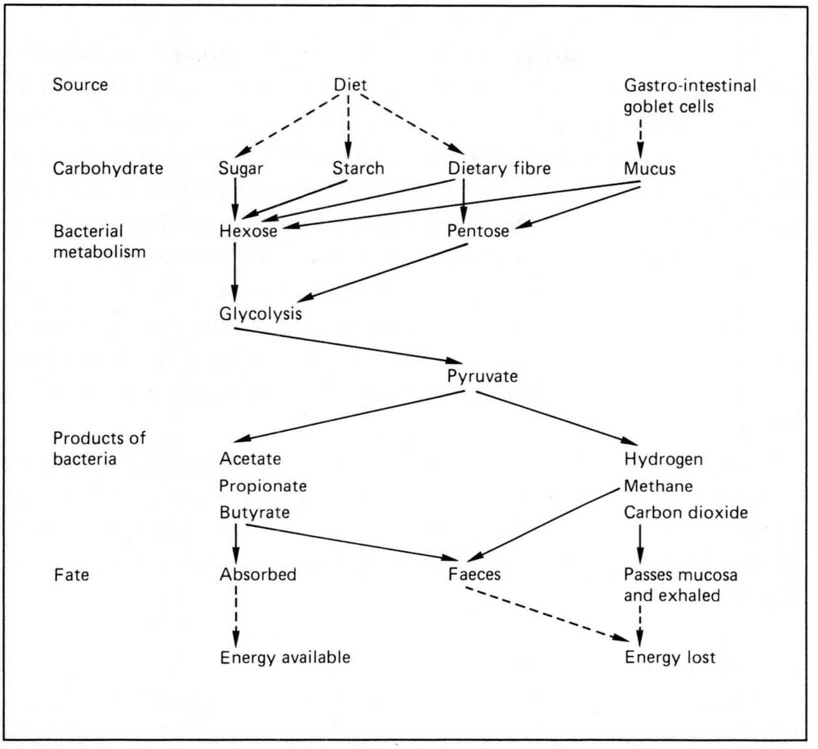

Fig. 4. Carbohydrate metabolism in the large intestine.

found that SCFA are rapidly absorbed with a profound influence on sodium and water transport [5]. The amount of the SCFA absorbed have been quantitated. In the sheep Faichney [80] used a continuous isotope infusion and estimated the mean production from the caecum alone to be up to 11.9% of total SCFA production for the whole animal. Similarly Allo et al. [3] arrived at 8% in the sheep and about 5% in deer.

SCFA (mostly from the rumen) are the most important energy source in ruminants, contributing 60–90% of all energy requirements [3]. Thus, the large intestine can provide about 8–10% [3, 80] when estimated by SCFA production in toto. When estimated in terms of energy intake Ulyatt and Macrae [232] found 4–9% of the energy consumed was lost in passage from ileum to faeces, matching other values ranging from 4 to 16% obtained previously [232].

Guinea-Pig

Studies in guinea-pigs have shown caecal SCFA concentrations to be in the range 45–100 m*M* with an acid pattern similar to the ovine rumen [96]. Cellulose was digested by caecal contents [144]. Absorption of acetate was more rapid in proximal than distal colon but propionate and butyrate absorption rates did not change when studied at perfusate pH 6.1 [191]. Changing luminal pH from 5 to 9 did not influence total absorption significantly in either proximal or distal colon [191], but clearance was increased in proportion to chain length in the distal colon [73]. Engelhardt and Rechkemmer [74] suggest that SCFA pass principally through paracellular pathways in proximal colon where size (the smaller the better) may be important, but in distal colon lipid solubility (the bigger the better) may be the major determinant of absorption.

Approximately 95–99% of SCFA produced in the colon are estimated to be absorbed there [73]. Absorbed butyrate is metabolised to the ketone bodies, acetoacetate and hydroxybutyrate, during passage through the mucosa [96]. No estimates of the energy contributed by these processes is available.

Beaver and Porcupine

Concentrations of SCFA in the caecum of the beaver amounted to 0.5 mEq/g of dry matter [106]. During passage through the large intestine concentrations fell so that very little SCFA was present in faeces. Unusually, butyrate was present at a higher concentration than propionate. It is wondered if this is related to the dietary intake of the beaver. About 30% of cellulose was digested and the absorbed SCFA estimated to contribute 19% of basal energy requirements [106].

In the porcupine Johnson and McBee [128] found a large caecum with SCFA present in the ratios acetate 74:propionate 12:butyrate 14. About 83% of acids produced there were absorbed directly from the caecum [144]. More was absorbed from the colon as concentrations fell as digesta passed caudally. About 16% of basal energy needs (range 5–33%) were estimated to be produced from the caecum in the porcupine [128, 144].

Horse

The horse is one of the most extensively studied monogastric herbivores. Some fermentation takes place in the stomach where SCFA concentrations rise to 20–40 m*M* but the most important site for microbial breakdown of carbohydrate is the large intestine [8]. There SCFA concentrations reach 90–140 m*M*, falling through the colon to 50-70 m*M* in distal colon [8], and about 50 m*M* in faeces [161]. Carbohydrate breakdown has been known for many years. Cellulolytic bacteria have been isolated [58] and total digestibility of cellulose may amount to 50% [131].

Absorption of SCFA has been studied in vitro and in vivo. In vitro absorption rates of 16–28 μmol/cm²/2.5 h were observed [8], a value comparable to rumen epithelium in vitro [227]. Acetate influenced the absorption of sodium, reducing it surprisingly [7]. Absorption seemed to be by passive non-ionic diffusion. In vivo falling luminal pCO_2 suggested that the process of absorption was [7]:

$$H_2O + CO_2 \rightarrow H_2CO_3 \rightarrow HCO^{3-} + H^+ + SCFA^- \rightarrow SCFA \text{ (absorbed)}.$$

The amounts of SCFA generated have been estimated in the caecum by addition of isotopically labelled acids. Glinsky et al. [88] found production rates of 3–5 mmol/min for acetate, about 1–2 mmol/min for propionate and 0.45–0.6 mmol/min for butyrate. They estimated 30% of digestible energy intake was represented by SCFA produced in the caecum. Another study has estimated daily SCFA production at 1.6 mol [9], faecal loss being about 75 mmol.

Rabbit

The rabbit has a complex large intestine of comparable size to the small bowel. Within this organ fermentation occurs producing concentrations of SCFA that reach 70–90 m*M* [177], and considerable breakdown of fibre occurs. Comparable studies in germ-free animals have shown reduced fibre metabolism [256]. Acetate and butyrate were absorbed from caecal sacs at rates that were not affected by changing pH from 6 to 7.4 [98, 137]. Absorption, however, could not take place against a concentration gradient [98]. During absorption in vitro considerable metabolism of the acids occurs in the gastro-intestinal wall, particularly from butyrate to produce ketone bodies and this mostly occurs in the proximal colon [97]. Butyrate metabolism to carbon dioxide occurred along the whole of the large intestine [97] indicating butyrate's potential as a mucosal energy source. In vivo it is believed that this ketone body production will be reduced [98].

A variety of methods have been used to estimate the contribution SCFA make to energy requirements. Early results suggest that 4–12% of maintenance energy came via SCFA absorption in the caecum [144]. In 1972, Hoover and Heitmann [107] considered that SCFA contributed at least 12% to energy needs. Using a radio isotope disappearance technique,

Parker [176] concluded that the caecum produced about 30% of maintenance energy requirements. He also demonstrated considerable inter-conversion between the acids, particularly of acetate to butyrate, within the caecum.

Rabbits practice coprophagy, thus improving their digestive efficiency. By day soft faecal pellets are passed and ingested and these contain more water, vitamins and protein than the hard pellets passed at night [99]. The concentration of SCFA is also higher in the soft, refected pellets being 170–290 μmol/g dry weight compared to 30–60 μmol/g at night. During the night it is estimated that 96% of the SCFA are absorbed during passage from caecum to rectum, but only 36% by day when gastric and small intestinal absorption can also be used [99].

Rat

A variety of studies have been undertaken on this omnivorous animal. Carbohydrate breakdown has been demonstrated in the caecum and colon. Glucose instillation into the large intestine resulted in a considerable excretion of labelled carbon dioxide in the expired air [27]. Germ-free animals did not demonstrate this phenomenon with glucose yet did with acetate instillation. Bond and Levitt [27] felt that insufficient oxygen was present to produce all this carbon dioxide so concluded that the glucose was metabolised to SCFA which were subsequently absorbed and metabolised. Fibre digestion dependent on an intact large bowel has been demonstrated too [68, 255]. Mucus carbohydrate is metabolised [112].

The concentration of SCFA in the caecum is high, being about acetate 100 m*M*:propionate 57 m*M*:butyrate 32 m*M* [194]. These concentrations fell with fasting and with passage down the colon. Dietary alterations or a small intestinal blind loop syndrome will alter the ratios of the SCFA [186, 229]. Though the rat colon is able to absorb hexose slowly [94, 230], it is likely that virtually all carbohydrates will be metabolised by the microflora. The SCFA produced are readily absorbed.

SCFA absorption is a passive process, the rate proportional to the concentration of the acids [5, 167]. At the same concentration acetate, propionate and butyrate are absorbed equally rapidly [15, 233]. Considerable quantities of bicarbonate appear in the lumen and this is thought to be the result of the exchange of ionized SCFA for bicarbonate or hydroxyl ions [15, 233]. The pCO_2 did not fall in studies of SCFA absorption [233]. Lowering luminal pH from 7 to a very unphysiological pH 2.9 increased absorption of acetate and simultaneously induced secretion of sodium, water and mucus [32]. The juxta-mucosal pH of the rat large intestine has been measured and found to be pH 6.5–7 [74, 157]. At this pH, SCFA will be almost wholly ionized.

The absorbed acids have various important roles. Firstly butyrate is the major energy source for colonic mucosal cells [199]. The metabolism of butyrate has been recognised for much longer [15, 194] but its importance only recently appreciated. Absorbed SCFA pass into the portal circulation and the liver then extracts about 75% of absorbed acetate and 85–90% of the propionate and butyrate that have been absorbed [195]. The propionate may be important in gluconeogenesis [195]. Rats on a high-fibre diet produced considerable quantities of SCFA in the proportion acetate 60:propionate 25:butyrate 15 [64]. On a high fibre diet, which had little or no glucose available for small intestinal absorption, arterial-portal glucose levels fell and propionate was a major source of gluconeogenesis. In rats weighing around 200 g portal blood carried 15 μmol acetate/min, 6 μmol propionate and 3 μmol butyrate to the liver [63b].

These sequential processes have been estimated to provide 10% of the animal's energy requirements, indicating the particular importance of the large intestine to the rat [254].

Pig

The pig colon is sometimes used as a model for the human colon. In this animal substantial quantities of carbohydrate pass the terminal ileum, including starch [57], lactose [134] and dietary fibre [211]. This carbohydrate is broken down [196] and the result is SCFA that are present at concentrations of 150–200 m*M* [44, 124], with molar proportions of acetate 66:propionate 22:butyrate 7 [211].

The SCFA are absorbed in vitro at a rate of 20–25 $\mu mol/cm^2/2.5$ h [6]. Absorption increases in more acid conditions with a change in pH 7.4–6.4 [49]. Total absorption amounted to 1.3 mEq of acetate per minute in perfusion studies, and it appeared that luminal hydration of carbon dioxide to produce hydrogen ions was an important factor [10].

Estimates of metabolisable energy yielded by this process have varied from 1.9 to 2.7% [196] upwards. Imoto and Namioka [124] measured SCFA production at 0.9–1 moles daily of which 0.7–0.8 mol were absorbed. This was calculated to yield about 10% of maintenance energy – an important amount in an omnivorous animal. The diet is important in determining the amount of energy produced [90]. A maize starch diet yielded 578 kcal in passage from terminal ileum to anus, 10.5% of the total

5,500 kcal absorbed by the whole gastro-intestinal tract [196]. However, 1,375 kcal out of 6,170 (22.3%) were obtained from a potato starch diet by metabolism and absorption in the large intestine [196]. This reflects the ability of the large intestine to augment small intestinal digestion and also the relative indigestibility of raw potato starch.

Man

The studies of Grove et al. [93] and Olmsted and Williams [244, 245] 50 years and more ago demonstrated the basic facts about SCFA and fibre breakdown in the human large intestine. However, their relevance has been largely ignored, the colon being considered as an organ where salt and water conservation is completed and as a basis for social convenience in regulating defecation [35]. Recently a gradual recognition of the complexity of large intestinal function and the interactions between microflora and host has occurred and will be discussed.

Carbohydrate intake in man reflects his omnivorous diet, with several novel carbohydrates also being ingested. The passage of carbohydrate to the large intestine has been studied using various techniques. Starch digestion varies with the vegetable source of the starch. Firstly measurements of starch excretion from the ileostomy of patients who were consuming their normal diet has yielded values in the range 1–2 g daily [154]. After specially prepared meals, losses of starch varied from 1 to 3% from cooked potatoes [40] and white bread [75], 4% from cornflakes [75] and up to 90% of that in uncooked bananas [76]. The extent and manner of cooking is also important as shown by Englyst and Cummings [77] who found starch malabsorption from potato to range from 3 to 12%. They have found some starch resistant to mammalian digestion in vivo and in vitro and it is known as 'resistant starch'. Both resistant and fully digestible starch are metabolised in the large bowel by the microflora, however [78]. Starch malabsorption has also been measured indirectly by a breath hydrogen technique with 10–20% of the carbohydrate of white bread escaping digestion [4], and up to 20% of starch from cooked potatoes also [231]. Direct measurements of starch passing the terminal ileum has yielded values of about 2–4 g when meals of 20–60 g of starch have been consumed [226].

Simple sugars have also been assessed in a similar manner. Ileostomists fed various foods absorb virtually all glucose [46, 76], fructose and sucrose [76]. Breath hydrogen studies have shown that large fructose loads (50 g) can be malabsorbed [189] as can lactose in normal (up to 8% of an oral lactose load) and lactose-intolerant people [28]. A study using terminal ileal intubation has shown that 2–4% of sucrose [26], but under 0.5% of lactose enters the colon [60], unless lactase deficiency is present when 20% or more of lactose is malabsorbed [60]. Lactulose is a synthetic disaccharide with a β configuration and hence resistant to human digestive enzyme degradation [83]. It and other poorly absorbed oligosaccharides including those of beans (stachyose and raffinose) pass unchanged into the colon [83].

Non-starch polysaccharides, usually referred to as dietary fibre, pass through the small bowel as well. Though Holloway et al. [105] found substantial breakdown in the small intestine, more recent studies have recovered these polysaccharides in or near their entirety at ileostomy stomas [46, 75]. Intakes of dietary fibre vary greatly from 13 g daily in Japan [136] to perhaps 150 g daily in Uganda [20].

Mucus represents a further source of carbohydrate for fermentation with its numerous side chains containing from 2 to 22 units of five different sugars [1]. The quantities of mucus secreted in the colon are not known. Some mucus enters from the small intestine and will also provide a source of carbohydrate for fermentation [226].

These various carbohydrates can be and are broken down in the colon. Starch is well metabolised, as shown by the rise of lactate and SCFA after it is instilled into the caecum at a time when faecal composition fails to change [84]. Similarly, sugars are broken down. Lactose, that failed to be absorbed in the small intestine and passed the terminal ileum, appeared in greatly reduced amounts in faeces [28]. People who have had a jejuno-ileal bypass for obesity absorbed 16–70% of an oral sucrose load in the small intestine. Of the sucrose entering the colon 58% was lost from the faecal stream [26].

Dietary fibre breakdown is now well established. Cellulose breakdown was described by Williams and Olmstedt [244] and confirmed by Hummel et al. [122]. Since then, measurements of cellulose breakdown in the human gastro-intestinal tract have ranged from 15 to 55% [222], through 43% [130] to 57% [164] on standard diets. When cellulose was added in amounts of up to 200 g to a diet, 70–75% was degraded [33]. Hemicelluloses are broken down [244] but to a greater extent, with 72–97% of pentosans being degraded in one study [222]. Similarly Ispaghula husk, a branched arabinoxylan, is almost completely degraded [187], as is pectin, a polyuronate [56].

Human large intestinal bacteria are capable of degrading these carbohydrates [208]. Starch led to an increase in the end products of fermentation [84], and was broken down in vitro [70, 102]. Simple sugars are also part of the culture media for intestinal bacteria [70], and their breakdown is well known [102]. Lactulose metabolism has been thoroughly examined [206]. The metabolism of non-starch polysaccharides has been reviewed by Salyers [207], and they are able to be broken down by many bacterial species. Finally mucus is also metabolised by bacteria [162, 236], and so are other glycoproteins [111]. If excess carbohydrate enters the colon lactic acid (lactate) becomes one of the major products of bacterial action, and concentrations rise in the stool [132, 241]. The lactate produced can be absorbed (both *d*- and *l*-isomers) but not as rapidly as SCFA [150].

Glucose absorption was long considered to take place in the normal large intestine and this led to the use of large intestinal infusions of glucose solutions for nutritional purposes. Though there was a slow loss of luminal glucose in a study 45 years ago, no rise in blood glucose was detected after the infusion [85]. This was examined again and Long et al. [143] found that $^{14}CO_2$ appeared after labelled glucose infusions. However, isotopically labelled glucose in the blood was particularly low. They concluded that the magnitude of the absorption was near zero and that the $^{14}CO_2$ was related to microbial activity, particularly as it disappeared on antibiotic treatment.

Concentrations of SCFA in the human large intestine attain values comparable to those found in the rumen and in the large intestine of other mammals. In the fasting small bowel concentrations are in the range <0.4 m*M* [41, 115, 116] to 2.5 m*M* [215], and in the terminal ileum concentrations of 0.2–4 m*M* for acetate have been described [169], values similar to those found in ileostomy effluent [75]. The concentration and distribution of SCFA in human faeces is summarised in table I. It would appear that concentrations of SCFA fall as more distal parts of the large intestine are examined [165].

SCFA absorption has also been studied. It is known to occur in the jejunum and ileum [59, 215, 216]. In the human large intestine a variety of techniques have been employed. A mixture of acids was instilled into the excluded colon of a patient and the acids were found to be absorbed at rates that increased with chain length [59]. An indirect method using a breath test for $^{14}CO_2$ was employed by Hoverstad et al. [117]. 50–80% of the instilled acid was recovered after placing labelled SCFA in the colon at colonoscopy.

Using a dialysis bag technique McNeil et al. [15] examined absorption in the rectum. Absorption of each of the three major acids, acetate, propi-

Table I. Short chain fatty acids (SCFA) and human faeces

Faecal loss of SCFA:	7–40 mmol daily [93] 7–20 mmol daily [54] 11 mmol daily [114]			
Individual acids:	Acetate 5.0 mmol daily [89, 114] Propionate 2.0 mmol Butyrate 1.8 mmol			
Total (range)	Acetate	Propionate	Butyrate	Reference
Faecal concentrations of SCFA, mmol/kg				
117 (79–164)	71	17	16	119
87–93	–	–	–	54
80.0 (61–120)	34	14	22	118
63.5 (32–92)	31	11	15	118
In vivo dialysis of faeces – concentrations of SCFA, mmol/kg				
	41	12	13	53
	46	17	15	203
	54	23	14	200

onate and butyrate, was established at a rate of approximately 8 μmol/cm²/h with a total concentration of 90–100 m*M*. Rates in more proximal large intestine comparable to animal studies were also found and these rates were up to 12 μmol/cm²/h [147, 152]. The rate of absorption in the rectum was related to concentration and for acetate and chloride an identical relationship between concentration and absorption rate was found [149]. SCFA were absorbed in the absence of luminal chloride without affecting the net absorptive rate [156] and no increase in absorption with respect to increasing chain length was found [159]. Bicarbonate accumulated in the lumen though calculations for change in pCO_2 based on bicarbonate and pH showed no consistent fall [147].

A perfusion technique examining propionate absorption found concentration-dependent absorption with a synchronous increase in luminal bicarbonate [205]. Again no increased absorption was found with increasing chain length. The rise in bicarbonate was associated with a fall in pCO_2 and the authors considered luminal hydration of carbon dioxide to bicarbonate to be the likely event [205]. In vitro colonic segments have been perfused [201] with solutions that contain 20 m*M* butyrate. The absorbed butyrate increased sodium absorption above control studies and were associated with a rise in bicarbonate secretion [201].

An attempt has been made by several authors to estimate the maximal absorptive capacity for SCFA. As well as absorptive rates measured by time some authors have measured absorptive rates using surface area. Those using time only, i.e. after total colonic perfusion, suggested 750–780 mmol daily [205]. Those using area produced rates of 8–12 μmol/cm^2/h [152, 155] but only estimates of colonic surface area exist, ranging from 1000 to 2000 cm^2 [17, 69]. Using the lower estimate for colonic surface area 190–290 mmol could be absorbed daily, but at the higher 380–580 mmol. In studies of SCFA absorption, sodium absorption was greatly exceeded by the acids that were absorbed from equimolar solutions [155, 205]. Daily maximum sodium absorption has been estimated and these estimates include 816 mmol [61, 175] suggesting that the figures derived above for SCFA absorption may be underestimates.

The amount of energy yielded by these processes has been studied on few occasions for man [50, 153, 246]. Though the potential energy sources are well recognised their quantitation is much more difficult. No data are available for the quantity of carbohydrate that passes the terminal ileum on a normal diet or on the amount of mucus carbohydrate secreted by the human colon. Indirect methods therefore have had to be employed to estimate fermentation, though the quantities of bacteria in the large intestine are now known [14].

The British diet contains about 20 g of dietary fibre [21], and about 5 g is present in the faeces daily [222], leaving approximately 15 g to be fermented each day. About 150–200 g of starch is consumed daily [23] and estimates of starch malabsorption vary up to 20%. At 10% this would produce 15–20 g more carbohydrate for fermentation. With a small amount of mucus glycoprotein this will amount to 30–40 g of carbohydrate that is fermented in the large intestine. Using the equation [163]:

34.5 mol hexose →
48 mol acetate + 11 mol propionate + 5 mol butyrate + methane + carbon dioxide,

about 3–400 mmol of SCFA could be generated. Faecal losses are small (table I). This will represent 6–9% of daily energy requirements (200 kcal). If the real malabsorption of starch is higher – e.g. 20% – then 12% of energy requirements will be provided by these large intestinal processes.

A second approach is based on the growth requirements of bacteria. Wolin [246] considered daily faecal bacterial loss to be 16 g dry weight. As the synthetic needs of bacteria amount to 1 mol ATP per 10.5 g dry weight, then 1.5 mol ATP are needed for this daily faecal loss. If 1 mol hexose yields 4 mol ATP then 350–400 mmol of hexose must be fermented. Using the same equation as above this would produce 650–700 mmol of SCFA. This is equivalent to 12–14% of energy requirements.

Using a variation of this approach [50] it was felt likely that 60 g of carbohydrate were fermented daily yielding about 600 mmol of SCFA. This is again equivalent to over 10% of daily energy requirements. Interestingly Ruppin et al. [205] estimated maximal possible yields from SCFA absorption at about 25%. It would appear that there is still surplus capacity within the large intestine to conserve energy.

Absorbed SCFA may also be an important link in explaining the 'energy gap' discussed by Grossklaus [92], and in explaining the role of the colon in salvage during small intestinal problems [190]. Further speculation into energy and diet in the Third World produces some interesting questions. Though faecal carbohydrate loss is not known in Uganda where dietary fibre intake may reach over 150 g daily, it is likely that substantial amounts are fermented. In addition the amount of fibre is likely to reduce starch absorption in the small intestine. What proportion of energy is likely to be provided by SCFA absorption under these circumstances? How important does large intestinal disease become? What happens to people with an ileostomy on a Third World diet, even though ileostomy adaptation may occur?

Nitrogen Metabolism

Nitrogen metabolism in the large intestine is complex and incompletely understood. Nonetheless it can be considered in the same manner as carbohydrate metabolism (fig. 5).

The sources of nitrogen are ileal discharge, urea breakdown and mucus, desquamated cells and intestinal enzymes. The quantity of nitrogen passing into the colon varies with the diet [37, 196], increasing if substantial quantities of vegetable matter are consumed. Most nitrogen is present as protein with only small quantities as amino acids [174]. Urea is also present but at concentrations comparable to blood levels [55, 86]. Mucus production by the colon has not been quantified. Chacko and Cummings [37] found just under 1 g of nitrogen in a day's ileostomy output when dietary nitrogen intake was minimal at 0.16 g, and this may help quantitate enzyme and mucus passage into the colon.

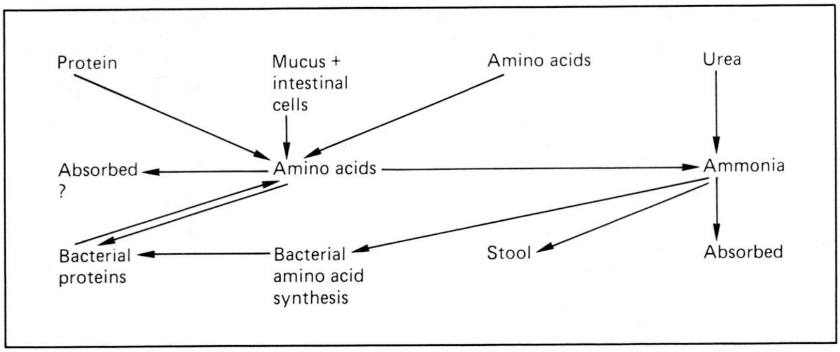

Fig. 5. Colonic nitrogen metabolism.

The large intestinal microflora is able to metabolise these various nitrogenous compounds. Protein breakdown is well recognised [101]. Though best described for the rumen microflora [38], it also occurs in the large intestine [193]. The amino acids produced have several potential fates. Firstly they can be utilized for bacterial protein synthesis [250]. Secondly, further bacterial metabolism can occur. This will produce ammonia and the carbon chain of the amino acid. For example leucine and valine will yield the SCFA isovalerate and isobutyrate which can be subsequently absorbed from the bowel [62, 235]. Amino acid could also be absorbed by the large intestinal mucosa [79, 197]. The ammonia produced is absorbed by the large intestine [34], or used for biosynthesis of amino acids that are subsequently incorporated into microbial protein [101].

Energy supplies within the colon greatly affect these various pathways. When abundant carbohydrate is present the microflora are able to use the various nitrogen compounds for protein synthesis themselves. However, as energy from carbohydrate becomes less then breakdown of nitrogenous products to produce energy will become dominant.

Urea hydrolysis is a more complex issue, well known to occur in relation to those parts of the gastro-intestinal tract containing microflora. The exact site and mechanism of urea hydrolysis remains unclear. In the rumen urea metabolism occurs in relation to the squamous epithelium [113] and it would appear that a mucosal or juxta-mucosal site accounts for large intestinal urea breakdown [2]. A substantial proportion of the urea synthesised each day is degraded to ammonia and carbon dioxide [247], the ammonia returning to the liver for ureagenesis.

Because of the many possibilities which exist in nitrogen metabolism within the large intestine, it is difficult to draw firm conclusions about the nutritional contribution of this luminal metabolic pool to the host. Nitrogenous products that are not absorbed are passed in faeces, and include principally microbial protein [224], ammonia [251] and some amines [172] with little free amino acid [174].

Though the effects of nitrogen metabolism will be reviewed in a similar way to carbohydrate metabolism, the information available for many animals is scanty. Only in man where hepatic encephalopathy is clinically significant have the more detailed studies been undertaken.

Ruminant Large Intestine

Nitrogen metabolism in the rumen is well understood, because of the economic value of supplying inorganic nitrogenous material which the microflora is able to convert into protein which can then be absorbed in the small intestine [101]. In the sheep Hecker and Grovum [95] found that ileal urea concentration was similar to blood levels. The gastro-intestinal tract in the sheep is an important source of urea degradation though this is likely to be mostly the rumen [45]. When sheep were fed four different diets some nitrogen conservation occurred in the large intestine [43]. Ileal flow varied from 4.1 to 5.9 g daily increasing with dietary nitrogen, but faecal loss was 3–3.6 g, so that 1–2 g were retained by the host animal. In a further study about 6% of dietary nitrogen was absorbed by the large intestine [218]. Carbohydrate is likely to be important, Ørskov et al. [171] described caecal starch infusion increasing faecal nitrogen from 5 to 9 g daily, presumably by encouraging bacterial growth.

Horse

The large intestine is an important (if not the most important) site for nitrogen absorption, with 30–50% of dietary protein being taken into the bloodstream there [192]. In this study the small intestinal absorption of protein was much less at 3–16%. Labelled bacterial protein introduced into the caecum is metabolised such that the tracer subsequently appears in caecal vein blood in two peaks [219]. The first peak consists of amino acids and ammonia at 1 h, the second of urea at 4 h [219]. The latter is presumably the result of labelled ammonia being incorporated by the liver into urea. Reitnour and Salsbury [193] found that after infusing protein into the caecum, nitrogen absorption was 83–98% of that obtained after feeding the same protein source orally. However, the nitrogen absorbed from the large intestine appeared more frequently as urea in the blood rather than in plasma protein fractions which occurred when the labelled nitrogen source was fed orally. This implies that the nitrogen is less readily available for protein synthesis after absorption from the large intestine. Most of the conservation of nitrogen occurs in the proximal colon [248].

Dog

The canine large intestine in vitro is able to absorb amino acids. Using animals in whom a small intestinal resection had been performed to induce greater absorption, Robinson et al. [197] found absorption rates to be one third of those of the small intestine: uptake seemed to be active and sodium-dependent in healthy dogs and similar results were found in mice but not rat, guinea-pig or man [197]. The canine large intestine has also been used for studying ammonia handling. Firstly, ammonia absorption occurs by passive non-ionic diffusion [185]. Secondly, in studies to determine the source of portal blood ammonia, 50% arose from the large intestine [240], of this two fifths came from urea metabolism, one tenth from glutamine metabolism and nearly one half from other sources [240].

Rabbit

A study comparing two diets, one supplemented with urea, showed no effect on growth as would occur in the ruminant [108]. In the gastrointestinal tract, the distal colon had lower concentrations of nitrogen, ammonia and amino acids than the caecum. Absorption of alanine and other amino acids was not able to be demonstrated in this study [108], and it was concluded that nitrogen conservation occurred by ammonia absorption with subsequent hepatic amino acid synthesis. In the rabbit coprophagy would be a useful and important source of amino nitrogen conservation.

Rat

Urea breakdown in the rat mostly occurs in the caecum where ammonia concentrations are much higher than in the ileum [63a]. Ammonia, produced from urea for example, is absorbed, and the absorption is enhanced by bicarbonate [82, 228]. Amino acids can also be absorbed in vitro though probably by passive processes [18, 79]. Dietary carbohydrate influences apparent nitrogen digestibility: potato starch reducing digestibility and increasing the proportion of bacterial protein in faeces when compared with rice starch or cellulose powder [158].

Pig

In common with other animals considerable quantities of nitrogen pass the ileum but are not found in the stool. This may amount to 25–38% of nitrogen for some wheats [126]. There has been a large variation in the extent of nitrogen metabolism found by different studies when the same diet has been consumed by the pig [196]. Furthermore, many variables affect faecal nitrogen excretion and presumably nitrogen metabolism within the large intestine. These have been shown to include fibre intake, starch intake, the type of starch and even the sugars eaten by the animal [196]. Though the pig is able to absorb microbial amino acids [170], Rerat [196] concluded that much of the nitrogen that is absorbed from the large intestine of the pig is poorly used for anabolic purposes, mostly appearing as urea. He felt that nitrogen supplied by these pathways was not efficient in nutritional terms [196].

Man

Because of the close relationship between the clinical consequences of hepatic encephalopathy (portosystemic encephalopathy) and large intestinal nitrogen metabolism [47], much more attention has been paid in man than animals to nitrogen metabolism and it has been the subject of recent reviews [237, 252].

Nitrogenous compounds passing the terminal ileum in ileostomists amount in total to 1–4 g daily [250]. The amount varies with dietary intake. When dietary protein was 75 g/day [22], 2.3–4 g of nitrogen was present in ileostomy effluent [39, 154], whereas on virtually protein-free diets under 1 g of nitrogen passed in the ileostomy effluent [37]. Studies of terminal ileal flow in healthy volunteers showed passage of 4–8 g of protein after single meals, whose protein content was not stated [225]. As well as protein, urea passes in ileal fluid. The concentration is similar to or slightly lower than that found in the blood [55] so that total amounts are likely to be under 1 g nitrogen daily [55]. Estimates of the contribution provided by mucus, shed epithelial cells and enzymes vary from 2 to 14 g daily [237].

The human colonic microflora is able to metabolise these various sources of nitrogen [145, 209, 237, 253]. Urea is known to be metabolised by many organisms and will be discussed below. Mucus breakdown is well recognised [209], and has been explored in some detail [109, 110]. The amino acids that result from this proteolysis are further metabolised or absorbed. They can be taken up by bacteria [237] and used for protein synthesis. Alternatively they are degraded by a variety of pathways to short chain fatty acids [101], ammonia [237], and various amines [129, 172]. Evidence that amino acids are absorbed by the human large intestine under normal conditions is lacking.

Ammonia has various roles in the ecology of the large intestine. Firstly it can be absorbed. Absorption appears to be passive, but pH-dependent, suggesting non-ionic diffusion as the principal mechanism of absorption [34, 67]. Non-ionic diffusion was felt to be about five times faster than ionic diffusion. Some studies have found only small changes in absorption rates when pH has changed [30], which may be explained by the finding of a pH microclimate near neutrality in the colon [157]. The absorbed ammonia seems to be used principally for urea synthesis, the extent of its nutritional contribution by the formation of amino acids in the liver being unknown [127]. Secondly, ammonia seems to be the preferred substrate for amino acid synthesis by some anaerobes [2].

Urea breakdown in relation to the gastro-intestinal tract, particularly the colon, amounts to about 20% of daily production [86, 238]. Because the colon seems to be relatively impermeable to urea [30, 247] the exact site and mechanism of this breakdown is under debate. The importance of this seems to have been thrown into relief by the recent study of Wrong et al. [253] who found that endogenous urea contributes little to faecal ammonia, a finding which matches that of Gibson et al. [87]. Clearly the lumen of the intestine is not the site of this urea breakdown, leaving the mucosa as the likely site.

In comparison to the variability of the amount of nitrogen that enters the large intestine, faecal losses are smaller and more constant. They average about 1–1.5 g [223] and about 60% is present as microbial protein [224]. The remainder is in partially destroyed bacterial components, ammonia and related to undigested dietary fibre. Faecal nitrogen is increased by feeding an energy supplement to the bacteria, for instance lactulose which gives a 2- to 3-fold increase [239]. When lactulose or dietary fibre are added to the large intestine [188] it must be assumed that the energy obtained by bacteria from the carbohydrate as SCFA are produced is used in part in cell division which requires the synthesis of protein.

In summary though the colon has the capacity for scavenging nitrogen and reducing faecal losses, the nutritional value of this is imprecise. Studies examining nitrogen metabolism in the colon under different dietary conditions may establish whether the nitrogen, principally absorbed as ammonia, can be used synthetically for human amino acid and subsequent protein synthesis, or is only used in the synthesis of urea.

Fat in the Large Intestine

Though the large intestine is able to absorb SCFA rapidly and medium chain fatty acids (octanoic acid) at a lesser rate [182], evidence that fat can be absorbed from the large bowel and then utilized is scanty. The amount of lipid passing the terminal ileum has not been well studied. Sambrook [211] found 10–25% of dietary fat passing an ileal re-entrant cannula but this was in studies which had faecal fat containing the equivalent of 7–42% of dietary fat intake. This is considerably more than occurs in normal human faeces. Human ileostomy fat losses were on average 5–7 g daily [154], with values over 6 g occurring in patients who have lost some of their small intestine. Mucosal lipid estimations have shown that when considerable quantities of fat enter the colon of man (steatorrhoea) mucosal lipid content is much increased [19]. Whether any is available for metabolism by the colonic epithelium cells or other tissues of the body is unknown. Most fat is likely to be present in the colon as calcium and magnesium soaps and probably unavailable for absorption.

Medium chain triglycerides may fill an intermediate role. In dogs and rabbits evidence of a relatively rapid absorption (under 30 min) of medium chain triglyceride by colonic epithelium exists [11, 66]. In the rat eight carbon acids and triglycerides can be absorbed from the caecum and the trioctanoate is partially metabolised within the caecum prior to absorption [238]. A single study in man was limited to the placing of medium chain triglyceride in the rectum, the least permeable region. Despite difficulties with keeping the mixture in the bowel up to 10% was absorbed from this short length of large intestine in 1 h [159].

Mucosal lipid may be added to luminal fat during passage through the large intestine and enter whatever metabolic pool of lipid exists there. Long chain fatty acids in the colon are metabolised to hydroxy-fatty acids and these induce intestinal secretion [250]. They may therefore negate any nutritional benefit obtained from fat by absorption.

One must conclude that, though interesting, any nutritional contribution from lipid in large intestine is speculative at best.

Vitamins and Minerals

Vitamin synthesis is one of the metabolic features of the large intestinal microflora and undoubtedly an important source in animals that practice coprophagy. In some animals administration of non-absorbable antibiotics leads to vitamin deficiency, an example being the development of biotin deficiency in rats [24].

Studies in man have shown that in some subjects it is very difficult to induce vitamin deficiency via dietary means. Examples include thiamine, riboflavine, biotin, folic acid and vitamin K which are presumably absorbed in adequate quantities after microbial synthesis. Other vitamins that are synthesised by the microflora but which do not appear to be absorbed by the mucosa include pyridoxine, niacin, riboflavine and vitamin B_{12}. The topic has been recently reviewed [250].

Studies of terminal ileal flow in man have been used to quantify salt and water absorption by the large intestine. Overall 1.5–2 litres of fluid enters the colon containing 190–280 mmol sodium, 100–240 mmol chloride and 8–15 mmol potassium. Average faecal losses are water 100 ml, sodium 3 mmol, chloride 1.5 mmol and potassium 10–15 mmol [72, 181, 250]. Thus net conservation of water in these electrolytes is equivalent to the daily oral intake [151].

In health calcium absorption occurs mostly in the small intestine though a proportion is absorbed from the colon normally [212]. However, dietary calcium restriction in vitamin D when given to rats stimulates colonic absorption of calcium [180]. Magnesium is mostly absorbed by the ileum and colon [42], a fact demonstrated by descriptions of magnesium poisoning following Epsom salt enemas [81].

Summary and Conclusions

The microflora in the large intestine anaerobically metabolises nutrients passing the terminal ileum. Carbohydrate metabolism is the most important in nutritional terms as anaerobic metabolism leaves end products, SCFA, that can be absorbed and used as an energy source. In many animals 10% and more of maintenance energy requirements are believed to be produced by this process. In man, it seems likely that a similar amount of energy is yielded. The nutritional potential of the process has not been fully explored and may represent a particularly valuable process in malnutrition. This concept needs further studies.

Nitrogen metabolism, along the same lines, recycles considerable quantities of nitrogen. However, the end product, ammonia, is much less readily utilizable in hepatic amino acid and protein synthesis. Therefore, the nutritional value of nitrogen metabolism is low, though in starvation potential benefits may be present. Again this is a topic that needs more examination. Fat, vitamins and minerals remain to be examined in detail.

References

1 Allen, A.: The structure of colonic mucus; in Bustos-Fernandez, Colon: structure and function, pp. 45–63 (Plenum, New York 1983).

2 Allison, M.J.: Biosynthesis of amino acids by ruminal microorganisms. J. Anim. Sci. *29:* 797–807 (1969).

3 Allo, A.; Oh, J.H.; Longhurst, W.M.; Connolly, G.E.: VFA production in the digestive systems of deer and sheep. J. Wildl. Mgmt *37:* 202–211 (1973).

4 Anderson, I.H.; Levine, A.S.; Levitt, M.D.: Incomplete absorption of the carbohydrate in all-purpose wheat flour. New Engl. J. Med. *304:* 891–892 (1981).

5 Argenzio, R.A.; Miller, N.; Engelhardt, W. von: Effect of volatile fatty acids on water and ion absorption from the goat colon. Am. J. Physiol. *229:* 997–1002 (1975).

6 Argenzio, R.A.; Southworth, M.: Site of organic acid production and absorption in the gastrointestinal tract of the pig. Am. J. Physiol. *228:* 454–460 (1975).

7 Argenzio, R.A.; Southworth, M.; Lowe, J.E.; Stevens, C.E.: Interrelationships of Na, HCO_3, and volatile fatty acid transport by equine large intestine. Am. J. Physiol. *233:* E469–E478 (1977).

8 Argenzio, R.A.; Southworth, M.; Stevens, C.E.: Sites of organic acid production and absorption in the equine gastrointestinal tract. Am. J. Physiol. *226:* 1043–1050 (1974).

9 Argenzio, R.A.; Stevens, C.E.: Cyclic changes in ionic composition of digesta in the equine intestinal tract. Am. J. Physiol. *228:* 1224–1230 (1975).

10 Argenzio, W.A.; Whipp, S.C.: Inter-relationship of sodium chloride, bicarbonate and acetate transport by the colon of the pig. J. Physiol., Lond. *295:* 365–381 (1979).

11 Bacques, C.; Dorier, A.: Etude expérimentale de l'absorption de glycérides chez le lapin et chez le chien par voie recto-colique. Annls pharm. fr. *31:* 665–677 (1973).

12 Baker, F.; Nasr, H.; Morrice, F.; Bruce, J.: Bacterial breakdown of structural starches and starch products in the digestive tract of ruminant and non-ruminant mammals. J. Path. Bact. *52:* 617–638 (1950).

13 Baldwin, R.L.; Wood, W.A.; Emery, R.S.: Conversion of glucose-C^{14} to propionate by the rumen microbiota. J. Bact. *85:* 1346–1349 (1963).

14 Banwell, J.G.; Branch, W.: Cummings, J.H.: The microbial mass in the human large intestine. Gastroenterology *80:* 1104 (1981).

15 Bar-Meir, S.; Ruppin, H.; Soergel, K.H.; Broor, S.; Wood, C.M.: Short-chain fatty acid transport by the rat colon in vitro. Gastroenterology *74:* 1005 (1978).

16 Beever, D.E.; Silva da Coelha, J.F.; Prescott, J.H.D.; Armstrong, D.G.: The effect in sheep of physical form and stage of growth on the sites of digestion of a dried grass. 1. Sites of digestion of organic matter, energy and carbohydrate. Br. J. Nutr. *28:* 347–356 (1972).

17 Billich, C.O.; Levitan, R.: Effects of sodium concentration and osmolality on water and electrolyte absorption from the intact human colon. J. clin. Invest. *48:* 1336–1347 (1969).
18 Binder, H.J.: Amino acid absorption in the mammalian colon. Biochim. biophys. Acta *219:* 503–506 (1970).
19 Binder, H.J.; Van Noorden, S.: The distribution of lipid in colonic mucosa. Proc. Soc. exp. Biol. Med. *131:* 1119–1123 (1969).
20 Bingham, S.; Cummings, J.H.: Sources and intake of dietary fiber in man; in Spiller, Kay, Medical aspects of dietary fiber, pp. 261–284 (Plenum, London 1980).
21 Bingham, S.; Cummings, J.H.; McNeil, N.I.: Intake and sources of dietary fiber in the British population. Am. J. clin. Nutr. *32:* 1313–1319 (1979).
22 Bingham, S.; Cummings, J.H.; McNeil, N.I.: Diet and health of people with an ileostomy. 1. Dietary assessment. Br. J. Nutr. *47:* 399–406 (1982).
23 Bingham, S.; McNeil, N.I.; Cummings, J.H.: The diet of individuals: a study of a randomly-chosen cross section of British adults in a Cambridgeshire village. Br. J. Nutr. *45:* 23–35 (1981).
24 Black, S.; McKibben, J.M.; Elvehjen, C.A.: Use of sulfaguanidine in nutrition experiments. Proc. Soc. exp. Biol. Med. *47:* 308–310 (1941).
25 Blackburn, T.H.; Hungate, R.E.: Succinic acid turnover and propionate production in the bovine rumen. Appl. Microbiol. *11:* 132–135 (1963).
26 Bond, J.H.; Currier, B.E.; Buchwald, H.; Levitt, M.D.: Colonic conservation of malabsorbed carbohydrate. Gastroenterology *78:* 444–447 (1980).
27 Bond, J.H.; Levitt, M.D.: Fate of soluble carbohydrate in the colon of rats and man. J. clin. Invest. *57:* 1158–1164 (1976).
28 Bond, J.H.; Levitt, M.D.: Quantitative measurement of lactose absorption. Gastroenterology *70:* 1058–1062 (1976).
29 Bornside, G.H.; Donovan, W.E.; Myers, M.B.: Intracolonic tensions of oxygen and carbon dioxide in germfree, conventional and gnotobiotic rats. Proc. Soc. exp. Biol. Med. *151:* 437–441 (1976).
30 Bown, R.L.; Gibson, J.A.; Fenton, J.C.B.; Snedden, W.; Clark, M.L.; Sladen, G.E.: Ammonia and urea transport by the excluded human colon. Clin. Sci. *48:* 279–287 (1975).
31 Boyne, A.W.; Campbell, R.M.; Davidson, J.; Cuthbertson, D.P.: Changes in composition of digesta along the alimentary tract of the sheep. Br. J. Nutr. *10:* 325–333 (1956).
32 Bustos-Fernandez, L.; Gonzalez, E.; Ledesmia, de Paolo, I.; Celener, D.; Ogawa de Furuya, K.: Organic anions induce colonic secretion. Am. J. dig. Dis. *21:* 329–333 (1976).
33 Canham, J.E.; Harding, R.S.; Consolazio, C.F.; Witt, N.F.: Gastrointestinal degradation of cellulose in the human. Fed. Proc. *24:* 314 (1965).
34 Castell, D.O.; Moore, E.W.: Ammonia absorption from the human colon. Gastroenterology *60:* 33–42 (1971).
35 Castro, G.A.: Digestion and absorption of specific nutrients; in Johnson, Gastrointestinal physiology, p. 126 (Mosby, St. Louis 1977).
36 Celesk, R.A.; Asano, T.; Wagner, M.: The size, pH and redox potential of the cecum in mice associated with various microbial floras. Proc. Soc. exp. Biol. Med. *151:* 260–263 (1976).

37 Chacko, A.; Cummings, J.H.: Effect of diet on nitrogen losses from the small bowel. Gut *27:* A619 (1986).
38 Chalupa, W.: Degradation of amino acids by the mixed rumen microbial population. J. Anim. Sci. *43:* 828–834 (1976).
39 Chapman, R.W.; Sillery, J.; Fontana, D.D.; Matthys, C.; Saunders, D.R.: Effect of oral dioctyl sodium sulfosuccinate on intake-output studies of human small and large intestine. Gastroenterology *89:* 489–493 (1985).
40 Chapman, R.W.; Sillery, J.K.; Graham, M.M.; Saunders, D.R.: Absorption of starch by healthy ileostomates: effect of transit time and of carbohydrate load. Am. J. clin. Nutr. *41:* 1244–1248 (1985).
41 Chernov, A.J.; Doe, W.F.; Gompertz, D.: Intrajejunal volatile fatty acids in the stagnant loop syndrome. Gut *13:* 103–106 (1972).
42 Chutkow, J.G.: Sites of magnesium absorption and excretion in the intestinal tract of the rat. J. Lab. clin. Med. *63:* 71–79 (1964).
43 Clarke, E.M.W.; Ellinger, G.M.; Phillipson, A.T.: The influence of diet on the nitrogenous components passing to the duodenum and through the lower ileum of sheep. Proc. R. Soc. B. *166:* 63–79 (1967).
44 Clemens, E.T.; Stevens, C.E.; Southworth, M.: Sites of organic acid production and patterns of digesta movement in the gastrointestinal tract of swine. J. Nutr. *105:* 759–768 (1975).
45 Cocimano, M.R.; Leng, R.A.: Metabolism of urea in sheep. Br. J. Nutr. *21:* 353–371 (1967).
46 Cohen, Z.; Wolever, T.W.S.; Thompson, L.U.; Jenkins, D.J.A.: Ileal losses of carbohydrate in man. Gastroenterology *84:* 1127 (1983).
47 Conn, H.O.; Lieberthall, M.: The hepatic coma syndrome and lactulose (Williams & Wilkins, Baltimore 1979).
48 Cook, G.C.: Tropical gastroenterology (Oxford University Press, Oxford 1980).
49 Crump, M.H.; Argenzio, R.A.; Whipp, S.C.: Effects of acetate on absorption of solute and water from the pig colon. Am. J. vet. Res. *41:* 1565–1568 (1980).
50 Cummings, J.H.: Short chain fatty acids in the human colon. Gut *22:* 763–779 (1981).
51 Cummings, J.H.: Cellulose and the human gut. Gut *25:* 805–810 (1984).
52 Cummings, J.H.; Branch, W.J.; Pomare, E.W.: Short chain fatty acids (SCFA) in human portal, hepatic and peripheral venous bloods. Gastroenterology *88:* 1358 (1985).
53 Cummings, J.H.; Hill, M.J.; Bone, E.S.; Branch, W.J.; Jenkins, D.J.A.: The effect of meat protein and dietary fibre on colonic function and metabolism. II. Bacterial metabolites in faeces and urine. Am. J. clin. Nutr. *32:* 2094–2101 (1979).
54 Cummings, J.H.; Hill, M.J.; Jenkins, D.J.A.; Pearson, J.R.; Wiggins, H.S.: Changes in fecal composition and colonic function due to cereal fiber. Am. J. clin. Nutr. *29:* 1468–1473 (1976).
55 Cummings, J.H.; Milton-Thompson, G.J.; Billings, J.A.; Misiewicz, J.J.: The flow rate and composition of ileal contents during fasting and in response to a liquid meal in man. Gut *17:* 817–818 (1976).
56 Cummings, J.H.; Southgate, D.A.T.; Branch, W.J.; Wiggins, H.S.; Houston, H.; Jenkins, D.J.A.; Jivraj, T.; Hill, M.J.: The digestion of pectin in the human gut and its effect on calcium absorption and large bowel function. Br. J. Nutr. *41:* 477–485 (1979).

57 Cunningham, H.M.; Friend, D.W.; Nicholson, J.W.G.: Observations on digestion in the pig using a re-entrant intestinal fistula. Can. J. Anim. Sci. *43:* 215–225 (1963).
58 Davies, M.G.: Cellulolytic bacteria in some ruminants and herbivores as shown by fluorescent antibody. J. gen. Microbiol. *39:* 139–141 (1965).
59 Dawson, A.M.; Holdsworth, C.D.; Webb, J.: Absorption of short chain fatty acids in man. Proc. Soc. exp. Biol. Med. *117:* 97–100 (1964).
60 Debongnie, J.C.; Newcomer, A.D.; McGill, D.B.; Phillips, S.F.: Absorption of nutrients in lactase deficiency. Dig. Dis. Sci. *24:* 225–231 (1979).
61 Debongnie, J.C.; Phillips, S.F.: Capacity of the human colon to absorb fluid. Gastroenterology *74:* 698–703 (1978).
62 Dehority, B.A.; Johnson, R.R.; Bentley, O.G.; Moxon, A.L.: Studies on the metabolism of valine, proline, leucine and isoleucine by rumen microorganisms in vitro. Archs Biochem. Biophys. *78:* 15–27 (1958).
63a Demigné, C.; Rémésy, C.: Evolution of the postnatal metabolism in the healthy or diarrhoeic calf. Ann. Rech. Vet. *10:* 23–31 (1979).
63b Demigné, C.; Rémésy, C.: Stimulation of absorption of volatile fatty acids and minerals in the cecum of rats adapted to a very high fiber diet. J. Nutr. *115:* 53–60 (1985).
64 Demigné, C.; Yacoub, C.; Rémésy, C.: Effects of absorption of large amounts of volatile fatty acids on rat liver metabolism. J. Nutr. *116:* 77–86 (1986).
65 Devroede, G.J.; Phillips, S.F.: Conservation of sodium, chloride and water by the human colon. Gastroenterology *56:* 101–109 (1969).
66 Dorier, A.; Perret, J.P.; Bacques, C.: Tolérance et conséquences métaboliques résultant de l'administration chronique de mélange de triglycérides saturés par voie recto-colique chez le lapin. Annls Nutr. Aliment. *30:* 549–579 (1976).
67 Down, P.F.; Agostini, L.; Murison, J.; Wrong, O.M.: The interrelations of faecal ammonia, pH and bicarbonate: evidence of colonic absorption of ammonia by nonionic diffusion. Clin. Sci. *43:* 101–114 (1972).
68 Dreyer, J.J.; Concannon, T.R.J.; Klerk, W.A. de: Digestibility of protein and dry matter in caecectomised and intact rats. S. Afr. med. J. *49:* 1661–1666 (1975).
69 Edmonds, C.J.; Pilcher, D.: Sodium transport mechanisms of the large intestine; in Burland, Samuel, Transport across the intestine, pp. 43–57 (Churchill, London 1972).
70 Edwards, C.A.; Duerden, B.I.; Read, N.W.: Metabolism of mixed human colonic bacteria in a continuous culture mimicking the human cecal contents. Gastroenterology *88:* 1903–1909 (1985).
71 Elsden, S.R.; Hitchcock, M.W.S.; Marshall, R.A.; Phillipson, A.T.: Volatile acid in the digesta of ruminants and other animals. J. exp. Biol. *22:* 191–202 (1946).
72 Emonts, P.; Vidon, N.; Bernier, J.-J.; Rambaud, J.-C.: Etude sur 24 heures des flux liquidiens intestinaux chez l'homme normal par la technique de la perfusion lente d'un marqueur non absorbable. Gastroentérol. clin. biol. *3:* 139–146 (1979).
73 Engelhardt, W. v.; Rechkemmer, G.: Absorption of inorganic ions and short-chain fatty acids in the colon of mammals; in Gilles-Baillier, Gilles, Intestinal transport, pp. 26–45 (Springer, Berlin 1983).
74 Engelhardt, W. v.; Rechkemmer, G.: Colonic transport of short-chain fatty acids and the importance of the microclimate; in Skadhauge, Heintze, Intestinal absorption and secretion, pp. 93–101 (MTP Press, Lancaster 1984).

75 Englyst, H.N.; Cummings, J.H.: Digestion of the polysaccharides of some cereal foods in the human small intestine. Am. J. clin. Nutr. *42:* 778–787 (1985).

76 Englyst, H.N.; Cummings, J.H.: Digestion of the carbohydrates of banana *(Musa paradisiaca sapientum)* in the human small intestine. Am. J. clin. Nutr. *44:* 42–50 (1986).

77 Englyst, H.N.; Cummings, J.H.: Digestion of polysaccharides of potato in the small intestine of man. Am. J. clin. Nutr. *45:* 423–431 (1987).

78 Englyst, H.N.; Macfarlane, G.T.: Breakdown of resistant and readily digestible starch by human gut bacteria. J. Sci. Food Agric. *37:* 699–706 (1986).

79 Evered, D.F.; Nunn, P.B.: Uptake of amino acids by mucosa of rat colon in vitro. Eur. J. Biochem. *4:* 301–304 (1968).

80 Faichney, G.J.: Production of volatile fatty acids in the sheep caecum. Aust. J. agric. Res. *20:* 491–498 (1969).

81 Fawcett, D.W.; Gens, J.P.: Magnesium poisoning following an enema of Epsom salt solution. J. Am. med. Ass. *123:* 1028–1029 (1943).

82 Feldman, G.A.; Cohen, R.M.; Stephenson, R.L.: Colonic ammonia absorption in vitro: dependence on bicarbonate secretion. Gastroenterology *88:* 1380 (1985).

83 Fleming, L.L.; Floch, M.M.: Digestion and absorption of fiber carbohydrate in the colon. Am. J. Gastroent. *81:* 507–511 (1986).

84 Flourie, B.; Florent, C.; Jouany, J.-P.; Thivend, P.; Etanchaud, F.; Rambaud, J.-C.: Colonic metabolism of wheat starch in healthy humans: effects on fecal output and clinical symptoms. Gastroenterology *90:* 111–119 (1986).

85 Garrer, A.H.; Groen, J.; Hallen, L.: The absorption of glucose from the human rectum. Acta med. scand. *107:* 1–10 (1941).

86 Gibson, J.A.; Park, N.J.; Sladen, G.E.; Dawson, A.M.: The role of the colon in urea metabolism in man. Clin. Sci. mol. Med. *50:* 51–59 (1976).

87 Gibson, J.A.; Sladen, G.E.; Dawson, A.M.: Protein absorption and ammonia production: the effects of dietary protein and removal of the colon. Br. J. Nutr. *35:* 61–65 (1976).

88 Glinsky, M.J.; Smith, R.M.; Spires, H.R.; Davies, C.L.: Measurement of volatile fatty acid production rates in the cecum of the pony. J. Anim. Sci. *42:* 1465–1470 (1976).

89 Gompertz, D.; Brooks, A.P.; Gaya, H.; Spiers, A.S.D.: Volatile fatty acids in the faeces of patients in 'germ-free' isolation. Gut *14:* 183–186 (1973).

90 Graham, H.; Hesselman, K.; Aman, P.: The influence of wheat bran and sugar-beet pulp on the digestibility of dietary components in a cereal-based pig diet. J. Nutr. *116:* 242–251 (1986).

91 Gray, G.M.: Carbohydrate absorption and hydrolysis; in Johnson, Physiology of the gastrointestinal tract, pp. 1063–1072 (Raven Press, New York 1981).

92 Grossklaus, R.: Energy gap? Nutr. Res. *3:* 595–604 (1983).

93 Grove, E.W.; Olmsted, W.H.; Koenig, K.: The effect of diet and catharsis on the lower volatile fatty acids in the stools of normal men. J. biol. Chem. *85:* 127–136 (1929).

94 Heaton, J.W.: Uptake of sugars by mucosa of rat colon. Am. J. dig. Dis. *17:* 7–16 (1972).

95 Hecker, J.F.; Grovum, W.L.: Absorption of water and electrolytes from the large intestine of sheep. Aust. J. biol. Sci. *24:* 365–372 (1971).

96 Henning, S.J.; Hird, F.J.R.: Concentrations and metabolism of volatile fatty acids in the fermentative organs of 2 species of kangaroo and the guinea-pig. Br. J. Nutr. *24:* 145–155 (1970).
97 Henning, S.J.; Hird, F.J.R.: Ketogenesis from butyrate and acetate by the caecum and the colon of rabbits. Biochem. J. *130:* 785–790 (1972).
98 Henning, S.J.; Hird, F.J.R.: Transport of acetate and butyrate in the hind-gut of rabbits. Biochem. J. *130:* 791–796 (1972).
99 Henning, S.J.; Hird, F.J.R.: Diurnal variations in the concentrations of volatile fatty acids in the alimentary tract of wild rabbits. Br. J. Nutr. *27:* 57–64 (1972).
100 Herschel, D.A.; Argenzio, R.A.; Southworth, M.; Stevens, C.E.: Absorption of volatile fatty acid, Na, and H_2O by the colon of the dog. Am. J. vet. Res. *42:* 1118–1124 (1981).
101 Hespell, R.A.; Smith, C.J.: Utilization of nitrogen sources by gastrointestinal tract bacteria; in Hentges, Human intestinal microflora in health and disease, pp. 167–187 (Academic Press, New York 1983).
102 Hill, M.J.: Metabolism of carbohydrates and glycosides; in Hill, Microbial metabolism in the digestive tract, pp. 31–41 (CRC Press, Boca Raton 1986).
103 Hill, M.J.; Drasar, B.S.: The normal colonic bacterial flora. Gut *16:* 318–323 (1975).
104 Hintz, H.F.; Hogue, D.E.; Walker, E.F.; Lowe, J.E.; Schryver, H.F.: Apparent digestion in various segments of the digestive tract of ponies fed with varying roughage-grain ratios. J. Anim. Sci. *32:* 245–248 (1971).
105 Holloway, W.D.; Tasman-Jones, C.; Lee, S.P.: Digestion of certain fractions of dietary fiber in humans. Am. J. clin. Nutr. *31:* 927–930 (1978).
106 Hoover, W.H.; Clarke, S.D.: Fiber digestion in the beaver. J. Nutr. *102:* 9–16 (1972).
107 Hoover, W.H.; Heitmann, R.N.: Effects of dietary fiber levels on weight gain, cecal volume and volatile fatty acid production in rabbits. J. Nutr. *102:* 375–380 (1972).
108 Hoover, W.H.; Heitmann, R.N.: Cecal nitrogen metabolism and amino acid absorption in the rabbit. J. Nutr. *105:* 245–252 (1975).
109 Hoskins, L.C.: Bacterial degradation of gastrointestinal mucins. II. Bacterial origin of faecal ABH(O) blood group antigen destroying enzymes. Gastroenterology *54:* 218–224 (1968).
110 Hoskins, L.C.: Ecological studies of intestinal bacteria: relation between the specificity of faecal ABO blood group antigen-degrading enzymes from enteric bacteria and the ABO blood group of the human host. J. clin. Invest. *48:* 664–673 (1969).
111 Hoskins, L.C.; Boulding, E.T.: Degradation of blood group antigens in human colon ecosystems. 1. In vitro production of ABH blood group-degrading enzymes by enteric bacteria. J. clin. Invest. *57:* 63–73 (1976).
112 Hoskins, L.C.; Zamcheck, N.: Bacterial degradation of gastrointestinal mucins. 1. Comparison of mucus constituents in the stools of germ-free and conventional rats. Gastroenterology *54:* 210–217 (1968).
113 Houpt, T.R.; Houpt, K.A.: Transfer of urea nitrogen across the rumen wall. Am. J. Physiol. *214:* 1296–1303 (1968).
114 Hoverstad, T.; Bjorneklett, A.: Short-chain fatty acids and bowel function in man. Scand. J. Gastroent. *19:* 1059–1065 (1984).

115 Hoverstad, T.; Bjorneklett, A.; Fausa, O.; Midtvedt, T.: Short-chain fatty acids in the small bowel bacterial overgrowth syndrome. Scand. J. Gastroent. *20:* 492–499 (1985).

116 Hoverstad, T.; Bjorneklett, A.; Midtvedt, T.; Fausa, O.; Bohmer, T.: Short-chain fatty acids in the proximal gastrointestinal tract of healthy subjects. Scand. J. Gastroent. *19:* 1053–1058 (1984).

117 Hoverstad, T.; Bohmer, T.; Fausa, O.: Absorption of short-chain fatty acids from the human colon measured by the $^{14}CO_2$ breath test. Scand. J. Gastroent. *17:* 373–378 (1982).

118 Hoverstad, T.; Carlstedt-Duke, B.; Lingaas, E.; Midtvedt, T.; Norin, K.E.; Saxerholt, H.; Steinbakk, M.: Influence of ampicillin, clindamycin and metronidazole on faecal excretion of short-chain fatty acids in healthy subjects. Scand. J. Gastroent. *21:* 621–626 (1986).

119 Hoverstad, T.; Carlstedt-Duke, B.; Lingaas, E.; Norin, E.; Saxerholt, H.; Steinbakk, M.; Midtvedt, T.: Influence of oral intake of seven different antibiotics on faecal short-chain fatty acid excretion in healthy subjects. Scand. J. Gastroent. *21:* 997–1003 (1986).

120 Howard, B.H.: Fermentation of pectin by rumen bacteria. Proc. Nutr. Soc. *20:* xxix (1961).

121 Howard, B.H.; Jones, G.; Purdom, M.R.: The pentosanases of some rumen bacteria. Biochem. J. *74:* 173–180 (1960).

122 Hummel, F.C.; Shepherd, M.L.; Macy, I.G.: Disappearance of cellulose and hemicellulose from the digestive tracts of children. J. Nutr. *25:* 59–70 (1943).

123 Hungate, R.E.: The rumen and its microbes (Academic Press, New York 1966).

124 Imoto, S.; Namioka, S.: VFA production in the pig large intestine. J. Anim. Sci. *47:* 467–478 (1978).

125 International Agency for Research on Cancer Intestinal Microecology Group: Dietary fibre, transit-time, faecal bacteria, steroids, and colon cancer in two Scandinavian populations. Lancet *ii:* 207–211 (1977).

126 Ivan, M.; Farrell, D.J.: Flow rates of components in digesta of pigs prepared with re-entrant cannulas in the proximal duodenum and terminal ileum, and fed semi-purified hard wheat, and soft wheat diets. Can. J. Physiol. Pharmacol. *54:* 891–897 (1976).

127 Jackson, A.A.: Amino acids: essential and non-essential? Lancet *i:* 1034–1038 (1983).

128 Johnson, J.L.; McBee, R.H.: The porcupine caecal fermentation. J. Nutr. *91:* 540–546 (1967).

129 Johnson, K.A.: The production of secondary amines by the human gut bacteria and its possible relevance to carcinogenesis. Med. Lab. Sci. *34:* 131–143 (1977).

130 Kelleher, J.; Walters, M.P.; Srinivasan, T.R.; Hart, C.; Findlay, J.M.; Losowsky, M.S.: Degradation of cellulose within the gastrointestinal tract in man. Gut *25:* 811–815 (1984).

131 Kern, D.L.; Slyter, L.L.; Weaver, J.M.; Jeffel, E.C.; Samuelson, G.: Pony cecum vs. steer rumen: the effect of oats and hay on the microbial ecosystem. J. Anim. Sci. *37:* 463–469 (1973).

132 Kern, F., Jr.; Singleton, J.W.; Struthers, J.E.: Fecal lactic acid in carbohydrate malabsorption. J. Lab. clin. Med. *64:* 874 (1964).

133 Kim, K.-I.; Benevenga, N.J.; Grummer, R.H.: Estimation of the fraction of the lactose in a high lactose diet available for fermentation in the cecum and colon of the rat. J. Nutr. *108:* 78–89 (1978).
134 Kim, K.-I.; Jewell, D.E.; Benevenga, N.J.; Grummer, R.H.: The fraction of dietary lactose available for fermentation in the caecum and colon of pigs. J. Anim. Sci. *46:* 1658–1665 (1978).
135 Kimmich, G.A.: Intestinal absorption of sugar; in Johnson, Physiology of the gastrointestinal tract, pp. 1035–1061 (Raven Press, New York 1981).
136 Kuratsune, M.; Honda, T.; Englyst, H.N.; Cummings, J.H.: Dietary fiber in the Japanese diet as investigated in connection with colon cancer risk. Ja. J. Cancer Res. (Gann) *77:* 736–738 (1986).
137 Leng, E.: Absorption of inorganic ions and volatile fatty acids in the rabbit caecum. Br. J. Nutr. *40:* 509–519 (1978).
138 Leng, R.A.: Formation and production of volatile fatty acids in the rumen; in Phillipson, Physiology of digestion and metabolism in the ruminant, pp. 406–421 (Oriel Press, Newcastle-upon-Tyne 1970).
139 Leng, R.A.; Leonard, G.J.: Measurements of the rates of production of acetic, propionic and butyric acids in the rumen of sheep. Br. J. Nutr. *19:* 469–484 (1965).
140 Levitt, M.D.: Production and excretion of hydrogen gas in man. New Engl. J. Med. *281:* 122–127 (1969).
141 Levitt, M.D.; Bond, J.H.: Volume composition and source of intestinal gas. Gastroenterology *59:* 921–929 (1970).
142 Lindquist, B.; Meeuwisse, G.W.; Melin, K.: Glucose-galactose malabsorption. Lancet *ii:* 666 (1966).
143 Long, C.L.; Geiger, J.W.; Kinney, J.M.: Absorption of glucose from the colon and rectum. Metabolism *16:* 413–418 (1967).
144 McBee, R.H.: Fermentation in the hindgut; in Clarke, Bauchop, Microbial ecology of the gut, pp. 185–222 (Academic Press, London 1977).
145 MacFarlane, G.T.; Cummings, J.H.; Allison, C.: Protein degradation by human intestinal bacteria. J. gen. Microbiol. *132:* 1647–1656 (1986).
146 McNair, A.; Gudmand-Hoyer, E.; Jarnum, S.; Orrild, L.: Sucrose malabsorption in Greenland. Br. med. J. *ii:* 19–21 (1972).
147 McNeil, N.I.: Short chain fatty acid absorption in the human large intestine; thesis, Cambridge (1980).
148 McNeil, N.I.: Bicarbonate production and anion absorption in the large intestine. Gastroenterology *79:* 1357–1358 (1980).
149 McNeil, N.I.: Human large intestinal absorption of short-chain fatty acids; in Kasper, Goebell, Colon and nutrition, pp. 55–58 (MTP Press, Lancaster 1982).
150 McNeil, N.I.: The absorption of lactate from the human large intestine; in Kasper, Goebell, Colon and nutrition, pp. 141–145 (MTP Press, Lancaster 1982).
151 McNeil, N.I.: Nutritional consequences of large intestinal function in health. Nutr. Hlth *2:* 111–114 (1983).
152 McNeil, N.I.: Differences in electrolyte handling through the human large intestine; in Skadhauge, Heintze, Intestinal absorption and secretion, pp. 111–116 (MTP Press, Lancaster 1984).
153 McNeil, N.I.: The contribution of the large intestine to energy supplies in man. Am. J. clin. Nutr. *39:* 338–342 (1984).

154 McNeil, N.I.; Bingham, S.; Cole, T.J.; Grant, A.M.; Cummings, J.H.: Diet and health of people with an ileostomy. 2. Ileostomy function and nutritional state. Br. J. Nutr. *47:* 407–415 (1982).
155 McNeil, N.I.; Cummings, J.H.; James, W.P.T.: Short chain fatty acid absorption by the human large intestine. Gut *19:* 819–822 (1978).
156 McNeil, N.I.; Cummings, J.H.; James, W.P.T.: Rectal absorption of short chain fatty acids in the absence of chloride. Gut *20:* 400–403 (1979).
157 McNeil, N.I.; Ling, K.L.E.; Wager, J.: Mucosal surface pH of the large intestine of the rat and of normal and inflamed large intestine in man. Gut *28:* 707–713 (1987).
158 Mason, V.C.; Palmer, R.M.: The influence of dietary carbohydrates and proteins on faecal nitrogen excretion in rats. Proc. Nutr. Soc. *32:* 82A–83A (1973).
159 Max, J.-P.; Rollin, P.; Drouin, P.; Debry, G.: Absorption rectale de triacylglycérols à chaînes moyennes chez l'homme. Gastroentérol. clin. biol. *6:* 581–584 (1982).
160 Meldrum, S.J.; Watson, B.W.; Riddle, H.C.; Bown, R.L.; Sladen, G.E.: pH profile of gut as measured by radiotelemetry capsule. Br. med. J. *ii:* 104–106 (1972).
161 Merritt, A.M.; Smith, D.A.: Osmolarity and volatile fatty acid content of feces from horses with chronic diarrhea. Am. J. vet. Res. *41:* 928–931 (1980).
162 Miller, R.S.; Hoskins, L.C.: Mucin degradation in human colon ecosystems. Fecal population densities of mucin-degrading bacteria estimated by a 'most probable number' method. Gastroenterology *81:* 759–765 (1981).
163 Miller, T.L.; Wolin, M.J.: Fermentation by saccharolytic intestinal bacteria. Am. J. clin. Nutr. *32:* 164–172 (1979).
164 Milton-Thompson, G.J.; Lewis, B.: The breakdown of dietary cellulose in man. Gut *12:* 853–854 (1971).
165 Mitchell, B.L.; Lawson, M.J.; Davies, M.; Kerr Grant, A.; Roediger, W.E.W.; Illmann, R.J.; Topping, D.L.: Volatile fatty acids in the human intestine: studies in surgical patients. Nutr. Res. *5:* 1089–1092 (1985).
166 Morrison, I.M.: The rate and products of degradation of xylans by rumen hemicellulases. Biochem. Soc. Trans. *3:* 992–994 (1975).
167 Mottaz, P.; Worbe, J.-F.: Transfert des acides gras volatiles dans la paroi du caecum isolé de rat. C.r. Séanc. Soc. Biol. *171:* 375–380 (1977).
168 Myers, L.L.; Jackson, H.D.; Packett, L.V.: Absorption of volatile fatty acids from the cecum of sheep. J. Anim. Sci. *26:* 1450–1458 (1967).
169 Newton, C.R.; Bennett, A.N.; Billings, J.A.; Milton-Thompson, G.J.: Ileal short chain fatty acid concentrations after a chemically defined meal. Archs Mal. Appar. dig. Mal. Nutr. *61:* 37C (1972).
170 Niiyama, M.; Deguchi, E.; Kagota, K.; Namioka, S.: Appearance of ^{15}N-labelled intestinal microbial amino acids in the venous blood of pig colon. Am. J. vet. Sci. *40:* 716–726 (1979).
171 Ørskov, E.R.; Fraser, C.; Mason, V.C.; Mann, S.O.: Influence of starch digestion in the large intestine of sheep on caecal fermentation, caecal microflora and faecal nitrogen excretion. Br. J. Nutr. *24:* 671–682 (1970).
172 Owens, C.W.I.; Albuquerque, Z.P.; Tomlinson, G.M.: In vitro metabolism of creatinine, methylamine and amino acids by intestinal contents of normal and uraemic subjects. Gut *20:* 568–574 (1979).

173 Packett, L.V.; Myers, L.L.; Jackson, H.D.: Gastrointestinal content and mucosal oxidation of volatile fatty acids in sheep. J. Anim. Sci. *25:* 402–405 (1966).
174 Padovan, W.; Owens, C.W.I.; Ferguson, R.: Creatinine and amino acid profiles of ileal and faecal fluids. Clin. Sci. *49:* 27P (1975).
175 Palma, R.; Vidon, N.; Bernier, J.J.: Maximal capacity for fluid absorption in human bowel. Dig. Dis. Sci. *26:* 929–934 (1981).
176 Parker, D.S.: The measurement of production rates of volatile fatty acids in the caecum of the conscious rabbit. Br. J. Nutr. *36:* 61–70 (1976).
177 Parker, D.A.; McMillan, R.T.: The determination of volatile fatty acids in the caecum of the conscious rabbit. Br. J. Nutr. *35:* 365–371 (1976).
178 Pazur, J.H.; Budovich, T.; Shuey, E.W.; Georgi, C.E.: The hydrolysis of xylan and xylooligosaccharides by ruminal enzymes. Archs Biochem. Biophys. *70:* 419–425 (1957).
179 Pazur, J.H.; Shuey, E.W.; Georgi, C.E.: The conversion of *D*-xylose into volatile organic acids by rumen bacteria. Archs Biochem. Biophys. *77:* 387–394 (1958).
180 Petith, M.M.; Schedl, H.P.: Intestinal adaptation to dietary calcium restriction: in vivo cecal and colonic calcium transport in the rat. Gastroenterology *71:* 1039–1042 (1976).
181 Phillips, S.F.; Giller, J.: The contribution of the colon to electrolyte and water conservation in man. J. Lab. clin. Med. *81:* 733–746 (1973).
182 Pihl, B.G.; Glotzer, D.J.; Patterson, J.F.: Absorption of medium chain fatty acids by the dog colon. J. appl. Physiol. *21:* 1059–1062 (1966).
183 Plotkin, G.R.; Isselbacher, K.J.: Secondary disaccharidase deficiency in adult celiac disease (non-tropical sprue) and other malabsorption states. New Engl. J. Med. *271:* 1033–1037 (1964).
184 Pomare, E.W.; Branch, W.J.; Cummings, J.H.: Carbohydrate fermentation in the human colon and its relation to acetate concentrations in venous blood. J. clin. Invest. *75:* 1448–1454 (1985).
185 Price, J.B.; Sawada, M.; Voorhees, A.B.: Clinical significance of intraluminal pH in intestinal ammonia transport. Am. J. Surg. *119:* 595–598 (1970).
186 Prizont, R.; Whitehead, J.S.; Kim, Y.S.: Short chain fatty acids in rats with blind loops. 1. Analysis of SCFA in small intestine, cecum, feces and plasma. Gastroenterology *69:* 1254–1264 (1975).
187 Prynne, C.J.; Southgate, D.A.T.: The effects of a supplement of dietary fibre on faecal excretion by human subjects. Br. J. Nutr. *41:* 495–503 (1979).
188 Rampton, D.S.; Cohen, S.L.; Crammond, V. de B.; Lilburn, M.F.; Rabet, J.Y.; Vince, A.J.; Wager, J.D.; Wrong, O.M.: Treatment of chronic renal failure with dietary fibre. Clin. Nephrol. *21:* 159–163 (1984).
189 Ravich, W.J.; Bayless, T.M.; Thomas, M.: Fructose: incomplete intestinal absorption in humans. Gastroenterology *84:* 26–29 (1983).
190 Read, N.W.: Diarrhoea: the failure of colonic salvage. Lancet *ii:* 481–483 (1982).
191 Rechkemmer, G.; Engelhardt, W. v.: Absorptive processes in different colonic segments of the guinea-pig and the effects of short-chain fatty acids; in Kasper, Goebell, Colon and nutrition, pp. 61–67 (MTP Press, Lancaster 1982).
192 Reitnour, C.M.; Baker, J.P.; Mitchell, G.E.; Little, C.O.: Nitrogen digestion in different segments of the equine gastrointestinal tract. J. Anim. Sci. *29:* 332–334 (1969).

193 Reitnour, C.M.; Salsbury, R.L.: Digestion and utilization of cecally infused protein by the equine. J. Anim. Sci. *35:* 1190–1193 (1972).
194 Remesy, C.; Demigne, C.: Partition and absorption of volatile fatty acids in the alimentary canal of the rat. Ann. Rech. Vet. *7:* 39–55 (1976).
195 Remesy, C.; Demigne, C.; Chartier, F.: Origin and utilization of volatile fatty acids in the rat. Reprod. Nutr. Dev. *20:* 1339–1349 (1980).
196 Rerat, A.: Digestion and absorption of carbohydrates and nitrogenous matters in the hindgut of the omnivorous nonruminant animal. J. Anim. Sci. *46:* 1808–1837 (1978).
197 Robinson, J.W.L.; Luisier, A.-L.; Mirkovitch, V.: Transport of amino acids and sugars by the dog colonic mucosa. Pflügers. Arch. *345:* 317–326 (1973).
198 Roediger, W.E.W.: Role of anaerobic bacteria in the metabolic welfare of the colonic mucosa in man. Gut *21:* 793–798 (1980).
199 Roediger, W.E.W.: Utilization of nutrients by isolated epithelial cells of the rat colon. Gastroenterology *83:* 424–429 (1982).
200 Roediger, W.E.W.; Heyworth, M.; Willoughby, P.; Piris, J.; Moore, A.; Truelove, S.C.: Luminal ions and short chain fatty acids as markers of functional activity of the mucosa in ulcerative colitis. J. clin. Path. *35:* 323–325 (1982).
201 Roediger, W.E.W.; Moore, A.: Effect of short-chain fatty acid on sodium absorption in isolated human colon perfused through the vascular bed. Dig. Dis. Sci. *26:* 100–106 (1981).
202 Roediger, W.E.W.; Truelove, S.C.: Method of preparing isolated colonic epithelial cells (colonocytes) for metabolic studies. Gut *20:* 484–488 (1979).
203 Rubinstein, R.; Howard, A.V.; Wrong, O.M.: In vivo dialysis of faeces as a method of stool analysis. iv. the organic anion component. Clin. Sci. *37:* 549–564 (1969).
204 Rubsamen, K.; Engelhardt, W. v.: Absorption of Na, H ions and short chain fatty acids from the sheep colon. Pflügers Arch. *391:* 141–146 (1981).
205 Ruppin, H.; Bar-Meir, S.; Soergel, K.H.; Wood, C.M.; Schmitt, M.G.: Absorption of short-chain fatty acids by the colon. Gastroenterology *78:* 1500–1507 (1980).
206 Sahota, S.S.; Bramley, P.M.; Menzies, I.S.: The fermentation of lactulose by colonic bacteria. J. gen. Microbiol. *128:* 319–325 (1982).
207 Salyers, A.A.: Energy sources of major fermentative anaerobes. Am. J. clin. Nutr. *32:* 158–163 (1979).
208 Salyers, A.A.: Breakdown of polysaccharides by human intestinal bacteria. J. environ. Path. Toxicol. *5:* 211–231 (1985).
209 Salyers, A.A.; O'Brien, M.: Cellular location of enzymes involved in chondroitin sulphate breakdown by Bacteroides thetaiotaomicron. J. Bact. *143:* 772–780 (1980).
210 Salyers, A.A.; Vercellotti, J.R.; West, S.E.H.; Wilkins, T.D.: Fermentation of mucin and plant polysaccharides by strains of Bacteroides from the human colon. Appl. environ. Microbiol. *33:* 319–322 (1977).
211 Sambrook, I.E.: Studies on digestion and absorption in the intestines of growing pigs. 8. Measurements of the flow of total lipid, acid-detergent fibre and volatile fatty acids. Br. J. Nutr. *42:* 279–287 (1979).
212 Sandstrom, B.; Cederblad, A.; Kivisto, B.; Stenquist, B.; Andersson, H.: Retention of zinc and calcium from the human colon. Am. J. clin. Nutr. *44:* 501–504 (1986).

213 Satter, L.D.; Esdale, W.J.: In vitro lactate metabolism by ruminal ingesta. Appl. Microbiol. *16:* 680–688 (1968).
214 Saunders, D.R.; Wiggins, H.S.: Conservation of mannitol, lactulose and raffinose by the human colon. Am. J. Physiol. *241:* G397–G402 (1981).
215 Schmitt, M.G.; Soergel, K.H.; Wood, C.M.: Absorption of short chain fatty acids from the human jejunum. Gastroenterology *70:* 211–215 (1976).
216 Schmitt, M.G.; Soergel, K.H.; Wood, C.M.; Steff, J.J.: Absorption of short chain fatty acids from the human ileum. Am. J. dig. Dis. *22:* 340–347 (1977).
217 Selvendran, R.R.: The plant cell wall as a source of dietary fiber: chemistry and structure. Am. J. clin. Nutr. *39:* 320–337 (1984).
218 Sklan, D.; Halevy, O.: Digestion and absorption of protein along the ovine gastrointestinal tract. J. Dairy Sci. *68:* 1676–1681 (1985).
219 Slade, L.M.; Bishop, R.; Morris, J.G.; Robinson, D.W.: Digestion and absorption of ^{15}N-labelled microbial protein in the large intestine of the horse. Br. vet. J. *127:* xi–xiii (1971).
220 Smith, A.C.; Podolsky, D.K.: Colonic mucin glycoproteins in health and disease. Clin. Gastroenterol. *15:* 815–832 (1986).
221 Southgate, D.A.T.: Chemical aspects (of dietary fibre); in Truelove, Heyworth, Topics in gastroenterology, vol. 6, pp. 13–38 (Blackwell, Oxford 1978).
222 Southgate, D.A.T.; Durnin, J.V.G.A.: Caloric conversion factors. An experimental reassessment of the factors used in the calculation of the energy value of human diets. Br. J. Nutr. *24:* 517–535 (1970).
223 Stephen, A.M.; Cummings, J.H.: The influence of dietary fibre or faecal nitrogen excretion in man. Proc. Nutr. Soc. *38:* 141A (1979).
224 Stephen, A.M.; Cummings, J.H.: The microbial contribution to human faecal mass. J. med. Microbiol. *13:* 45–56 (1980).
225 Stephen, A.M.; Haddad, A.C.; Phillips, S.F.: The effect of lactulose and dietary fiber on colonic metabolism of nitrogen. Gastroenterology *84:* 1323 (1983).
226 Stephen, A.M.; Haddad, A.C.; Phillips, S.F.: Passage of carbohydrate into the colon. Direct measurements in humans. Gastroenterology *85:* 589–595 (1983).
227 Stevens, C.E.; Stettler, B.K.: Transport of fatty acid mixtures across rumen epithelium. Am. J. Physiol. *211:* R264–271 (1966).
228 Swales, J.D.; Tange, J.D.; Wrong, O.M.: The influence of pH, bicarbonate and hypertonicity on the absorption of ammonia from the rat intestine. Clin. Sci. *39:* 769–779 (1970).
229 Thomsen, L.L.; Tasman-Jones, C.; Lee, S.P.; Roberton, A.M.: Dietary factors in the control of pH and volatile fatty acid production in the rat caecum; in Kasper, Goebell, Colon and nutrition, pp. 47–51 (MTP Press, Lancaster 1982).
230 Thomson, A.B.R.; McIntyre, Y.; MacLeod, J.; Keelan, M.: Adaptation of colonic uptake of hexoses and lipids following ileal resection: effect of variation in the fat content of the diet. Digestion *35:* 89–94 (1986).
231 Thornton, J.R.; Dryden, A.; Kelleher, J.; Losowsky, M.S.: Does super efficient starch absorption promote diverticular disease? Br. med. J. *292:* 1708–1710 (1986).
232 Ulyatt, M.J.; MacRae, J.C.: Quantitative digestion of fresh herbage in sheep. 1. The sites of digestion of organic matter, energy, readily fermentable carbohydrate, structural carbohydrate and lipid. J. agric. Sci. *82:* 295–307 (1974).

233 Umesaki, Y.; Yajima, T.; Yokokura, T.; Mutai, M.: Effect of organic acid absorption on bicarbonate transport in rat colon. Pflügers Arch. *379:* 43–47 (1979).
234 Valdivieso, V.D.; Schwabe, A.D.: Absorption of medium chain lipids from the rat cecum. Am. J. dig. Dis. *11:* 474–479 (1966).
235 van den Hende, C.; Oyeart, W.; Bouckaert, J.H.: Metabolism of glycine, alanine, valine, leucine and isoleucine by rumen bacteria. Res. vet. Sci. *4:* 382–389 (1963).
236 Vercellotti, J.R.; Salyers, A.A.; Bullard, W.S.; Wilkins, T.D.: Breakdown of mucin and plant polysaccharides in the human colon. Can. J. Biochem. *55:* 1190–1196 (1977).
237 Vince, A.J.: Metabolism of ammonia, urea and amino acids, and their significance in liver disease; in Hill, Microbial metabolism in the digestive tract, pp. 83–105 (CRC Press, Boca Raton 1986).
238 Walser, M.; Bodenlos, L.J.: Urea metabolism in man. J. clin. Invest. *38:* 1617–1626 (1959).
239 Weber, F.L.: The effect of lactulose on urea metabolism and nitrogen excretion in cirrhotic patients. Gastroenterology *77:* 518–523 (1979).
240 Weber, F.L.; Veach, G.L.: The importance of the small intestine in gut ammonium production in the fasting dog. Gastroenterology *77:* 235–240 (1979).
241 Weijers, H.A.; Kamer, J.H. van de; Dicke, W.K.; Ijsseling, J.: Diarrhoea caused by deficiency of sugar splitting enzymes. 1. Acta paediat., Stockh. *50:* 55–71 (1961).
242 Weijers, H.A.; Kamer, J.H. van de; Mossel, D.A.A.; Dicke, W.K.: Diarrhoea caused by deficiency of sugar splitting enzymes. Lancet *ii:* 296–297 (1960).
243 Wheeler, W.E.; Noller, C.H.: Gastrointestinal tract pH and starch in feces of ruminants. J. Anim. Sci. *44:* 131–135 (1977).
244 Williams, R.D.; Olmsted, W.H.: The effect of cellulose, hemicellulose and lignin on the weight of the stool: a contribution to the study of laxation in man. J. Nutr. *11:* 433–450 (1936).
245 Williams, R.D.; Olmsted, W.H.: The manner in which food controls the bulk of the feces. Ann. intern. Med. *10:* 717–727 (1936).
246 Wolin, M.J.: Fermentation in the rumen and human large intestine. Science *213:* 1463–1468 (1981).
247 Wolpert, E.; Phillips, S.F.; Summerskill, W.H.J.: Transport of urea and ammonia production in the human colon. Lancet *ii:* 1387–1390 (1971).
248 Wootton, J.F.; Argenzio, R.A.: Nitrogen utilization within equine lrge intestine. Am. J. Physiol. *229:* 1062–1067 (1975).
249 Wright, D.E.: Pectic enzymes in rumen protozoa. Archs Biochem. Biophys. *86:* 251–254 (1960).
250 Wrong, O.M.; Edmonds, C.J.; Chadwick, V.S.: The large intestine: its role in mammalion nutrition and homeostasis (MTP Press, Lancaster 1981).
251 Wrong, O.M.; Metcalfe-Gibson, A.; Morrison, R.B.I.; Ng, S.T.; Howard, A.V.: In vivo dialysis of faeces as a method of stool analysis. 1. Technique and results in normal subjects. Clin. Sci. *28:* 357–375 (1965).
252 Wrong, O.M.; Vince, A.: Urea and ammonia metabolism in the human large intestine. Proc. Nutr. Soc. *43:* 77–86 (1984).
253 Wrong, O.M.; Vince, A.J.; Waterlow, J.C.: The contribution of endogenous urea to faecal ammonia in man, determined by ^{15}N labelling of plasma urea. Clin. Sci. *68:* 193–199 (1985).

254 Yang, M.G.; Manoharan, K.; Mickelsen, O.: Nutritional contribution of volatile fatty acids from the cecum of rats. J. Nutr. *100:* 545–550 (1970).
255 Yang, M.G.; Manoharan, K.; Young, A.K.: Influence of degradation of dietary cellulose in cecum of rats. J. Nutr. *97:* 260–263 (1969).
256 Yoshida, T.; Pleasants, J.R.; Reddy, B.S.; Wostmann, B.S.: Efficiency of digestion in germ-free and conventional rabbits. Br. J. Nutr. *22:* 723–737 (1968).
257 Zijlstra, J.B.; Beukema, J.; Wolthers, B.G.; Byrne, B.M.; Groen, A.; Dankert, J.: Pretreatment methods prior to gas chromatographic analysis of volatile fatty acids from faecal samples. Clinica chim. Acta *78:* 243–250 (1977).

N.I. McNeil, MD, MA, MRCP, Department of Medicine,
Faculty of Clinical Sciences, The Rayne Institute,
University Street, London WC1E 6JJ (UK)

Wld Rev. Nutr. Diet., vol. 56, pp. 43–55 (Karger, Basel 1988)

Nutrition and Respiration

Michael M. Rothkopf, Jeffrey Askanazi

Medical Service, Veterans Administration Medical Center, East Orange, N.J.;
Department of Anesthesiology, Albert Einstein College of Medicine,
Bronx, N.Y., USA

Contents

Malnutrition may either be a cause or consequence of ventilatory impairment. An awareness of the relationship between nutritional status and pulmonary function has clinical relevance for the treatment of chronic lung disease and the management of critical illness.

Malnutrition as a Cause of Chronic Lung Disease

The impact of protein/calorie deficiency on lung function has been studied in both the laboratory and clinical environments. The relationship of malnutrition to the development of chronic lung disease has been addressed in a number of studies. The first, a study of prolonged fasting in normal volunteers by Benedict et al. [1] examined the physiological effects produced by a restricted diet that resulted in a 10% weight loss. In that experiment, basal metabolic rate declined some 15–20%. Oxygen consumption declined by a mean of 18% and minute ventilation by 12%. The minute volume decrease was produced by reductions of both respiratory rate and tidal volume. It was not accompanied by a rise in PCO_2, however, suggesting that the ventilatory drive was adjusted based on CO_2 production rather than O_2 consumption.

The second major study of starvation was performed during the tragic conditions of the Warsaw Ghetto during World War II [2]. The Jewish physicians within the ghetto recorded the observations made on themselves and their starving patients with attention to the physiologic and pathologic sequelae of their internment. They described a series of clinical events which was termed hunger disease. Weight loss greater than 50% of preinternment weight was associated with three progressive degrees of illness: (1) fat depletion; (2) withering, and (3) terminal cachexia.

Advanced hunger disease was characterized metabolically by a decreased basal metabolic rate (BMR), respiratory quotient (RQ) and impaired glucose metabolism. The respiratory system was found to be significantly affected. Decreases in diaphragmatic excursion, minute ventilation, respiratory rate and the depth of ventilation were observed. There was an increased incidence of bronchitis, pneumonia, and TB. On autopsy a striking incidence of emphysema was found in young adult patients.

The development of emphysema in young patients without known risk factors deserves further attention. Unfortunately, much of the work performed by the Warsaw Ghetto physicians has been lost and only a piecemeal accounting exists. No record of pulmonary function or exercise tolerance was found. However, autopsy material was prepared and reported on by Drs. Joseph Stein and Henryk Fenigstein. They stated that of 370 cases where detailed lung study was conducted 50 (13.8%) revealed emphysema. Twenty of these cases were patients under 40 years of age. The pathologists stated: 'Although the changes were present mostly in young adults they resembled those of emphysema of old age.' Histology was performed in only five of these cases and each of these showed emphysematous changes.

The classic study of Keys et al. [3] in which subjects underwent a 24-week period of semistarvation reaffirms the findings of the other two studies in relation to decreased minute ventilation, tidal volume and respiratory rate coincident with malnutrition. Keys et al. [3] also demonstrated that these subjects exhibited diminished respiratory efficiency during work. These three studies of essentially normal individuals subjected to a spectrum of malnutrition from fasting to death by starvation provide the foundation for the study of malnutrition and chronic lung disease. In each, calorie deprivation was associated with a decrease in minute ventilation, tidal volume, and respiratory rate. When allowed to continue, malnutrition led to an increased incidence of pulmonary infections and eventually to the premature development of chronic lung disease. We will examine a number of possible explanations for this relationship.

Lung Expansion. Since a decreased minute ventilation has been uniformly reported in malnutrition, this might contribute to the development of lung disease. A decline in minute ventilation, tidal volume, and respiratory rate reduces total lung expansion. As lung segments must be expanded periodically to prevent atelectasis, it is conceivable that the reduction in tidal volume and respiratory rate would promote the development of atelectasis, and eventually segmental collapse in the lung. This reduces the available functional airway, increasing the physiologic shunt. Since anatomic dead space remains unchanged, the efficiency of ventilation would be reduced. This results in an increased work of breathing which increases energy consumption by the respiratory muscles.

Atelectasis and segmental collapse generally progress to pneumonia if not reversed. Since malnourished individuals are known to have deficiencies in cellular and humoral immunity, such pulmonary infections could be particularly severe. Thus, the simple reduction in lung expansion occurring as a consequence of malnutrition can have far-reaching effects of respiratory physiology and disease.

Malnutrition has other effects on both the lung parenchyma and the respiratory muscles. Parenchymal effects of malnutrition include: alterations of the injury and repair process, insufficient protein, collagen and surfactant synthesis, abnormal alveolar defenses, and abnormal prostaglandin and leukotriene metabolism. Respiratory muscle alterations relate to changes in energy consumption and metabolism.

Injury and Repair. The reported alterations in the lung's injury and repair process in malnourished patients pose a serious threat to the delicate lung infrastructure. By disrupting the balance of protein breakdown and resynthesis, such changes have the potential to induce chronic lung disease.

The lung matrix is a dynamic structure which is constantly undergoing removal and replacement of elastin and collagen. Proteinases and collagenases remove damaged elastin, fibronectin, and collagen. This proteolytic activity is kept in check by counterbalance systems such as the anti-proteinase, α_1-antitrypsin. This balance insures that only a graded amount of

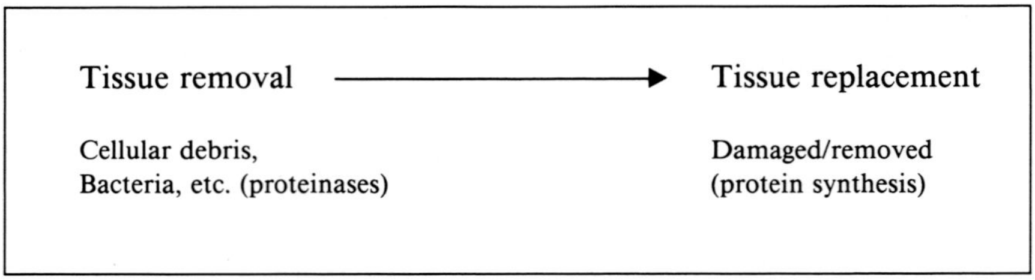

Fig. 1. Tissue equilibrium in the lung. Following infection or inflammation, enzyme activation occurs, removing dead tissue and bacteria. These enzymes are kept in check by circulating antiproteinases (e.g. α_1-antitrypsin) so that protein removal is limited to the area of injury. After removal, tissue replacement occurs.

tissue breakdown occurs. Elastin and collagen synthesis is then promptly activated to restore the structural integrity.

In malnutrition, both sides of this equation are abnormal (fig. 1). Neutrophil migration and elastase activity is increased resulting in an increase in proteolytic activity. The circulating antiproteinases are depleted. This is probably because, like other circulating proteins in starvation, they are consumed as fuel. Instead of a graded, controlled removal of damaged matrix, unopposed destructive activity ensues. Normally, such enhanced destruction would be matched by increased synthesis of elastin, collagen and the other elements of the lung matrix. However, in malnutrition protein synthesis and fibril cross-linking are impaired, resulting in a weakened and structurally abnormal lung matrix.

Airway Compliance. The abnormalities in injury and repair do not fully explain the changes in lung mechanics observed in malnutrition. Sahebjami [9, 10] and others have described changes in surface recoil in malnourished laboratory animals. Lung pressure-volume curves become abnormal during malnutrition and are restored after refeeding. This is apparently related to a decrease in the production of pulmonary surfactant, which has been shown to decline with malnutrition.

Surfactant, dipalmitoyl phosphatidylcholine, is synthesized in the granular alveolar pneumocyte. Once manufactured, surfactant is stored in the lamellar bodies of these cells and secreted onto the alveolar surface. Starved animals have been found to have decreased granular pneumocyte lamellar bodies and mitochondria suggesting a decrease in surfactant production.

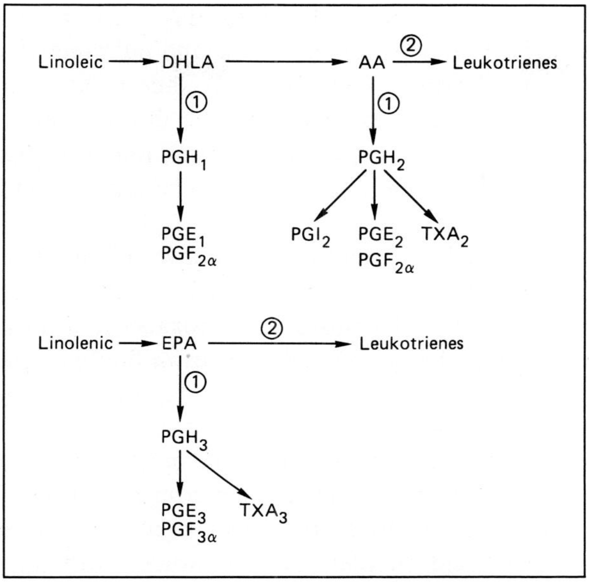

Fig. 2. Fatty acid metabolites. The cyclooxygenase pathway (1) converts eicosanoids to prostaglandins whereas the lipooxygenase pathway (2) produces leukotrienes. The physiologic effect of each metabolite varies depending on the parent eicosanoid.

Pulmonary Immune Response. In addition to the direct effects of malnutrition on lung mechanics, malnutrition has profound effects on both the cellular and humoral arms of the immune system. Malnourished individuals have a higher incidence of spontaneous and postoperative infections and are considered compromised hosts. Moreover, malnutrition inhibits alveolar defense mechanisms.

A decrease in the number of alveolar macrophages and lung phagocytic activity has been shown in malnourished laboratory animals. Pulmonary clearance of bacteria was found to be severely impaired in starvation. Recently, bacterial adherence to respiratory epithelium was found to be increased in malnourished patients, suggesting a link between nutritional status and the degree of bacterial colonization.

Fatty Acid Metabolites. Recently, we have explored the role of nutritional impact on prostaglandin and leukotriene production in the lung (fig. 2). These products of fatty acid (FA) metabolism are potent modulators of inflammation throughout the body. In the lung they exert additional effects on bronchial smooth muscle, vascular tone and pulmonary secretions. For example, prostaglandins PGD_2 and PGF_{2a} and leukotrienes C, D, and E_4 are potent bronchoconstrictors while the thromboxanes and leukotrienes B_4 and C, D, and E_4 are powerful pro-inflammatory agents. PGE_2 and prostacyclin, on the other hand, are bronchodilators and anti-inflammatory.

The prostaglandins and leukotrienes listed above are products of essential FA metabolism. Linoleic acid is converted to arachidonic acid which then forms prostaglandins (including thromboxanes and prostacyclin) in the cyclooxygenase pathway and leukotrienes in the lipoxygenase pathway. Prostaglandins derived from linoleic acid are designated by the subset 2 and leukotrienes by the subset 4 (fig. 2).

The availability of linoleic acid plays a key role in the production of these substances. Hageman and Hunt showed that administration of linoleic acid resulted in an increased production of PGE_2 and prostaglandin metabolites. Such linoleic acid supplementation would exert an anti-inflammatory effect provided that it did not result in additional production of the pro-inflammatory prostaglandins and leukotrienes. Our own experience with cystic fibrosis patients has taught us that there is a therapeutic window for these substances. Dosages must be large enough to stimulate PGE_2 and prostacyclin but less than that required to produce thromboxane. This situation is not unlike the effect of aspirin on bleeding time.

FA other than linoleic may play a role as immune modulators. Linolenic acid has been considered by some as an essential FA because of its extensive incorporation into membranes of the neonate. It is structurally distinct from linoleic acid predominantly because of the existence of a double bond 3 carbons from the N-terminal. This structure is designated N-3 or ω-3. When linolenic acid is substituted for linoleic eicosapentanoic acid is formed instead of arachidonic. The resulting prostaglandins and leukotrienes are chemically different from those derived from linoleic acid. Linolenate-derived prostaglandins are designated by the subset 3 and leukotrienes by the subset 5 (fig. 2). Remarkably, the slight difference in structure of linoleic and linolenic acid metabolites affects their role in inflammation. For example, thromboxanes A_3 and B_3 are physiologically inert and leukotriene B_5 is markedly less chemotactic than its arachidonic acid counterpart, B_4. However, PGE_3 appears to be similar in anti-inflammatory and bronchodilatory activity to PGE_2 and prostacyclin PGI_3 is equipotent to PGI_2. Thus, the net effect of substituting linolenic acid for linoleic appears to strongly favor an anti-inflammatory effect. This work has important implications for the interaction between malnutrition and chronic lung disease.

Respiratory Musculature. Respiratory muscle failure in malnourished patients occurs because of depletion of muscle glycogen and amino acids. Felig and Wahren [4] have shown that work in a selected group of skeletal muscles depletes glycogen from not only the working muscle, but from resting muscle groups as well. Thus, glycogen stores are mobilized on a whole-body basis for use by the working muscle. This global utilization of muscle glycogen does not spare the respiratory musculature. Therefore, starvation or stress depletes respiratory muscles of fuel stores which leads to exhaustion (i.e. decreased endurance).

In the absence of a readily available fuel source, working muscle has the capacity to utilize intracellular amino acids for fuel. This eventual breakdown of muscle protein progressively weakens the muscles as contractile fiber proteins are consumed. With weakening and diminished endurance of the respiratory musculature, alveolar hypoventilation ensues. Such inefficient ventilation increases the work of breathing, thereby increasing muscle energy demands. The increased need for fuel in the absence of an available fuel source leads to rapid depletion of muscle proteins.

The respiratory muscles become progressively weaker in this scenario and eventually atelectasis develops. As noted above, the decrease in lung expansion is thought to play an active role in the production of pulmonary infection and ongoing lung inflammation. This perpetuates the vicious cycle of lung inflammation, abnormal lung response to infection and injury, and permanent lung damage (fig. 3).

Chronic Lung Disease as a Cause of Malnutrition

The chronic lung patient has long been recognized as a patient in nutritional risk. Clinical observations, such as those of Fowler and Godlee [13] in 1898, documented the accompaniment of emaciation with emphysema.

Dornhost [14] discussed a change in body composition apparently brought on by chronic lung disease in which 'thinness' was a prominent

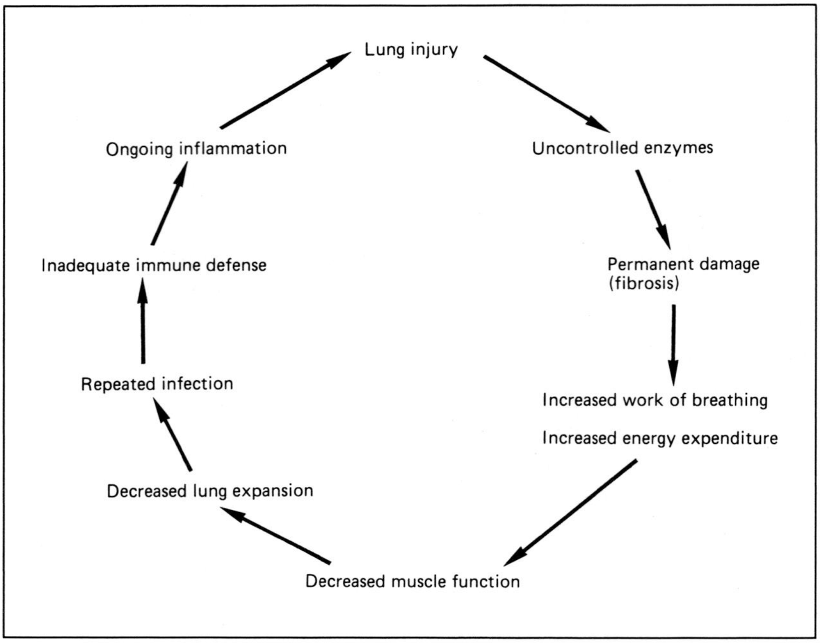

Fig. 3. Feedback cycle of lung injury and malnutrition. The decrease in circulating antiproteinases leads to uncontrolled enzyme activity in the lung. Fibrosis ensues which increases energy demand, further unbalancing the energy equilibrium. Lung expansion is decreased which promotes infection. Nutritional deficiency hampers immune defenses which amplifies the effect of infection, producing ongoing inflammation and injury.

feature. Filley et al. [15] described the clinical subtypes of chronic obstructive bronchopulmonary disease (COPD) as pink puffers (PP) and blue bloaters (BB). The former group was characterized by a thin appearance and a history of 'major weight loss'. The mean weight in this group was 129.3 lb, 14 lb less than the BB group and some 25 lb below their ideal body weight. It is interesting to note that both groups of COPD patients had an increase in BMR and VO_2. Moreover, during exercise, the PP group showed a greater increase in VO_2 which was associated with diminished tolerance.

The VA Cooperative Study of pulmonary function related severity of pulmonary disease to weight loss. Four hundred and eighty-seven patients with clinical and physiologic evidence of chronic lung disease were followed for 4 years. Survival was found to correlate with the degree of ventilatory disturbance. Of particular interest was the finding that body weight also correlated with the FEV_1. Patients with FEV_1 less than 0.5 had the lowest weights (mean 124) although they were comparable to the other groups in height and age. Practically all patients (96%) gave a history of respiratory tract infections with a significant number (33.3%) reporting 5 or more per year.

Vendenburgh et al. [17] examined weight loss accompanying COPD in 71 patients over a 7-year period. All patients had established COPD (chronic bronchitis or emphysema) but no other known pulmonary pathology. Twenty-nine patients with comparable lung disease but no weight loss were also followed. COPD patients with weight loss were found to have a significantly lower survival rate than COPD patients without weight loss (49 vs 76%). Patients who lost weight were found to have a reduced caloric intake, many falling below their estimated requirements. This is even more striking when one takes into account the fact that energy expenditure is often underestimated in COPD patients. Studies on indirect calorimetry on these patients demonstrated significant elevation in measured energy expenditure, in excess of that predicted by such methods as the Harris-Benedict equation.

Several authors have studied the effects of the increased work of breathing in COPD. In a series of articles, Cherniak [20, 21] and associates showed the COPD patients demonstrated increased oxygen consumption of the respiratory musculature. Recently, Rochester et al. [22] showed that the increased work load of the respiratory musculature led to diminished muscle efficiency and an increase in the energy cost of breathing.

This situation, in which energy requirements are enhanced in the face of diminished caloric intake, would certainly be expected to cause muscle wasting. As stated previously, all working muscle groups would be affected to some extent.

As the respiratory muscle weakens, the efficiency of ventilation declines further until alveolar hypoventilation with CO_2 retention ensues. Accompanying this decline in ventilation one would anticipate the development of atelectasis and later pneumonia. If by this point the patient is already malnourished, decreased immune response would worsen the course of pulmonary infection and, similar to the starved individual discussed above, antiprotease activity might be inefficient and incapable of controlling the enzymes activated by the infection. Eventually, this would further worsen pulmonary function leading to even greater work for the respiratory musculature and the vicious cycle would continue.

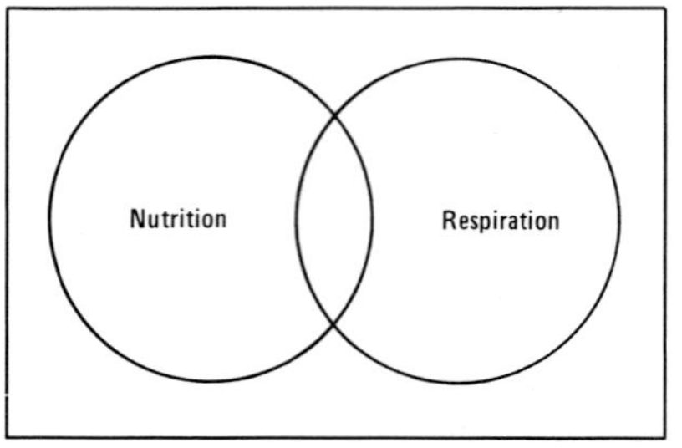

Fig. 4. Overlapping spheres of influence. Nutritional and respiratory status are linked. Dysfunction in one area may produce disease in the other.

Clinical Applications

From the work accomplished to date, it is apparent that pulmonary function should be evaluated in malnutrition and that nutritional status should be considered in chronic lung disease. There is an overlap between these two distinct entities where one may produce the other (fig. 4). Once triggered, a feedback cycle of worsened pulmonary function producing increased energy consumption and worsened nutritional status may prove fatal.

Adequate nutritional intervention would appear to be the key to breaking the feedback cycle and promoting recovery. This is particularly true during stress states, such as pulmonary infection, when energy requirements may increase further.

Much has been learned regarding the type of nutritional support best utilized by the patient with chronic lung disease. Although attention to energy and nitrogen balance remains the basic goal, the types of fuel or protein sources may alter respiratory muscle function.

The choice of fuel sources for working muscle has recently been clarified by Newsholme [23], Rochester [24, 25] and others. From this information, it appears that respiratory muscle, particularly the diaphragm, uses both glucose and FA for fuel. This is because diaphragm is made up of mostly (60%) type I, slow twitch, muscle fibers which utilize both substrates. The remaining type II, fast twitch, fibers mainly consume stored muscle glycogen. As the muscle works, both blood-derived and stored energy are utilized. However, when muscle glycogen is depleted, exhaustion ensues.

Increased FA utilization slows glycogen depletion and would be expected to enhance muscle endurance. During FA metabolism, slow twitch fibers rely less on stored muscle glycogen and, thus, they exhibit a slowed progression to exhaustion. It has recently been shown that the enhanced FA metabolism in the respiratory muscles improves pulmonary function (FEV_1, FVC) and increases exercise endurance.

Fuel consumption produces CO_2 at rates which vary with the fuel source. This is usually expressed in terms of the RQ (CO_2 production/O_2 consumption). Carbohydrate fuels produce a greater quantity of CO_2 per mole of oxygen than FA. A rise in CO_2 production would lead to a rise in PCO_2 which, in turn, would stimulate ventilation. Thus, CO_2 production and ventilatory work are closely related. High carbohydrate loads would therefore appear to be inappropriate for patients at risk for pulmonary decompensation.

Chronic bronchitic patients lose responsiveness to PCO_2 stimulation as the levels gradually rise. However, they still show reductions in PCO_2 when converted to a high fat intake. Patients under stress of critical illness or on artificial ventilation also exhibit a decrement in CO_2 production during FA metabolism which would be expected to reduce their need for ventilatory support. High carbohydrate intakes have been shown to have the opposite effect on such patients, leading to worsened ventilatory status. This fact teaches us a valuable lesson: too much nutritional support can be as bad as too little. When choosing a fuel source for the patient with a compromised respiratory system, a mixture of glucose and FA calories should be provided. The caloric intake should approximate, but not exceed, the patient's energy requirements.

Amino acid utilization also affects ventilatory status. Concentrated amino acid infusions stimulate ventilatory drive and response to PCO_2 independent of caloric intake. While minute ventilation increases, CO_2 production does not, implying that the effect of amino acids is not related to an increased requirement for CO_2 elimination. Certain amino acids (i.e. leucine, isoleucine, and valine) may have a greater effect in this regard. These could act as ventilatory stimulants and would be useful in the management of patients with diminished ventilatory drive.

Conclusion

Nutritional and respiratory status are functionally linked so that each depends on the other to maintain equilibrium. Derangements in either impact on the other in a vicious cycle that results in further deterioration. It is possible for starvation to produce chronic lung disease and for chronic lung disease to produce malnutrition. Between these points a spectrum exists of diminished function and abnormal metabolism. The astute clinician must recognize this situation in order to properly avert its pitfalls. Numerous areas remain open for investigation within this area.

References

1 Benedict, F.A.: A study of prolonged fasting (Carnegie Institute, Washington 1915).

2 Winick, M. (ed.): Hunger disease: studies by the Jewish physicians of the Warsaw Ghetto (Wiley & Sons, New York 1979).

3 Keys, A.; et al. (Minnesota Experiment): The biology of human starvation (University of Minnesota Press, Minneapolis 1950).

4a Felig, P.; Wahren, J.: Fuel homeostasis in exercise. New Engl. J. Med. *293:* 1078–1084 (1975).

4b Ahlborg, G.; et al.: Splanchnic and peripheral glucose and lactate metabolism during and after prolonged arm exercise. J. clin. Invest. *77:* 690–699 (1986).

5 Martin, T.R.; et al.: The effects of severe protein-calorie malnutrition on antibacterial defense mechanisms in the rat lung. Am. Rev. resp. Dis. *128:* 1013–1019 (1983).

6 Niederman, M.S.; et al.: Nutritional status and bacterial binding in the lower respiratory tract in patients with chronic tracheostomies. Ann. intern. Med. *100:* 795–800 (1984).

7 Kulapongs, P.; et al.: Defective local leukocyte mobilization in children with kwashiorkor. Am. J. clin. Nutr. *30:* 367–370 (1977).

8 Kerr, J.S.; et al.: Nutritional emphysema in the rat: influence of protein depletion and impaired lung growth. Am. Rev. resp. Dis. *131:* 644–650 (1985).

9 Sahebjami, H.; et al.: Effects of starvation and refeeding on lung mechanics and morphometry. Am. Rev. resp. Dis. *119:* 443–451 (1979).

10 Sahebjami, H.: Nutrition and the pulmonary parenchyma. Clin. Chest Med. *7:* 111–126 (1986).

11 Gail, D.B.; et al.: Influence of fasting on the lung. J. appl. Physiol. *42:* 88–92 (1977).

12 Martin, T.R.; et al.: The effects of severe protein-calorie malnutrition on antibacterial defense mechanisms in the rat lung. Am. Rev. resp. Dis. *128:* 1013–1019 (1983).

13 Fowler, J.; Goodlee, R.: Emphysema and the lungs; in Diseases of the lungs (Longmans, Green, London 1898).

14 Dornhost, A.: Respiratory insufficiency. Lancet *268:* 1185–1187 (1955).

15 Filley, G.; et al.: Chronic obstructive bronchopulmonary disease. Am. J. Med. *44:* 26–28 (1968).

16 Renzetti, A.D.; et al.: The VA Cooperative Study of pulmonary function. Am. J. Med. *41:* 115–129 (1966).

17 Vandenburgh, E.; et al.: Weight changes in the terminal stages of chronic obstructive lung disesae. Am. Rev. resp. Dis. *95:* 556–565 (1947).

18 Openbrier, D.; et al.: Nutritional status and lung function in patients with emphysema and chronic bronchitis. Chest *83:* 17–22 (1983).
19 Brain, S.R.; et al.: The prevalence and determinants of nutritional changes in chronic obstructive pulmonary disease. Chest *86:* 558–563 (1984).
20 Cherniak, R.M.: The oxygen consumption and efficiency of the respiratory muscles in health and emphysema. J. clin. Invest. *38:* 494–499 (1959).
21 Levison, M.; Cherniak, R.M.: Ventilatory cost of exercise in chronic obstructive pulmonary disease. J. appl. Physiol. *25:* 21–27 (1968).
22 Rochester, D.F.; et al.: The respiratory muscles in chronic obstructive pulmonary disease. Bull. Eur. Physiopathol. Resp. *15:* 951–975 (1979).
23 Newsholme, E.A.: The regulation of extracellular and intracellular fuel supply during sustained exercise. Ann. N.Y. Acad. Sci. *301:* 81–91 (1977).
24 Rochester, D.F.; et al.: Metabolism of the working diaphragm. Am. Rev. resp. Dis. *119:* 101–106 (1979).
25 Rochester, D.F.: Malnutrition and the respiratory muscles. Clin. Chest Med. *7:* 91–99 (1986).
26 Askanazi, J.; et al.: Respiratory change induced by large glucoise loads of total parenteral nutrition. J: Am. med. Ass. *243:* 1444–1446 (1980).
27 Askanazi, J.; et al.: Nutrition and the respiratory system. Crit. Care Med. *10:* 163–172 (1982).
28 Weissman, C.; et al.: Amino acids and respiration. Ann. intern. Med. *98:* 41–44 (1983).
29 Askanazi, J.; et al.: Treatment of cystic fibrosis with long-term home TPN. Nutr. Int. (in press).
30 Skeie, B.; et al.: Long-term parenteral nutrition and exercise tolerance in cystic fibrosis. Crit. Care Med. (in press).
31 Skeie, B.; et al.: Intravenous fat emulsions and lung function. Crit. Care Med. (in press).

Michael M. Rothkopf, MD, Medical Service (111),
Veterans Administration Medical Center, East Orange, NJ 07019 (USA)

Wld Rev. Nutr. Diet., vol. 56, pp. 56–92 (Karger, Basel 1988)

Iron and Folate Nutriture during Life Cycle

Lynn B. Bailey, James J. Cerda

Food Science and Human Nutrition Department and the Department of Medicine, University of Florida, Gainesville, Fla., USA

Contents

Introduction

Iron and folate are two essential nutrients that are often deficient in diets of population groups. Both are required for the normal functioning of the hematopoietic system as well as numerous critical metabolic processes. A deficiency of either will result in anemia with the associated physiological consequences.

Periods of rapid growth and development as during pregnancy, early childhood, and adolescence increase the requirement for both iron and folate. An increase in the prevalence of deficiency is associated with these periods of the life cycle. Changes in iron and folate status in the aged may occur due to a combination of physiological factors such as reduction in nutrient intake coupled with drug and alcohol use. The purpose of this paper is to review the basics of iron and folate nutriture in conjunction with a discussion of how the physiological changes during the life cycle may affect the requirement for these two nutrients.

Iron Nutriture

Form in Food, General Functions, and Status Assessment

A review of iron interactions, measurements, and bioavailability in foods has been previously reported [1]. Iron is present in food as either inorganic iron or heme iron. The availability of dietary iron for absorption is as important a factor as overall total iron content in determining nutritional adequacy [2]. Non-heme iron bioavailability is greatly enhanced by the presence of ascorbic acid and meat and may be inhibited by factors including tea, coffee, bran, and fiber [1]. Meat contains heme iron which is more available for absorption than non-heme iron and is not influenced by inhibitors [2].

The important role of iron in oxygen metabolism is well recognized and associated with its requirement for hemoglobin, myoglobin and cytochrome synthesis. Sometimes overlooked when considering the metabolic role of iron is its essentiality in specific enzymes which may be sensitive to an iron deficiency. For example, a reduction in the iron-dependent mitochondrial oxidases has been associated with a decrease in work capacity in experimental animals [3].

The recognition of iron deficiency and assessment of iron status depends on three laboratory tests [3]. The first is plasma ferritin which provides a simple and reliable estimate of iron stores, provided inflammation has been excluded. In the normal adult, 1 μg ferritin is equivalent to about 120 μg iron/kg. The second measure is transferrin saturation which is a gauge of iron supply to tissues. When the value is less than 16%, normal erythropoiesis is impaired. The third measurement is red cell protoporphyrin, an increase in which usually indicates a deficient iron supply in the developing red cell. This measurement takes 2–3 weeks to become abnormal in contrast to the more rapid changes in transferrin saturation. These three measurements coupled with the hemoglobin concentration make it possible to distinguish specific categories of iron deficient individuals: those who are iron-replete, those with depleted iron stores (decreased ferritin), those with iron deficiency but no anemia (decreased ferritin and transferrin saturation with increased red cell protoporphyrin), and those with iron deficiency anemia (the indices of iron deficiency plus a decrease in hemoglobin).

Status during Life Cycle

Pregnancy. Iron deficiency during pregnancy is a common problem due to the marked increase in its requriement. During the latter half of pregnancy, the total volume of red cells and their hemoglobin content increases dramatically [5]. If iron is readily available approximately 0.5 g will be utilized to augment maternal erythropoiesis [5].

The iron that is directed to the fetus and placenta (exclusive of maternal hemoglobin in the placenta) amounts to ~0.2–0.3 g. Therefore if iron is readily available, iron utilization induced by pregnancy with a single fetus amounts to about 0.8 g and with multiple fetuses to more. Prorated on a daily basis this equals ~6 mg/day to which must be added 1 mg for gut and other losses [4]. Blood loss during delivery can induce a significant drain on iron stores. Average blood loss is estimated to be 500–600 ml, which constitutes ~250 mg of iron or ½ the average amount added to the maternal circulation as hemoglobin during pregnancy.

This relatively large amount of iron may be obtained from either maternal iron stores or diet. The iron stores of women however are seldom large enough (average ~300 mg) to supply all the iron that is needed. Food rarely provides sufficient iron to permit 6–7 mg to be absorbed each day since diets typically contain 6 mg/1,000 cal, most of which is not absorbed.

Data collected in the second National Health and Nutrition Examination Survey (1976–1981) (NHANES II) provide limited information on iron status of pregnant women [5]. For the 61 pregnant women aged 20–44 years for which serum ferritin was analyzed, the prevalence of two or three abnormal values using a ferritin model technique was 25%. For the 91 women aged 20 through 44 years for which mean cell volume (MCV) was analyzed, the prevalence of two or three abnormal values using a MCV model was 10.7%. These data were obtained from women in various months of pregnancy.

Bailey et al. [6] reported that 12% of a group of adolescent and adult pregnant women had deficient transferrin saturation levels. The majority of the subjects were in the second trimester of pregnancy. There were no differences in mean values between adolescent and adult women. These data are in line with the prevalence estimate based on the MCV model from the NHANES II Survey [5].

A dietary supplement of 30 mg of iron as ferrous fumarate or ferrous gluconate taken during the last 4–5 months of pregnancy protects existing iron stores. The Committee on Maternal Nutrition of the National Research Council recommends that during the second and third trimesters 30–60 mg of iron be taken daily [4]. In addition, attention should be given to increasing the dietary intake of the more bioavailable forms of heme iron found in meat products and iron consumed in conjunction with ascorbic acid.

Infancy. Pregnancy is period of increased need for dietary iron. However, the consequences of iron deficiency affect the mother far more than the fetus [7–9]. Suboptimal iron endowment at birth is rarely a cause of subsequent iron deficiency. In the fetus, the ratio of iron to body weight remains relatively constant throughout pregnancy at an average level of 75 mg/kg [7]. The bulk of the infant's iron endowment at birth is represented by hemoglobin iron; 1 g of hemoglobin contains 3.4 mg of elemental iron [3]. As a result, the amount of iron in the body at the time of birth depends on the blood volume and the hemoglobin concentration. Any complications of pregnancy or the perinatal period that result in fetal blood loss will compromise the infant's iron endowment.

Unless extreme, the presence of maternal iron deficiency does not appear to compromise the iron endowment of the fetus. The hemoglobin concentration in the cord blood of infants born to anemic iron-deficient mothers does not differ from that of infants born to iron-sufficient mothers until maternal hemoglobin values fall below 6 g/dl. With extreme maternal iron deficiency anemia, the placenta is small and the cord blood hemoglobin concentration is reduced [8].

Employing plasma ferritin concentrations as an index of iron sufficiency, Rios et al. [9] were unable to document any correlation between plasma ferritin concentrations in mothers with high and low values and the plasma ferritin concentrations of their infants at birth or at 1.5 months of age (table I). Therefore, it may be concluded that except in the most unusual circumstances, maternal iron deficiency by itself does not result in iron deficiency anemia in the infant, either at birth or later in the first year of life. Factors such as rate of growth relative to birth weight, initial iron endowment that has been compromised by blood loss, and infant nutrition seem to be far more important in determining the later appearance of anemia.

After birth there are profound changes in metabolism and in the rate of erythropoiesis. They can be conveniently divided into 3 stages. (1) The first

Table I. Different parameters in two groups of mothers and their newborns divided according to the predelivery plasma ferritin. From ref. [9]

Parameters	Maternal		Newborn	
	group A	group B	group A	group B
Hemoglobin, g/dl	11.6	13.0	15.5	16.1
Transferrin saturation, %	12.0	22.5	53.7	61.2
Plasma ferritin, ng/ml	6.4	18.0	100.5	117.0

stage, encompassing the first 6–8 weeks of life, is marked by a decline in the concentration of hemoglobin from the highest to the lowest levels observed during any period of development. This decline is attributed to an abrupt decrease in erythropoiesis in response to increased postnatal delivery of oxygen to the tissues. Storage iron is augmented. (2) At about 2 months of age, the concentration of hemoglobin (Hgb) has fallen to its lowest point and the rate of erythropoiesis is increased. Storage iron gradually decreases. (3) The third stage is characterized by an increased dependence on dietary iron. A rapid rate of growth and the low iron content of either breast milk or unsupplemented cow's milk products predispose the infant to the depletion of iron stores. If iron stores are exhausted, then the rise in concentration of hemoglobin that started during the second stage can be either curtailed or reversed. Not until the third stage is additional iron likely to be effective in augmenting the concentration of hemoglobin.

The effect of breast feeding on the iron status of infants during the first 9 months of life was evaluated by Siimes et al. [10]. The maintenance of iron status indicators as well as hematological indices were comparable between the breast-fed infants and infants receiving iron-fortified infant formula. The increase in hemoglobin for both the breast-fed and the control group is illustrated in figure 1.

Therefore, when 6-month-old infants who are breast-fed are contrasted with infants receiving iron-fortified formula, the rate of iron accumulation, the transferrin saturation and hemoglobin values are identical. It appears safe to conclude from these and other data that the exclusively breast-fed infant does not require any form of iron supplementation during the first 6 months of life. In addition, maternal iron supplementation dur-

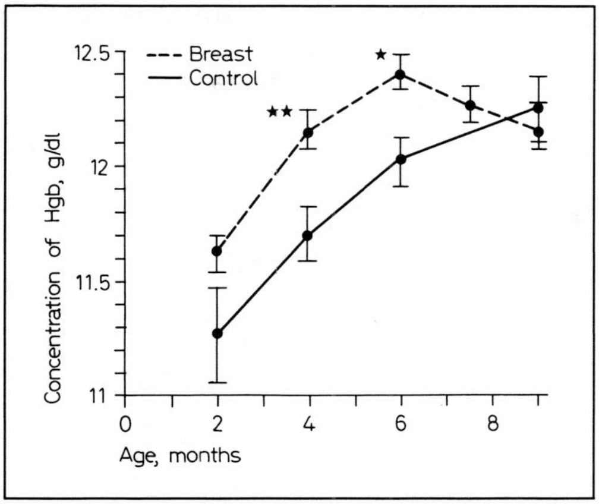

Fig. 1. Concentration of hemoglobin in formula and breast-fed infants. From ref. [10].

ing breast feeding has not been shown to have any effect on the infant's iron nutrition as illustrated by these data reported by Siimes et al. (table II) [10].

Both breast milk and cow's milk have relatively low contents of iron as shown in table III [1]. The iron content of breast milk gradually falls from about 0.5 mg/l during the first month after birth to about 0.3 mg/l between 4 and 6 months of age [1]. The iron content in unfortified infant formula ranges between 0.5 and 1 mg/l. Expressed in terms of kilocalories, both human milk and cow's milk average less than 1 mg iron per 1,000 kcal in contrast to the 6 mg/1,000 kcal in the average mixed diet of developed countries. Despite the small amount of iron in milk, differences in percentage absorbed can have an important impact. An average of 50% of the iron in breast milk is absorbed compared to only 10% from cow's milk.

Iron fortified cow's milk formulas contain between 11 and 12 mg iron per liter as iron sulfate or iron gluconate which is 15–20 times higher than that in unfortified milk. The mean absorption is about 4% [1]. Although the percentage of iron absorbed is less than half that of iron in unfortified formula, the absolute amount is approximately 6 times greater. The introduction of solid foods may compromise the unique bioavailability of iron from human milk. It would seem prudent when solid foods are introduced that these foods be a good source of iron in order to compensate for this reduction in iron bioavailabilty. Iron-fortified infant cereal appears to be a

Table II. Iron status according to laboratory values in exclusively breast-fed infants at 9 months. From ref. [10]

	Group I	Group II
Maternal iron dose, mg/day	66	266
Hemoglobin, g/dl	12.1	12.1
Transferrin saturation, %	16.0	21.0
Serum ferritin, μg/l	26.0	27.0

Table III. Iron content of infant food. From ref. [11]

Food		Content	% absorbed
Breast milk	1 month after birth	0.5 mg/l	5
	4–6 months after birth	0.3 mg/l	
Unfortified cows' milk		0.5–1.0 mg/l	10
Iron-fortified cows' milk formulas		11–12 mg/l	4
Iron-fortified dry infant cereal		45 mg/100 g	4

logical first food. The level of fortification is about 10 times greater than the iron present in whole grain products.

Prevalence estimates of iron deficiency for very young infants are scarce. This young age group was not included in the NHANES II Survey. However, studies in the USA have shown that the prevalence of overt iron-deficiency anemia is 5–15% in American infants and children 9–36 months old [5].Data from NHANES II indicate that iron deficiency has a relatively high prevalence in young children, i.e. 1–2 years (9.2–9.4%) (fig. 2). Although iron-deficiency is most prevalent among the poor, owing to feeding practices and dietary inadequacy of foods rich in iron, which tend to be expensive, it does cut across socioeconomic barriers.

Iron deficiency is particularly frequent during the second year of life because of exhaustion of transplacental iron reserves, rapid growth, and consumption of large amounts of iron-poor milk. The Committee on Nutrition of the American Academy of Pediatrics recommends that iron-

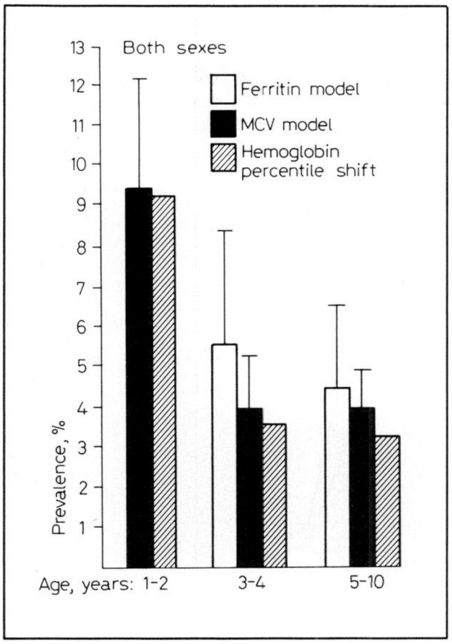

Fig. 2. Prevalence of impaired iron status in early life: NHANES II.

fortified cow's milk formulas should be considered for infants who are not breast-fed [12]. This is sufficient to meet iron requirements during the first year of life. Other dietary staples for infants can also be enriched with iron. Infant cereals containing 45 mg of iron per 100 g of cereal, are well accepted and can prevent nutritional iron deficiency.

In 1972, the US Department of Agriculture implemented the Special Supplemental Food program for Women, Infants and Children (WIC). This program provides nutritious food supplements for eligible pregnant women, infants, and children from low-income families. Iron-fortified milk formulas and cereals are provided during the first year of life.

In a study reported recently in the *New England Journal of Medicine,* the disappearance of iron deficiency anemia in a high-risk infant population given supplemental iron was documented [13]. Two groups of children were compared – the first group of ~ 300 was studied in 1971 in inner-city New Haven. Evaluation of these children who ranged in age from 9 to 36 months revealed a high prevalence of iron deficiency. This initial evaluation took place in 1971 prior to the implementation of the WIC program.

In 1984, a second group, of the same size and same age range, who were ethnically and demographically similar to the 1971 cohort, were eval-

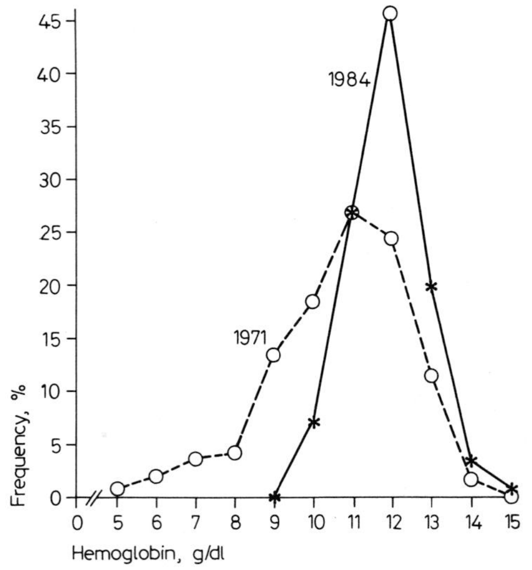

Fig. 3. Distribution of hemoglobin values in 258 infants in 1971 and 324 infants in 1984. All subjects were between 9 and 36 months of age when studied. From ref. [12].

uated. The authors reported a remarkable decrease in the prevalence of anemia in the 1984 cohort as compared with the 1971 cohort, and documented that severe iron-deficiency anemia had disappeared in this population (fig. 3). The marked improvement was attributed to the nutritional supplementation with iron-fortified foods provided by the WIC program.

Moderate or severe anemia was present in many of the children in 1971, and 23% had hemoglobin levels below 9.8 g/dl. In 1984, severe anemia was not found and only 1% of the children had hemoglobin levels below 9.8 g/dl. The difference in mean hemoglobin levels between groups 1 and 2 (0.7 g/dl) was statistically significant.

There was an observed increase in mean hemoglobin level (0.7 g/dl) which is similar to that reported in groups of infants, children and women with low or low normal hemoglobin levels who were given iron therapy. This study demonstrates near disappearance of nutritional anemia in an inner-city population of poor infants and children between 1971 and 1984.

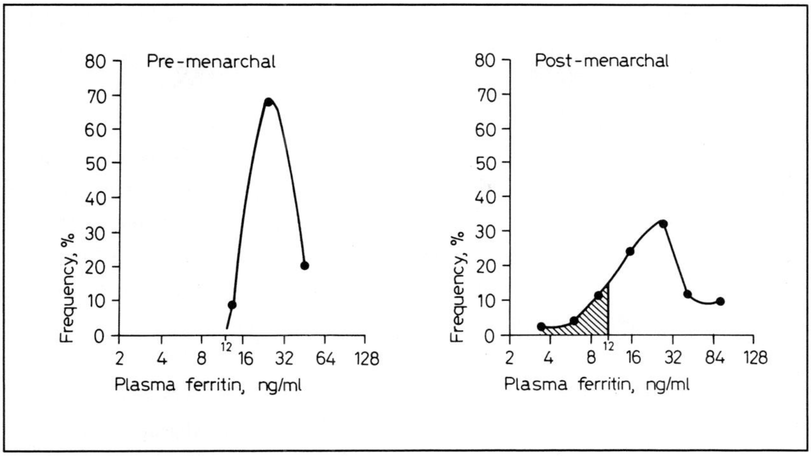

Fig. 4. Frequency distribution curves for pre- and post-menarchal adolescent females. From ref. [14].

Adolescence. Acceleration of growth, particularly during the years of sexual maturation, imposes increased requirements of iron primarily for the production of hemoglobin [11]. For example, during the peak year of the adolescent growth spurt, boys gain an average of 10 kg. This can be calculated to require a net increase of about 300 mg of iron merely to maintain a constant concentration of hemoglobin in the expanding blood volume. However, the concentration of hemoglobin also increases between 0.5 g and 1.0 g/dl per year at this age. An increase in hemoglobin concentration of 0.5 g/dl in a representative 55 kg adolescent boy requires a net increase of ~ 350 mg of iron during his year of peak growth [11].

In adolescent girls, iron needs are also large, but they do not peak as sharply as in boys because the maximum yearly weight gain is somewhat less than in boys and because the concentration of hemoglobin in girls increases only slightly during this period. The average weight gain of 9 kg/year in girls requires about 280 mg iron for the maintenance of a constant concentration of hemoglobin [11].

Bailey et al. [14] evaluated iron stores in adolescents by measuring plasma ferritin concentration. The median iron stores of boys and girls were estimated to be 350 and 280 mg, respectively. Of the boys, 3% had ferritin values less than 12 ng/ml compared to 10% of the girls. Postmenarchal girls had lower ferritin levels than premenarchal girls (fig. 4). None of the premenarchal girls had ferritin levels below 12 ng/ml, in contrast to 15% of the postmenarchal girls. These data suggest that adolescent girls are at a greater risk of iron deficiency than are boys and that menstrual blood loss is a significant factor in determining iron status.

Linear regression analysis was used by this group to model changes on biochemical variables as a function of age. Transferrin saturation levels for females declined as age increased in contrast to the increase in transferrin saturation in males. The decrease in percentage transferrin saturation with age in the female adolescents may be partially explained by the onset of menstruation which precedes the growth spurt [15].

Old Age. Lynch et al. [16] reviewed iron metabolism and requirements in the elderly. The effect of age on the quantity of storage iron has been investigated and the findings suggest that iron requirements decrease with age. Hepatic non-heme iron concentration has been reported for various ages using a liver necropsy technique in Malasians and Singaporeans [17]. After the neonatal period, liver iron concentrations in males remained low until puberty followed by a progressive rise. In women, the low levels persisted until after the menopause followed by a gradual increase until levels similar to those in the men were reached. The highest level of total liver iron content was found in subjects of both sexes between the age of 60 and 79 years. Similar data have been observed in other populations [18–23]. Stainable bone marrow iron and serum ferritin concentrations have also been found to increase with age [23–30].

Garry et al. [30] compared the serum ferritin levels of a group (n = 280) of free-living healthy elderly (60–93 years) men and women with levels in a group (n = 271) of young (20–39 years) subjects. Ferritin levels were significantly higher in the elderly group as compared to the younger subjects. The geometric means for ferritin levels in the elderly men and women were 145 and 104 ng/ml, respectively, compared to 85 and 37 ng/ml for the young men and women. Only 1% of the young group had ferritin levels higher than 200 ng/ml as compared to 35 and 15% of the elderly men and women, respectively.

The rate of excretion primarily determines iron requirements in the elderly since growth, pregnancy and menstrual losses are no longer influencing factors. Finch used a radioisotopic method (^{55}Fe) to measure the change in specific activity in the blood over a prolonged time in men and women of different ages [31]. He reported a mean iron exchange rate of 0.64 mg in elderly (59–77 years) non-menstruating women compared to

1.22 mg in younger (32–44 years) menstruating women. In elderly (57–84 years) men, the iron exchange rate was found to be 0.61 mg compared to 0.95, 0.90, and 1.02 mg for three groups of younger men [31, 32]. These data suggest that iron loss in older women and men is no greater than in younger individuals and may be less.

The Recommended Dietary Allowance (RDA) for adult men and post-menopausal women is 10 mg. This is based on an estimated daily loss of 1 mg and adjusted for 10% efficiency of absorption [33]. Dietary intake data from both national and regional surveys indicate that the dietary iron intake for the aged individual is adequate [16, 30, 34–40]. The most recent comprehensive national survey is from the US Department of Health, Education and Welfare and Nutrition Examination Survey (NHANES II) [16]. The mean dietary iron intake in this survey for both men and women exceeded the 1980 RDA of 10 mg (table IV) [33].

Table IV. Mean energy and iron intakes for males and females reported in NHANES II (1976–1980). From ref. [5]

Age years	Males			Females		
	energy		iron mg/1,000 kcal	energy		iron mg/1,000 kcal
	kcal	mg		kcal	mg	
6–11 (months)	1,001	12.8	12.8	991	12.9	13.0
1–2	1,311	8.7	6.6	1,262	8.5	6.7
3–5	1,628	10.5	6.5	1,508	9.5	6.3
6–8	1,981	12.5	6.3	1,807	10.8	6.0
9–11	2,183	14.4	6.6	1,857	11.4	6.2
12–14	2,430	15.9	6.5	1,813	10.8	5.9
15–17	2,817	17.4	6.2	1,731	9.9	5.7
18–24	3,040	17.8	5.8	1,687	10.6	6.3
25–34	2,734	17.3	6.3	1,643	10.9	6.6
35–44	2,424	16.1	6.6	1,579	11.2	7.1
45–54	2,361	16.2	6.9	1,439	10.4	7.3
55–64	2,071	14.8	7.1	1,401	10.7	7.6
65–74	1,828	14.1	7.7	1,295	10.2	7.9

A review of data in table IV indicates that iron density in the diet increases with age to intakes that exceed 7 mg/1,000 kcal. This provides an explanation for maintenance of adequate iron intakes when caloric intakes are reduced. Bailey et al. [41] found that the average iron intake of a group of elderly persons in Florida met the RDA even when calorie intake was low. The mean daily dietary iron intake of institutionalized elderly men and women was reported to be 16.9 and 12.7 mg, respectively, by Gregor [42]. Garry et al. [30] found average dietary intakes of 15.2 and 12.4 mg for free-living elderly men and women, respectively, in Albuquerque. Iron density was 7.2 mg, and 7.7 mg/1,000 kcal for men and women respectively which agrees with data from the NHANES II Survery [16].

Data from a United States Department of Agriculture Food Consumption Survey carried out in 48 states was based on the average of 3 days intake [16]. Approximately 90% of men and women over the age of 50 consumed 70% or more of the RDA for iron. These data suggest that the overall average intake of dietary iron in the older population is adequate.

The question of an age effect on serum iron concentration arose following the report of Pirrie [43] that there were lower serum iron levels in elderly versus young adults. However, these findings have not been confirmed by other authors [30]. In fact, Garry et al. [30] found higher serum iron and serum ferritin levels in elderly versus young subjects. In addition, serum ferritin levels increase if inflammation is present and may not accurately reflect body iron stores [44]. This fact emphasizes the point that health status should be evaluated when measuring iron parameters in the elderly.

Data from studies in various parts of the USA illustrate the fact that iron deficiency appears to be uncommon in the elderly [45, 46]. Bailey et al. [46] found a 14% incidence of anemia [hemoglobin (Hb) $<$ 12 g/dl] in an elderly predominately Black population from low-income households in Florida. However, no subject had a serum iron level below 50 μg/dl or a transferrin saturation of less than 15% which led to the conclusion that there was no evidence of iron deficiency in these elderly subjects. In a study conducted with the elderly in rural Utah 14% of men and 3% of women had low Hb levels and none were in the deficient range based on Ten-State Nutrition Survey (TSNS) norms [34, 47]. Only a small proportion had low serum iron levels. In Corvallis, Oregon, an assessment study of elderly men and women showed that while 20% of men had Hb values below 14 g/dl, only 1% of women had levels below 12 g/dl [48]. Serum iron values were low in 4% of the men and none of the women and transferrin saturations were low in only 1% of the women and none of the men, again suggesting that iron deficiency was rare. The effect of oral iron supplementation and food iron fortification in anemic elderly subjects in the Boston area was reported by Gershoff et al. [49]. Following the fortification trial, both control (no fortification) and fortification groups showed a 0.4-g/dl rise in Hb. Three months of administration of ferrous sulfate to those whose Hb levels remained below 13 g/dl was without effect.

The iron status of a group (n = 280) of healthy elderly from Albuquerque was assessed and compared to that of younger adults (n = 271). Only two elderly men and four elderly women had low (< 16%) transferrin saturation levels. Ferritin levels were normal (> 12 ng/ml) in all elderly individuals and higher than that of the healthy young adults. Extrapolation of data from surveys of hospitalized elderly has resulted in the erroneous conclusion that iron deficiency anemia is a major problem in the elderly [50, 51]. In these elderly patients, infection, chronic diseases, and neoplasms may be the most frequent cause of anemia. Care should be taken in the clinical setting to correctly diagnose the cause of the anemia.

The widespread use of iron supplements by the elderly results from the misconception that iron deficiency is prevalent and that supplemental iron will improve one's health and sense of well-being [52]. Studies carried out in both the USA and Sweden suggest that some elderly take large quantities of supplemental iron [53, 54]. The potential toxic side effects of large doses of supplemental iron should be recognized [55, 56]. Arbitrary iron supplementation by the average iron-replete elderly individual is at the very least wasteful and unnecessary.

Folate Nutriture

Form in Food, General Functions, and Status Assessment

Folate is a generic term for this water-soluble vitamin that exists in many different forms. Pteroylglutamic acid (PteGlu) $C_{19}H_{19}N_7O_6$ (MW 441.40) is the synthetic pharmaceutical form of the vitamin. The major subunits of the molecule are the pteridine moiety linked by a methylene bridge to para-aminobenzoic acid, which is joined by peptide linkage to glutamic acid (fig. 5). Pteroylglutamic acid becomes biochemically active after it has undergone reduction to become tetrahydrofolate. In addition to being reduced, various one-carbon adducts may be linked to tetrahydrofo-

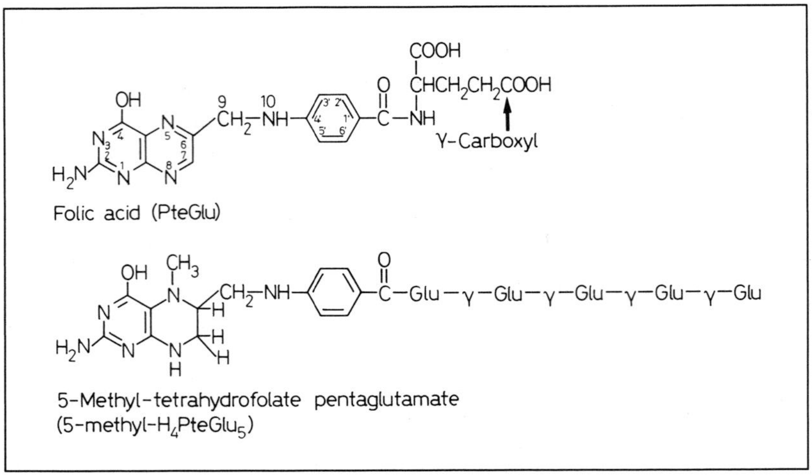

Fig. 5. Structures of folic acid and 5-methyl-tetrahydrofolate pentaglutamate.

late at the N-5, N-10 or 5,10 position and the number of glutamate residues may vary. In almost all forms of dietary folate, the double bonds on the pyrazine ring of the pteridine moiety are reduced, and a methyl or formyl group is attached at the N-5 or N-10 position [57]. The vitamin can exist as the monoglutamate form with one glutamic acid residue or as the polyglutamate form which is the major dietary form.

Our knowledge of folate content of food is incomplete. Early reports of food folate composition are considered invalid since the essentiality of adding ascorbic acid to the assay was not recognized. More recently Perloff and Butrum [58] reported the folate composition of a wide variety of foodstuffs. There is current research emphasis on developing new and better analytical techniques to more accurately quantitate food folate. However, much of the current inconsistency observed between laboratories may reflect inherent variability in the concentration of folate in the same food source. In foods that have been well characterized, in relation to their folate content, most of the vitamin (>90%) is present as polyglutamates with five or more glutamate residues added in γ-carboxyl linkage to the single glutamic acid found in PteGlu [59, 60]. Concentrated food sources

Fig. 6. Reactions involved in one-carbon metabolism.

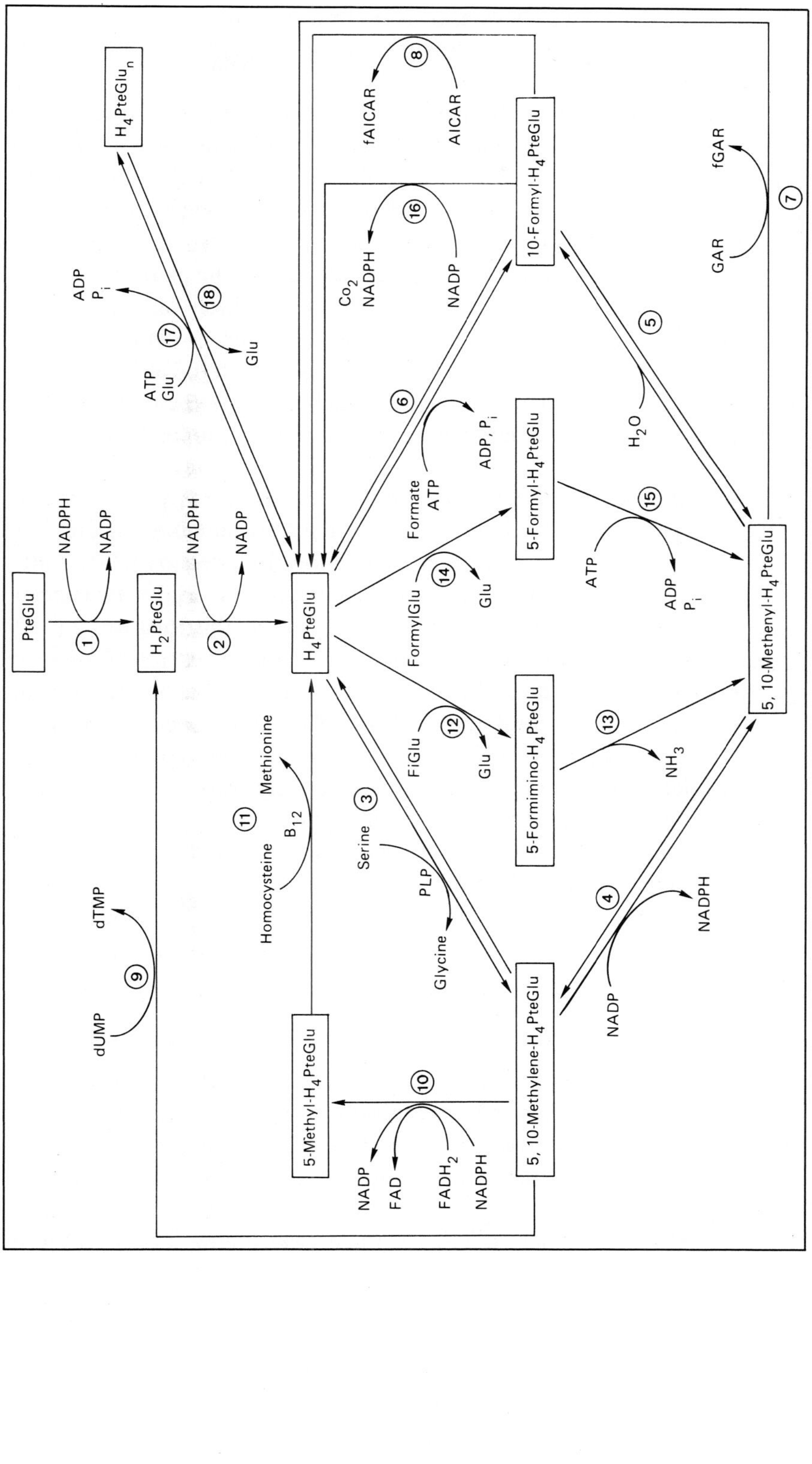
PteGlu
H_2PteGlu
H_4PteGlu
$H_4PteGlu_n$
5-Methyl-H_4PteGlu
5, 10-Methylene-H_4PteGlu
5-Formimino-H_4PteGlu
5-Formyl-H_4PteGlu
10-Formyl-H_4PteGlu
5, 10-Methenyl-H_4PteGlu
NADPH
NADP
ATP
Glu
ADP
P_i
Co_2
fAICAR
AICAR
GAR
fGAR
Formate
ADP, P_i
H_2O
FormylGlu
FiGlu
NH_3
Serine
PLP
Glycine
Homocysteine
B_{12}
Methionine
dUMP
dTMP
FAD
$FADH_2$
1 2 3 4 5 6 7 8 9 10 11 12 13 14 15 16 17 18

6

include green leafy vegetables and liver. Legumes may also contribute a significant amount of folate to the diet. Except for liver, animal foods are poor sources of folate.

The primary metabolic function of folate is in one-carbon metabolism [61]. Folate coenzymes serve as acceptors and donors of one carbon units in a variety of reactions involved in amino acid and nucleotide metabolism. The one carbon units can be at the oxidation levels of methanol, formaldehyde and formate, but not carbon dioxide. These reactions (fig. 6) known as one carbon metabolism illustrate the cyclic nature of folate metabolism. Such transfers are essential in the synthesis of nucleic acids and in the normal metabolism of amino acids, hence a folate deficiency can lead to alterations in the pattern of cell replication [62]. For example, one specific pathway affected in a folate deficiency is the conversion of deoxyuridylate to thymidylate which is required for duplication of DNA chains and cell division.

The progressive stages of folate deficiency as recently presented by Herbert [63] are illustrated in figure 7. Megaloblastic anemia is a late finding in the progressive stages of folate depletion. In assessing folate status prior to the development of anemia, one can measure serum folate concentration as an early indicator of depletion. However, this measure quickly fluctuates with recent dietary intake and used alone gives no information regarding tissue folate stores. In contrast, the red cell folate concentration is considered to be the best indicator of folate status since it has been shown to parallel tissue folate changes as evidenced here by reduction in the liver folate concentration. The reduced concentration of red cell folate is followed by hypersegmentation of neutrophils, macrocytosis and megaloblastic anemia. The folate in the red blood cell represents what was incorporated at the time of erythropoiesis and very little, if any, folate is transferred across the mature erythrocyte membrane. Hematological manifestations do not appear until after 3–4 months of folate deprivation [62].

Status during Life Cycle

Pregnancy. The increased requirement for folate in pregnancy arises from the markedly accelerated cell multiplication involved in the enlargement of the uterus, development of the placenta, expansion of blood volume and growth of the fetus. Many studies have demonstrated a steady fall in serum folate levels throughout pregnancy. The best study is probably that from Aberdeen in which 2,754 women were followed (table V) [64].

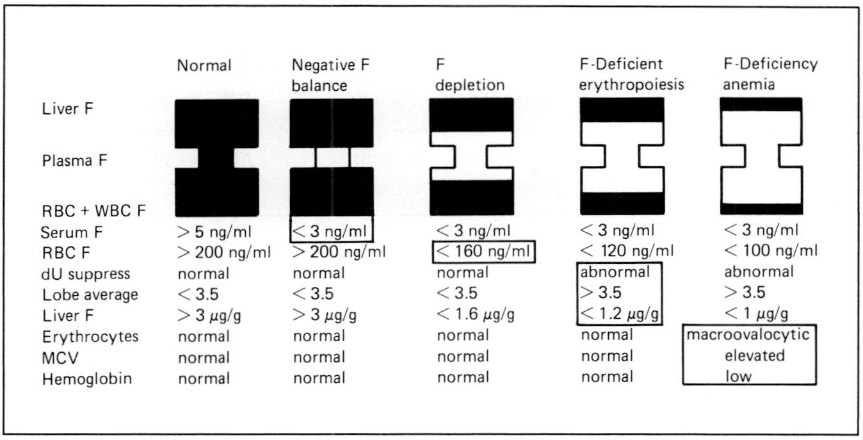

Fig. 7. Progressive stages of folate deficiency. From ref. [63].

Table V. Serum folate concentration in the complete population study. From ref. [64]

Gestation	Primigravidae		Multigravidae	
	number of women	mean serum folate, ng/ml	number of women	mean serum folate, ng/ml
Booking	1,061	6.60	1,693	6.72
30 weeks	665	5.15	1,060	4.94
36 weeks	305	4.45	477	4.17
Puerperium	482	3.67	772	3.51

The progressive reductions in serum levels were reported at 4 different stages. The authors attributed much of the fall of serum folate to hemodilution.

Pregnancy induces an increase in blood volume that begins late in the first trimester and expands relatively rapidly during all of the second trimester. Throughout the last few weeks of normal pregnancy, blood volume is relatively constant. Early in pregnancy more plasma than red cells is added to the maternal circulation, but late in pregnancy the reverse is true [4].

Table VI. Percent of low serum or RBC folate levels in pregnant women: NHANES II, 1976–1980. From ref. [66]

Group		Serum folate < 3 ng/ml		RBC folate < 140 ng/ml	
		number of persons	percent	number of persons	percent
Pregnant		51	20	42	21
Non-pregnant		411	15	347	12
Parity	0–2 births	313	13	264	11
	3+ births	149	22	125	16

Red blood cell (RBC) folate levels have been quantitated during pregnancy by a number of researchers. Chanarin [65] reported a progressive fall in RBC folate during pregnancy and near term ~30% of the women had low RBC folate levels. Folate status of ~300 pregnant women from low socioeconomic background was assessed by Bailey et al. [6]. All of the subjects were initial registrants for prenatal visits to Maternal and Infant Care Clinics in Florida and the majority (67%) were in their second trimester of pregnancy. 30% of this group had RBC folate concentrations < 140 ng/ml (fig. 8) which is in agreement with the data of Chanarin [65]. These data cannot be explained by hemodilution since only red cells were assayed and they indicate declining levels of folate available to the developing erythron, and presumably other tissues in pregnancy.

Prevalence estimates from NHANES II are inconclusive due to small sample size [66]. However, with this in mind, approximately 20% of the pregnant women included had either low serum or red blood cell folate levels as compared to ~13% for either measurement in non-pregnant women (table VI). These data also suggest that increased parity increased the risk of folate deficiency [66].

Possible complications of folate deficiency that have been implicated during pregnancy include megaloblastic anemia, prematurity, low birth weights and neural tube defects. Megaloblastic anemia complicating pregnancy is common where nutrition is inadequate, as in large parts of Africa, India and Latin American countries [65]. There is a high frequency of

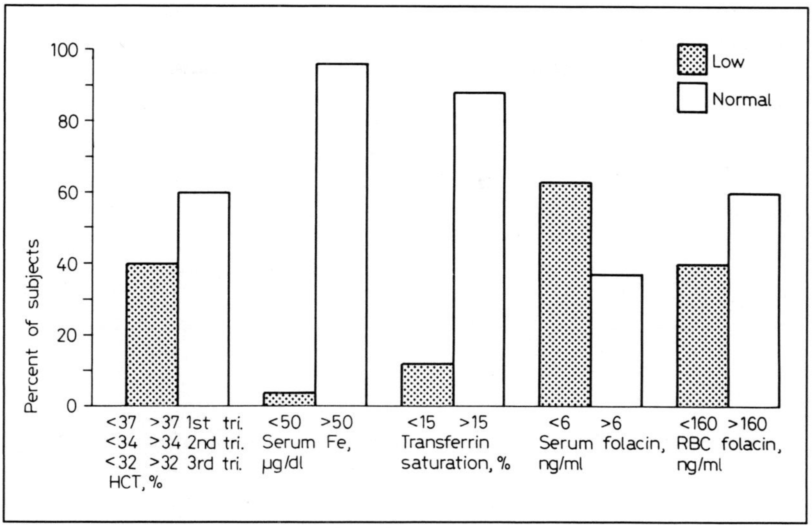

Fig. 8. Prevalence of low folate and iron blood levels in pregnant women. From ref. [6].

megaloblastic hematopoiesis in marrow aspirates which is far higher than the frequency of diagnosis based on peripheral blood examination. The explanation probably lies in the dominant role played by iron deficiency during anemia in pregnancy. Iron deficiency can conceal evidence of a mild megaloblastic process. The megaloblastosis may only become apparent in late pregnancy when there may be insufficient time for its consequence to appear in the peripheral blood. Suspicion of megaloblastic anemia may be aroused by the presence of anemia that fails to respond to iron therapy. Symptoms are non-specific, for example tiredness and rarely soreness of the mouth and a sore tongue may be present [65].

Baumslag et al. [67] showed that folate added to an iron supplement increased birth weight in folate deficient African women but had no effect when given to well-nourished Caucasian women. There were 19 low birth weight infants in the iron group but only 4 in the folate-iron supplement group (table VII). These observations have been confirmed by others. Iyengar et al. [68] also reported higher infant weights following folate supplementation in India. The supplements appeared to have contributed to higher birth weights of infants by bringing about changes in the placenta (table VIII). Not only were the placentas of the folic acid supplemented

Table VII. Reduction of incidence of prematurity by folic acid supplementation in pregnant Bantu women. From ref. [67]

Treatment	Weight of newborn		
	over 5 lb	under 5 lb	
Iron only	44	19	63
Iron + folic acid	61	4	65
Total	105	23	128

Table VIII. Effect of folic acid supplement on birth weight of infants. From ref. [68]

Group	Number	Birth weight, g
No supplement	52	2,567
Iron supplement (30 mg elemental/day)	96	2,650
Folic acid (200–500 μg/day) + iron	134	2,890

Table IX. Differences between folic acid supplement group and the control group, with respect to gestational age, birth weight, placental weight and content of RNA and DNA. From ref. [69]

		N	Mean	Significance	% diff.
Gestational age	+ folic acid	20	281	n.s.	0.2
	– folic acid	16	281		
Birth weight	+ folic acid	20	3,610	$p < 0.01$	12.7
	– folic acid	16	3,203		
Placental weight	+ folic acid	20	459	$p < 0.1$	11.9
	– folic acid	16	410		
Placental RNA	+ folic acid	19	822	$p < 0.1$	14.4
	– folic acid	15	718		
Placental DNA	+ folic acid	19	712	n.s.	11.1
	– folic acid	15	641		

group heavier, they also had more DNA and protein. Rolschau et al. [69] from Denmark also found a positive association between birth and placental weight in folate supplemented (5 mg) mothers (table IX). The beneficial effects on birth weight seen in the these studies suggests that the effect was due to improved nutrition via enhanced placenta size.

There is particular interest in folate in early pregnancy and indeed before conception takes place, in view of the possible relationship between folate and the occurrence of neural tube defects (NTD), the most common of which is spina bifida [70–75]. Smithells et al. [70] conducted a folate supplementation study in pregnant women who had previously delivered a baby with a neural tube defect. The supplement contained 360 μg of folate as well as other vitamins and minerals. The control group consisted of women who either refused to take the supplement or who were already pregnant and were not taking supplements.

Of the 429 infants born to women who took the supplement during the specified period, 3 (0.7%) had a neural tube defect as compared to 24 (4.7%) of the infants born to women who did not take the supplement. The risk to the women who had taken the supplement was only slightly greater than the risk to women in the general population who had not had a child with NTD.

Laurence [73] conducted a small trial in Southern Wales with folic acid alone. A non-significant decrease in the recurrence risks was seen among women who had been randomly assigned to receive 4 mg of folic acid daily compared with those who had taken a placebo.

Both of these studies have been criticized [74]. The study by Smithells was not a randomized placebo controlled study and the experimental group may have been affected by changes in dietary habits associated with participating in the study. In addition, one cannot rule out the possibility that other vitamins and minerals in the supplement may have influenced pregnancy outcome. Molloy et al. [75] found no difference in serum folate concentration in mothers whose infants were born with neural tube defects compared to the control group. These reports have generated sufficient interest for the British Medical Research Council to fund a large multinational clinical trial which is currently in progress, and for the National Institutes of Health to solicit a contract for a case controlled study to investigate the possible effect of periconceptional, nutritional status and vitamin supplementation on the incidence of neural tube defects.

The frequent findings, especially in deprived populations, of biochemical and cytological changes suggesting maternal folate deficiency have

Table X. Plasma, red blood cells (RBC), and milk folate levels (ng/ml) of lactating mothers before and after folate administration. From ref. [81]

	Plasma	RBC	Milk
Before PteGlu	6.0	251	130
After PteGlu (1 mg/day, 4 weeks)	42.0	390	137

resulted in the trend toward routine folic acid supplementation during pregnancy. The optimal dosage of folic acid supplements is controversial. If the goal is to raise the blood folate levels to the normal non-pregnant range in a population where megaloblastic anemia is rare, then as little as 100 μg of folic acid is adequate [65]. If however, pregnant women belong to a population where megaloblastic anemia is more common, 100 μg of folic acid may be inadequate. For pregnant women in a population with a high incidence of megaloblastic anemia, 125 μg was insufficient but 350 μg maintained the serum for most pregnant women in the non-pregnant range [65].

If the goal is to eradicate from all obstetric populations megaloblastic anemia due to folate deficiency, higher doses of folic acid might be given. Folic acid in a daily dose of 1 mg orally can be expected to produce hematologic remission in undelivered women with severe megaloblastic anemia. Therefore, a supplement of 200–400 μg of folic acid per day throughout the latter half of pregnancy should protect most pregnant women from anemia due to folate deficiency [4].

The RDA for pregnant women is 800 μg or twice that of non-pregnant women [18]. This is the amount contained in most prenatal vitamin supplements given in this country. Nutrition education is important as it relates to the selection of folate-dense foods. For example, the folate intake during pregnancy can be increased substantially by the consumption of fortified breakfast cereal [77].

Infancy. There are numerous reports that blood levels of folate are higher during early infancy than in adults [78–80]. These data (fig. 9) which illustrate this are from the NHANES II Survey [66]. One can easily see that if norms established for adults are applied to blood levels during infancy, prevalence estimates for deficiency are likely to be underesti-

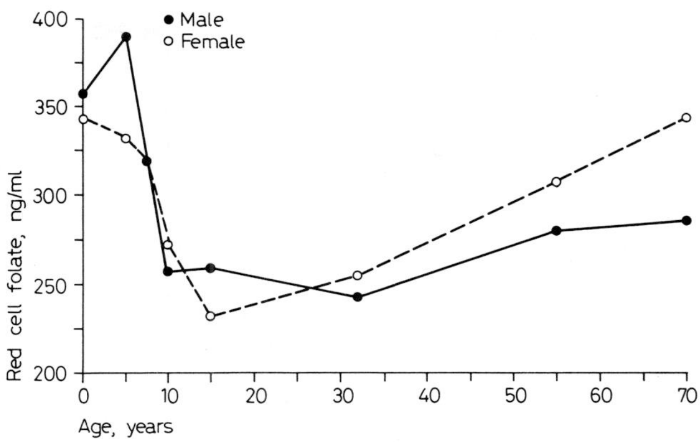

Fig. 9. Mean red cell folate levels by age and sex: NHANES II.

mated. These higher blood levels are present at birth indicating fetal sequestering during in utero development and are maintained at high levels for approximately 3 months by either breast-feeding or feeding folate supplemented infant formula.

Smith et al. [80] evaluated the effect of folate supplementation during pregnancy and lactation on maternal blood, milk, and infant blood folate levels at 6–12 weeks postpartum. Maternal folate blood levels were higher in lactating women taking supplements versus controls. There were no differences in milk folate concentration or infant blood levels between supplemented and unsupplemented groups.

Tamura et al. [81] reported similar findings as illustrated in table X. Milk folate was the same regardless of whether the mothers received folate supplements; however, maternal blood folate levels were compromised. These results indicate that human milk folate levels are maintained at the expense of maternal reserve and that folate supplementation during lactation may be of value for preserving maternal reserves.

The RDA for the lactating mother is 500 μg [76]. It seems advisable to recommend maternal supplementation to maintain optimal maternal folate status since milk folate concentrations appear to be maintained at the expense of maternal body stores.

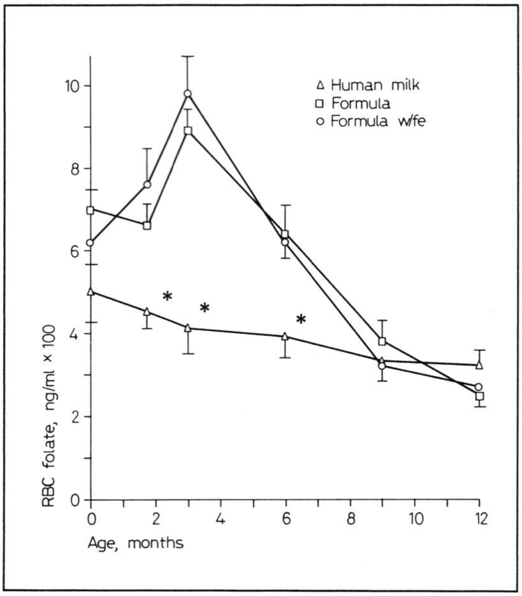

Fig. 10. Red blood cell levels of formula-fed and breast-fed infants during the first year of life. From ref. [82].

Smith et al. [82] recently reported data related to folate status of infants studied longitudinally from birth to 1 year (fig. 10). Infants were fed either human milk, a standard cow-milk infant formula or the same formula with added iron. Solid foods were introduced after 3 months. The mean folate content of human milk was 85 μg/l, Enfamil 162 μg/l and Enfamil plus iron 158 μg/l. At 6 weeks and 3 months formula fed infants had folate intakes and blood concentrations significantly greater than human milk infants. With the introduction of solid foods, decreases in blood folate concentration paralleled decreases in milk folate intake.

Breast milk or fortified infant formula is an important dietary source of folate during the first year. Both types of feeding during early infancy provide more than sufficient folate to maintain blood folate concentration above acceptable limits.

Adolescence. Adolescence is a period of rapid growth and development, and it is obvious that folate requirements may be elevated during this period of the life cycle. Bailey et al. [15, 83] evaluated the folate and

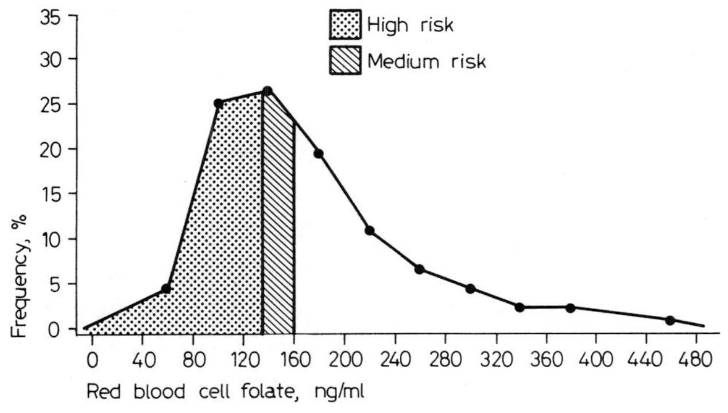

Fig. 11. Frequency distribution curve of red blood cell folate levels from urban black adolescents. From ref. [15].

Table XI. Differences between sexual maturity rating for serum folacin as determined by Duncan's multiple range tests[1]. From ref. [15]

	Serum folacin concentration for black males and females			
Sexual maturity rating	2	3	4	5
Serum folacin, ng/ml	11.5	11.5	7.9	7.5

[1] Means connected by same line indicate no difference ($p < 0.05$).

iron status including hematological parameters in a group of approximately 400 adolescent males and females. A unique aspect of this study was the assessment of folate status in relation to biological age versus age in years. This was accomplished by categorizing each subject into a sexual maturity category using Tanner's Sexual Maturation guidelines. [84, 85].

Approximately 40% of the adolescents had low (< 140 ng/ml) red blood cell folate concentrations which coexisted with poor iron status (fig. 11). Serum folate levels were found to decrease with an increase in sexual maturation as indicated by the decreasing mean serum folate level as the adolescents matured sexually (table XI).

The RDA for folate during adolescence is 400 μg or the same as that for an adult [76]. It was established that this high prevalence of folate inadequacy was associated with infrequent consumption of folate-dense foods which is quite typical of adolescent eating habits [86].

Old Age. The effect of alcohol on folate absorption and metabolism is of concern in the elderly since it is now recognized that 2–10% of individuals over the age of 60 in the USA are alcoholics [87, 88]. 15–20% of elderly patients admitted to general hospital wards or nursing homes have been found to be chronic alcoholics [87]. In a series of 121 consecutive patients admitted to two New York City hospitals over a 10-year period with megaloblastic anemia due to folate deficiency associated with alcoholism, 17.4% were over the age of 60 and 9.2% were over 65 [89]. Potential causes of folate deficiency in alcoholism include poor diet, intestinal malabsorption, and defective metabolism due to associated liver disease. Malabsorption of radiolabelled folate has been documented in two studies of malnourished alcoholics [90, 91]. Data from one study suggests that folate malabsorption in chronic alcoholism results from a synergistic effect of folate deprivation and ethanol toxicity on transport processes in the mucosa [92].

Drugs other than alcohol interfere with folate absorption or utilization. The use of anticonvulsant drugs (Phenytoin, Dilantin®, barbiturates or Primidone/Mysoline®) may lead to the development of folate deficiency in individuals exposed to their action over a long period of time [93]. Sulfasalazine which is used for the treatment of inflammatory bowel disease impairs folate absorption and may cause megaloblastic anemia [94]. The potential effect of these and other drugs on folate absorption and metabolism in the aged is not clear.

Several groups have investigated the effect of aging per se on folate absorption. Bhamthumnavin et al. [95] found no difference in the intestinal transport of radiolabeled monoglutamyl folate in everted gut sacs prepared from rats of various ages. Since the majority of dietary folate is in the polyglutamate form, the relevance of these data may be questioned. Hurdle and Williams [96] found no difference in the increase in serum folate following an oral dose of monoglutamyl folate in aged and young control human subjects. The data are difficult to interpret since tissues were not presaturated and no flushing dose was administered.

Kesavan and Noronha [97] investigated the effect of age on mucosal conjugase activity in rats using an everted-sac technique. Conjugase enzyme activity was significantly lower in the aged animals and polyglutamyl folate was absorbed less efficiently in the older animals. Baker et al. [98] reported that the rise in serum folate following the oral ingestion of polyglutamyl folate was significantly less in aged human subjects than the rise observed in young controls. In contrast, absorption of monoglutamyl folate was comparable in both age groups as was the absorption of other water-soluble vitamins.

Bailey et al. [99] recently compared the absorption of both radiolabelled mono- and polyglutamyl folate between healthy young and aged subjects using an in vivo triple-lumen perfusion technique. Conjugase enzyme activities were compared following jejunal biopsy in both age groups. No difference was found in the luminal disappearance, urinary recovery or conjugase enzyme activities between age groups. It was concluded that age per se had no effect on folate absorption.

Chronic folate deficiency results in changes in the intestinal epithelial cells similar to the megaloblastic changes in the bone marrow [100, 101]. Atrophy of the intestinal villi and impairment of the enzymatic functions of the cells have also been reported [102]. Once these morphological and functional changes in the intestinal epithelium have occurred, the ability of the intestine to absorb folate is impaired resulting in further depletion of the vitamin. Elsborg [103] demonstrated in elderly subjects that folate malabsorption was reversible following folate supplementation in folate-deficient elderly subjects.

There are not extensive data available on the dietary intake of folate in the elderly. Major national food intake surveys including those performed by the USDA and both the TSNS and NHANES surveys have not included calculated dietary folate intakes. In Canada, the daily folate intake of elderly (> 65 years) men and women averaged 151 and 130 μg respectively [104]. In the USA data from several recent regional surveys are of interest [41, 53]. Bailey et al. [99] found that the average folate intake was higher in groups of elderly from middle- and upper-income households when compared to groups from low-income households (table XII). Approximately 65% of a group of elderly from a densely populated low-income area in Dade County, Florida, consumed less than 200 μg of folate each day. In contrast, approximately 40% of middle-upper income groups in Florida and Albuquerque consumed less than 200 μg [41, 53].

Socioeconomic factors such as income, educational level, social interaction, shopping frequency, cooking, refrigeration and storage facilities, may particularly affect nutritional status and in this case folate intake. For

Table XII. Folacin intake data for elderly Florida and New Mexico residents

		n	Daily intake[1] µg/day	% with dietary intake 200 µg	Reference
Urban low income (Dade County)		128	192	65	46
Rural and urban low income (Alachua County)		173	184	61	41
Middle and high income (retirement community, N. Fla.)		40	217	45	unpublished
Urban middle and high income (Gainesville)		30	250	37	unpublished
Middle and high income (Albuquerque, NM)	Men	125	240	37	53
	Women	145	210	43	53

[1] Values represent mean values for folacin studies and median values for Albuquerque study.

example, the shopping frequency for low-income eldely living in Dade County, Florida, was less than twice per month. As determined by 24-hour food recall, only 17% of this group indicated that they consumed fresh vegetables and only 30% consumed citrus fruit [46]. Food preparation habits included boiling vegetables for several hours and discarding the cooking water. Folate supplements were not taken by any subjects in the Florida studies in contrast to 30% of subjects in Albuquerque. Those taking supplements in the Albuquerque study had an average of 48% higher plasma folate levels and 49% higher red blood cell folate levels.

Estimates of dietary folate intakes are low compared to the RDA regardless of socioeconomic status. However, intakes below the RDA standard in the middle and upper-income groups were associated with blood folate levels above the accepted norm. One explanation for this discrepancy is that folate values in food-nutrient data bases are incomplete. This of course may result in a substantial underestimation of dietary intakes of folate. Also, actual bioavailability of the vitamin from the diet may be somewhat higher than the percentage assumed in setting the RDA of

400 μg. Another possibility is that the current folate RDA may be unrealistically high.

There are very litte data available at the present time regarding folate status of the elderly in the USA. In the TSNS, the percent of the population with serum and red cell levels below accepted norms was not reported [34]. In the NHANES I survey, only folate in serum was measured [105]. Of the 369 persons aged 65–74 years, approximately 6% had serum folate below 3.0 ng/ml. In NHANES II only a small sub-sample of the population surveyed had blood folates analyzed and individuals over the age of 74 years were not included. Several smaller folate status assessment studies have been conducted on selected elderly population subgroups in the USA [41, 53, 60, 106]. The biochemical data substantiate the conclusion that elderly from low-socioeconomic households are at particular risk of developing a folate deficiency. In a densely populated urban poverty area of Florida (Miami), 60% of a predominately black group of elderly had red cell folate concentration less than 140 ng/ml [60]. In a separate study of elderly from low income households in Alachua County, Fla., Bailey et al. [41] found that 31% had deficient (< 140 ng/ml) red cell levels. In contrast, Wagner et al. [106] reported that only 6% of a white elderly group living in a middle and upper income retirement community in Florida had deficient (< 140 ng/ml) red cell folate levels. A similar prevalence (6% of group with red blood cell level < 140 ng/ml) was found in a highly educated, nutrition-conscious white elderly group in Albuquerque, New Mexico [unpublished findings].

Institutionalized elderly individuals may be at risk of folate deficiency due to a number of factors including chronic diseases, multiple medications, and poor dietary intake. Baker et al. [107] reported a higher prevalence of low (< 5 ng/ml) serum folate levels in institutionalized versus non-institutionalized elderly (19.5 and 9%, respectively). Similar findings have been reported by numerous other investigators in countries other than the USA [108–112]. Magnus et al. [113] reported that institutionalized elderly in Norway had significantly lower serum and red cell folate levels than younger healthy persons. This finding was also reported by other investigators [114, 115]. Folate deficiency was recently reported to occur in 22% of a group of institutionalized elderly in Canada and prophylactic administration of folate among long-term nursing home type patients was recommended [116]. Factors contributing to the high prevalence of deficiency in institutionalized elderly include poor diet, drug use, and chronic disease.

Summary

Physiological changes associated with the life cycle affect requirements for the essential nutrients iron and folate. Folate deficiency is often associated with pregnancy and is best assessed by progressive reductions in red blood cell folate concentrations. The rapid cell division associated with the growth and development of the fetus is primarily responsible for the marked elevation in folate requirements during this period of the life cycle. Folate supplementation is recommended throughout pregnancy. During infancy either folate-fortified infant formula or breast milk provide sufficient folate for the infant and at the expense of the lactating mother in the breast-fed infant. Accelerated growth and development during adolescence increases the requirement for folate and poor food selection habits increase the risk of developing a folate deficiency. The elderly often live alone with a restricted income which limits dietary folate intake. This often coexists with multiple drug use including alcohol which could have a negative influence on folate status.

Iron requirements are markedly elevated during pregnancy and iron supplements are recommended to protect body stores. Infant iron status is primarily affected by dietary iron intake which is best supplied by either breast milk or iron-fortified infant formula. Iron deficiency is common during the second year of life and during adolescence. In contrast, the requirements of the elderly are reduced and iron deficiency is rarely associated with old age.

References

1 Smith, K.T.: Effects of chemical environment on iron bioavailability measurements. Food Tech. *37:* 115–120 (1983).
2 Monson, E.R.; Balintfy, J.L.: Calculating dietary iron bioavailability: refinement and computerization. J. Am. diet. Ass. *80:* 307–311 (1982)
3 Finch, C.A.; Cook, J.D.: Iron deficiency. Am. J. clin. Nutr. *39:* 471–477 (1984).
4 Hytten, F.E.; Thomson, A.M.: Maternal physiological adjustments. Maternal nutrition and the course of pregnancy, pp. 41–47 (Community on Maternal Nutrition, Food Nutrition Board, Natn. Res. Council, National Academy of Sciences, Washington 1971).
5 Expert Scientific Working Group: Summary of a report on assessment of the iron nutritional status of the United States population. Am. J. clin. Nutr. *42:* 1318–1330 (1985).
6 Bailey, L.B.; Mahan, C.S.; Dimperio, D.: Folacin and iron status in low-income pregnant adolescents and mature women. Am. J. clin. Nutr. *33:* 1997–2001 (1980).

7 Oski, F.A.: Iron deficiency. Pediat. Clins N. Am. *32:* 493–497 (1985).
8 Singla, P.N.; Chand, S.; Agawal, K.N.: Cord serum and placental tissue iron status in maternal hypoferremia. Am. J. clin. Nutr. *32:* 1462–1465 (1979).
9 Rios, E.; Lipschitz, P.A.; Cook, J.D.; Smith, N.J.: Relationship of maternal and infant iron stores as assessed by determination of plasma ferritin. Pediatrics, Springfield *55:* 694–699 (1975).
10 Siimes, M.A.; Salmenpera, L.; Perkeentupa, J.: Exclusive breast-feeding for 9 months: risk of iron deficiency. J. Pediat. *104:* 196–199 (1984).
11 Dallman, P.R.; Siimes, M.A.; Stekel, A.: Iron deficiency in infancy and childhood. Am. J. clin. Nutr. *33:* 86–118 (1980).
12 Vasquez-Seoane, P.; Windom, R.; Pearson, H.A.: Disappearance of iron-deficiency anemia in a high-risk infant population given supplemental iron. New Engl. J. Med. *313:* 1239 (1985).
13 Committee on Nutrition: Iron balance and requirements in infancy. Pediatrics, Springfield *43:* 134–142 (1969).
14 Bailey, L.B.; Gingsburg, J.G.; Wagner, P.; Voyes, W.; Christakis, G.; Dinning, J.: Serum ferritin as measure of iron stores in adolescents. J. Pediat. *101:* 774–776 (1982).
15 Bailey, L.B.; Wagner, P.A.; Christakis, G.J.: Folacin and iron status and hematological findings in Black and Spanish American adolescents from urban low-income households. Am. J. clin. Nutr. *35:* 1023–1032 (1982).
16 Lynch, S.R.; Finch, C.A.; Monsen, E.R.; Cook, J.D.: Iron status of elderly Americans. Am. J. clin. Nutr. *36:* 1032–1045 (1982).
17 Loh, T.T.; Chang, L.L.: Hepatic iron status in Malaysians and Singaporeans. Southeast Asian J. trop. Med. publ. Hlth *II:* 131–136 (1980).
18 Sturgeon, P.; Shoden, A.: Total liver storage iron in normal populations of the USA. Am. J. clin. Nutr. *24:* 469–474 (1971).
19 Weinfeld, A.: Storage iron in man. Acta med. scand. *177:* suppl. 427, pp. 1–155 (1964).
20 Shah, B.; Belonje, B.: Liver storage iron in Canadians. Am. J. clin. Nutr. *29:* 66–69 (1976).
21 Celada, A.; Heneras, V.; DeCastro, S.: Liver iron storage in Spanish aging population. Am. J. clin. Nutr. *33:* 2662–2664 (1980).
22 Gautier de Defaiz, H.; Puente, R.; Vidal, B.; Perenz, B.; Vidal, H.: Liver storage iron in normal population in Cuba. Am. J. clin. Nutr. *33:* 133–136 (1980).
23 Benzie, R.: The influence of age upon the iron content of bone marrow. Lancet *i:* 1074–1075 (1963).
24 Burkhardt, R.: Iron overload of bone marrow and bone; in Kief, Iron metabolism and its disorders, pp. 264 (Excerpta Medica, Amsterdam 1975).
25 Cook, J.D.; Finch, C.A.; Smith, N.: Evaluation of the iron status of a population. Blood *48:* 449–455 (1976).
26 Valberg, L.S.; Sorbie, J.; Ludwig, J.; Pelletier, O.: Serum ferritin and the iron status of Canadians. Can. med. Ass. J. *114:* 417–421 (1976).
27 Leyland, M.J.; Harris, H.; Brown, P.J.: Iron status in a general practice and its relationship to morbidity. Br. J. Nutr. *41:* 291–295 (1979).
28 Ovist, E.; Norden, A.; Olofsson, T.: Serum ferritin in the elderly. Scand. J. clin. Lab. Invest. *40:* 609–613 (1980).

29 Casale, G.; Bonora, C.; Migliavacca, A.; Zurita, I.E.; Nicola, P. de: Serum ferritin and aging. Age Aging *10:* 119–122 (1981).
30 Garry, P.J.; Goodwin, U.S.; Hunt, W.C.: Iron status and anemia in the elderly: new findings and a review of previous studies. J. Am. Geriat. Soc. *31:* 389–399 (1983).
31 Finch, C.A.: Body iron exchange in man. J. clin. Invest. *38:* 392–396 (1959).
32 Green, R.; Charlton, R.W.; Steflel, H.; Bothwell, T.; Mayet, F.; Adams, B.; Finch, C.; Layrisse, M.: Body iron excretion in man. A collaborative study. Am. J. Med. *45:* 336–353 (1968).
33 Food and Nutrition Board: Recommended dietary allowances (National Academy of Sciences, Washington 1980).
34 Ten State Nutrition Survey 1968–70. No. V Dietary (US Dept. of Health, Education, Welfare, Center for Disease Control, Atlanta 1972).
35 O'Hanlon, P.; Kohrs, M.B.: Dietary studies of older Americans. Am. J. clin. Nutr. *31:* 1257–1269 (1978).
36 Kohrs, M.B.; O'Neal, R.; Preston, A.; Eklund, D.; Abrahams, O.: Nutritional status of elderly residents in Missouri. Am. J. clin. Nutr. *31:* 2186–2197 (1978).
37 Yearick, E.S.; Wang, M.S.L.; Pisias, S.J.: Nutritional status of the elderly: dietary and biochemical findings. J. Geront. *35:* 663–671 (1980).
38 US Dept. Ag. Science and Education Administration: Food and nutrient intakes of individuals in 1 day in the United States, Spring 1979. Preliminary report No. 2 (US Dept. of Agriculture, Washington 1980).
39 US Dept. Ag. Science and Education Administration: Food and nutrient intake of individuals in 1 day in Hawaii, Winter 1978. Preliminary report No. 5 (US Dept. of Agriculture, Washington 1981).
40 Garry, P.J.; Goodwin, J.S.; Hunt, W.C.; Hooper, E.M.; Leonary, A.G.: Nutritional status in a healthy elderly population: dietary and supplemental intakes. Am. J. clin. Nutr. *36:* 319–331 (1982).
41 Bailey, L.B.; Wagner, P.A.; Jernigan, J.A.; Nickens, C.; Brazzi, G.: Folacin and iron status of an elderly population. Fed. Proc. *41:* 951 (1982).
42 Greger, J.L.: Dietary intake and nutritional status in regard to zinc of institutionalized aged. J. Geront. *32:* 549–553 (1977).
43 Pirrie, R.: The influence of age upon serum iron in normal subjects. J. clin. Path. *5:* 10–15 (1952).
44 Lipschitz, D.A.; Cook, J.D.; Finch, C.A.: A clinical evaluation of serum ferritin as an index of iron stores. New Engl. J. Med. *290:* 1213–1216 (1974).
45 Health and Nutrition Examination Survey United States, 1971–1974: Dietary intake source data. No. (PHS) 79–1221 (DHEW, Maryland 1979).
46 Bailey, L.B.; Wagner, P.A.; Christaksis, G.J.; Araujo, P.E.; Appledorf, N.; Davis, C.G.; Masteryanni, J.; Dinning, J.S.: Folacin and iron status and hematological findings in predominantly black elderly persons from urban low-income households. Am. J. clin. Nutr. *32:* 2346–2353 (1979).
47 Fisher, S.; Hendricks, D.G.; Mahoney, A.W.: Nutritional assessment of senior rural Utahns by biochemical and physical measurements. Am. J. clin. Nutr. *32:* 667–672 (1978).
48 Yearick, E.S.; Wang, M.S.L.; Pisias, S.J.: Nutritional status of the elderly: dietary and biochemical findings. J. Geron. *35:* 663–671 (1980).

49 Geishoff, S.N.; Brusis, O.A.; Nino, N.V.; Huber, A.M.: Studies of the elderly in Boston. I. The effects of iron fortification on moderately anemic people. Am. J. clin. Nutr. *30:* 226–234 (1977).
50 Harant, Z.; Goldberger, J.V.: Treatment of anemia in the aged: a common problem and challenge. J. Am. Geriat. Soc. *23:* 127–131 (1975).
51 Lawson, I.R.: Anemia in a group of elderly patients. Geront. clin. *2:* 87–101 (1960).
52 Hale, W.E.; Stewart, R.B.; Cerda, J.J.; Marks, R.G.; May, E.E.: Use of nutritional supplements in an ambulatory elderly population. J. Am. Geriat. Soc. *30:* 401–403 (1982).
53 Garry, P.J.; Goodwin, J.S.; Hunt, W.C.; Hooper, E.M.; Leonard, A.G.: Nutritional status in a healthy elderly population: dietary and supplemental intakes. Am. J. clin. Nutr. *36:* 319–331 (1982).
54 Reizenstein, P.; Ljunggren, G.; Smedby, B.; Agenas, I.; Penchansky, M.: Overprescribing iron tablets to elderly people in Sweden. Br. med. J. 962–963 (1979).
55 Edwards, C.Q.; Solnick, M.N.; Kushner, J.P.: Hereditary hemochromatosis: contributions of genetic analyses. Prog. Hemat. *12:* 43–71 (1981).
56 Bothwell, T.N.; Charlton, R.W.; Cook, J.D.; Finch, C.A.: Iron metabolism in man (Blackwell, Oxford 1979).
57 Butterworth, C.E.; Santini, R.; Frommeyer, W.B.: The pteroylglutamate components of American diets as determined by chromatographic fractionation. J. clin. Invest. *42:* 1929–1939 (1963).
58 Perloff, B.P.; Butrum, R.R.: Folacin in selected foods. J. Am. diet. Ass. *70:* 161–172 (1977).
59 Halsted, C.N.: The intestinal absorption of folates. Am. J. clin. Nutr. *32:* 846–855 (1979).
60 Huskisson, Y.J.; Retief, F.P.: Folaatinhound van voedsel. S. Afr. med. J. *44:* 362–366 (1970).
61 Brody, T.; Shane, B.; Stokstad, R.: Folic acid; in Handbooks of vitamins, nutritional, biochemical and clinical aspects, pp. 459–496 (Dekker, New York 1984).
62 Herbert, V.: Biology of disease megaloblastic anemias. Lab. Invest. *52:* 3–19 (1985).
63 Herbert, V.: Proc. of 13th Int. Congr. (in press, 1986).
64 Hall, M.H.; Pirani, B.B.K.; Cambell, D.: The cause of the fall in serum folate in normal pregnancy. Br. J. Obstet. Gynec *83:* 132–136 (1976).
65 Chanarin, I.: Folate and cobalamin. Clin. Haematol. *14:* 629–641 (1985).
66 Senti, F.R.; Pilch, S.M.: Analysis of folate data from the second National Health and Nutrition Examination Survey. J. Nutr. *115:* 1398–1402 (1985).
67 Baumslag, N.; Edelstein, T.; Mety, J.: Reduction of incidence of prematurity by folic acid supplementation in pregnancy. Br. med. J. *i:* 16–17 (1970).
68 Iyengar, L.; Rajalakshmi, K.: Effect of folic acid supplement on birth weights of infants. Am. J. Obstet. Gynec *122:* 332–336 (1975).
69 Rolschau, J.; Date, J.; Kristoffersen, K.: Folic acid supplement and intrauterine growth. Acta obstet. gynec. scand. *58:* 343–346 (1979).
70 Smithells, R.W.; Sheppard, S.; Schorah, C.J.; Seller, M.J.; Nevin, N.C.; Harris, R.; Read, A.P.; Fielding, D.W.: Possible prevention of neural-tube defects by periconceptional vitamin supplementation. Lancet *i:* 339–340 (1980).

71 Smithells, R.W.; Sheppard, S.; Shorah, C.J.; Seller, M.J.; Nevin, N.C.; Harris, R.; Read, A.P.; Fielding, D.W.: Apparent prevention of neural tube defects by periconceptional vitamin supplementation. Archs Dis. Childh. *56:* 911–918 (1981).

72 Smithells, R.W.; Nevin, N.C.; Seller, M.J.; Harris, R.; Fielding, D.W.; Schorah, C.J.; Sheppard, S.; Read, A.P.; Walker, S.; Wild, J.: Further experience of vitamin supplementation for prevention of neural tube defect recurrences. Lancet *i:* 1027–1031 (1983).

73 Laurence, K.M.: Prevention of neural tube defects by improvement in maternal diet and preconceptional folic acid supplementation. Prog. clin. biol. Res. *163B:* 383–388 (1985)..

74 Elwood, J.M.: Can vitamins prevent neural tube defects? Can. med. Ass. J. *129:* 1088–1092 (1983).

75 Molloy, A.M.; Kirke, P.; Hillary, I.: Maternal serum folate and vitamin B_{12} concentrations in pregnancies associated with neural tube defects. Archs Dis. Childh. *60:* 660–665 (1985).

76 Committee on Dietary Allowances, Food and Nutrition Board: Recommended dietary allowances (Natn. Academy of Sciences, Washington 1980).

77 Thenen, S.W.: Folacin content of supplemental foods for pregnancy. J. Am. diet. Ass. *30:* 237–241 (1981).

78 Ek, J.; Magnus, E.M.: Plasma and red cell folacin in cow's milk fed infants and children during the first 2 years of life: the significance of boiling pasteurized cow's milk. Am. J. clin. Nutr. *33:* 1220–1224 (1980).

79 Matoth, Y.; Pinkas, A.; Sroks, C.: Studies on folic acid in infancy. III. Folates in breast-fed infants and their mothers. Am. J. clin. Nutr. *16:* 356–359 (1965).

80 Smith, A.M.; Picciano, M.F.; Deering, R.H.: Folate supplementation during lactation: maternal folate status, human milk folate content and their relationship to infant folate status. J. Pediat. Gastroenterol. Nutr. *2:* 622–628 (1983).

81 Tamura, T.; Yoshimura, Y.; Arakawa, T.: Human milk folate and folate status in lactating mothers and their infants. Am. J. clin. Nutr. *33:* 193–197 (1980).

82 Smith, A.M.; Picciano, M.F.; Deering, R.H.: Folate intake and blood concentrations of term infants. Am. J. clin. Nutr. *41:* 590–598 (1985).

83 Bailey, L.B.; Wagner, P.A.; Christakis, G.J.: Folacin and iron status of adolescents from low-income rural households. Nutr. Res. *2:* 397–407 (1982).

84 Marshall, W.A.; Tanner, J.M.: Variations in pattern of pubertal changes in girls. Archs Dis. Childh. *44:* 291–303 (1969).

85 Marshall, W.A.; Tanner, J.M.: Variations in pattern of pubertal changes in boys. Archs Dis. Childh. *45:* 13–23 (1970).

86 Bailey, L.B.; Wagner, P.A.; Davis, C.C.; Dinning, J.S.: Food frequency related to folacin status in adolescents. J. Am. diet. Ass. *84:* 801–804 (1984).

87 Schuckitt, M.A.; Pastor, P.A.: The elderly as an unique population: alcoholism. Alcohol. clin. exp. Res. *2:* 31–38 (1978).

88 Zimberg, S.: Alcohol and the elderly, in Peterson, Whittington, Payne, Drugs and the elderly, pp. 28–40 (Thomas, Chicago 1979).

89 Rosenberg, I.N.; Bowman, B.B.; Cooper, B.A.; Halsted, C.N.; Lindenbaum, J.: Folate nutrition in the elderly. Am. J. clin. Nutr. *36:* 1060–1066 (1982).

90 Halsted, C.N.; Griggs, R.C.; Harris, V.W.: The effects of alcoholism on the absorption of folic acid (^{3}H-PGA) evaluated by plasma levels and urine excretion. J. Lab. clin. Med. *69:* 116–131 (1967).

91 Halsted, C.H.; Robles, E.A.; Mezey, E.: Decreased jejunal uptake of folic acid (^{3}H-PGA) in alcoholic patients: roles of alcohol and nutrition. New Eng. J. Med. *285:* 701–706 (1971).
92 Halsted, C.N.; Robles, E.A.; Mezey, E.: Intestinal malabsorption in folate-deficient alcoholics. Gastroenterology *64:* 526–532 (1973).
93 Waxman, S.; Corcino, J.J.; Nerbert, V.: Drugs, toxins, and dietary amino acids affecting vitamin B_{12} on folic acid absorption or utilization. Am. J. Med. *48:* 599–608 (1970).
94 Franklin, J.L.; Roseberg, I.N.: Impaired folic acid absorption in inflammatory bowel disease: effects of salicylazosulfapyridine (azulfidine). Gastroenterology *64:* 517–525 (1973).
95 Bhanthumnavin, K.; Wright, J.R.; Halsted, C.H.: Intestinal transport of tritiated folic acid (^{3}HPGA) in the everted gut sac of different aged rats. Johns Hopkins med. J. *135:* 152–160 (1974).
96 Hurdle, A.D.F.; Williams, T.C.P.: Folic acid deficiency in elderly patients admitted to hospital. Br. med. J. *ii:* 202–205 (1966).
97 Kasavan, V.; Noronka, J.M.: Folate malabsorption in aged rats related to low levels of pancreatic folyl conjugase. Am. J.clin. Nutr. *37:* 262–267 (1983).
98 Baker, H.; Jaslow, S.; Frank, O.: Severe impairment of dietary folate utilization in the elderly. J. Am. Geriat. Soc. *26:* 218–221 (1978).
99 Bailey, L.B.; Cerda, J.J.; Bloch, B.S.; Busby, J.; Vargas, L.; Chandler, C.J.; Halsted, C.H.: Effect of aging on folate absorption and conjugase enzyme activities in humans. Fed. Proc. *43:* (1984).
100 Bianchi, A.; Chipman, D.; Dreskin, A.; Rosensweig, N.S.: Nutritional folic acid deficiency with megaloblastic changes in the small-bowel epithelium. New Eng. J. Med. *282:* 859–861 (1970).
101 Veeger, W.; Tan Thije, O.J.; Nellemans, N.; Mandema, E.; Nieweg, H.O.: Sprue with a characteristic lesion of the small intestine associated with folic acid deficiency. Acta med. scand. *177:* 493–502 (1965).
102 Berg, N.O.; Dahlquist, A.; Lindberg, K.; Norden, A.: Morphology dipeptidases and dissacharidases of small intestinal mucosa in vitamin B_{12} and folic acid deficiency. Scand. J. Haematol. *9:* 167–173 (1972).
103 Elsborg, L.: Reversible malabsorption of folic acid in the elderly with nutritional folate deficiency. Acta haemat. *55:* 140–147 (1976).
104 Nutrition Canada: Food consumption patterns report (Department of National Health and Welfare, Ottawa 1977).
105 Lowenstein, F.W.: Nutritional status of the elderly in the United States of America, 1971–1974. J. Am. Coll. Nutr. *1:* 1165–1177 (1982).
106 Wagner, P.A.; Bailey, L.B.; Krista, M.L.; Jernigan, J.A.; Robinson, J.D.; Cerda, J.J.: Comparison of zinc and folacin status in elderly women from differing socioeconomic backgrounds. Nutr. Res. *1:* 565–599 (1981).
107 Baker, H.; Frank, O.; Thind, I.S.; Jaslow, S.P.; Louria, D.P.: Vitamin profiles in elderly persons living at home or in nursing homes, versus profile in healthy young subjects. J. Am. Geriat. Soc. *27:* 444–450 (1979).
108 Read, A.E.; Gough, K.R.; Pardoe, J.L.; Nicholas, A.: Nutritional studies on the entrants to an old people's home, with particular perference to folic acid deficiency. Br. med. J. *ii:* 843–848 (1965).

109 Hurdle, A.D.F.; Picton Williams, T.C.: Folic acid deficiency in elderly patients admitted to hospital. Br. med. J. *ii:* 202–205 (1966).
110 Batata, M.; Spray, G.H.; Bolton, F.G.; Higgins, G.; Wollner, L.: Blood and bone marrow changes in elderly patients, with special reference to folic acid, vitamin B_{12}, iron and ascorbic acid. Br. med. J. *ii:* 667–669 (1967).
111 Elwood, P.C.; Shinton, N.K.; Wilson, C.I.D.; Sweetnam, P.; Franzer, A.C.: Haemoglobin, vitamin B_{12} and folate levels in the elderly. Br. J. Haematol. *21:* 557–563 (1971).
112 Morgan, A.G.; Kelleher, B.E.; Losowsky, M.S.; Droller, H.; Middleton, R.W.W.: A nutritional survey in the elderly: haematological aspects. Int. J. Vitam. Nutr. Res. *43:* 461–471 (1973).
113 Magnus, E.M.; Bache-Wiig, J.E.; Aanderson, T.R.; Melbostad, E.: Folate and vitamin B_{12} (cobalamin) blood levels in elderly persons in geriatric homes. Scand. J. Haematol. *28:* 360–366 (1982).
114 Meindoks, H.; Dvorsky, R.: Serum folate and vitamin B_{12} levels in the elderly. J. Am. Geriat. Soc. *18:* 317–326 (1970).
115 Webster, S.G.P.; Leeming, J.T.: Erythrocyte folate levels in young and old. J. Am. Geriat. Soc. *27:* 451–454 (1979).
116 Infante-Rivard, C.; Kueger, M.; Gascon-Baree, M.; Rivard, G.E.: Folate deficiency among institutionalized elderly. J. Am. Geriat. Soc. *34:* 211–214 (1986).

Lynn B. Bailey, PhD, Food Science and Human Nutrition Department and the Department of Medicine, University of Florida, Gainesville, FL 32611 (USA)

Wld Rev. Nutr. Diet., vol. 56, pp. 93–172 (Karger, Basel 1988)

Interrelationships Among Alcohol Abuse, Obesity, and Type II Diabetes Mellitus: Focus on Native Americans

Mary E. Mohs, Tina K. Leonard, Ronald R. Watson

Department of Family and Community Medicine, University of Arizona, Health Science Center, Tucson, Ariz., USA

Contents

Introduction

Obesity, alcohol abuse, and type II diabetes mellitus are all diet-related conditions having multiple etiologic factors which encompass a wide range of nature and nurture affectors. Genetic constitution, environmental forces, and experiences are factors in the development of and exacerbation of each of these conditions. Alcohol abuse and obesity are also related to type II diabetes mellitus through the physiological mechanisms of organ damage, and alteration of glucose and insulin metabolism accompanied by development of glucose intolerance. The question of what relative importance the genetic and environmental components may have in accounting for the etiology and expression of these diet-related conditions has been addressed by several lines of research.

This article reviews the way(s) in which genetic inheritance, cultural and socioeconomic factors, early life experience, and other environmental forces may interrelate with alcohol abuse, obesity, and type II diabetes mellitus as well as how these health problems may interrelate with each other. The central focus is on diabetes mellitus, with the roles of obesity and alcohol intake discussed only as they may relate to diabetes etiology or progression.

The Native American population has quite diverse genetic and cultural milieus. However, many Native American groups have higher type II diabetes mellitus incidence and prevalence rates than those seen among the general American population. The disproportionately high rates among Native Americans have developed in the past four and a half decades and have occurred concomitant with increased obesity prevalence and alcoholism incidence. Several Native American subpopulations have been well-studied in terms of genetic makeup and/or environmental factors in relation to one or more of these three conditions. This is particularly true for several tribes in Oklahoma and Arizona concerning type II diabetes mellitus and obesity. It is also true of several tribes in various parts of the North American continent concerning alcohol abuse. Altered dietary and exercise patterns have been implicated in the generally higher obesity, alcohol abuse, and diabetes mellitus rates seen among Native Americans. Some genetic constitutions, adapted to generations of feast-famine cycles or, in the case of far-north hunters, to an almost carbohydrate-free diet, may be interacting with these changing life-style patterns to affect the development of obesity and type II diabetes mellitus. Differential development of organ damage and resulting rates at which metabolic disturbances occur with alcohol intake may also be related to genetic makeup. The current state of the literature concerning these possibilities and others is explored. The review cites studies of the general population as well as those done specifically with Native American groups. Thus, most if not all of the findings are applicable to the population as a whole. The focus, however, is mainly on Native Americans and how the interrelationships affect them.

The article's scope is as follows. Trends of the past half-century and recent rates of the three conditions among the Native American population are reviewed. Some studies done on mixed European-Native American communities are also highlighted. Possible synergisms between genetic makeup and cultural changes in the development of the three conditions are discussed. The areas of research exploring the possible role of genetics in each of the three conditions, and the nature versus nurture aspects of these health problems are addressed. The physiological roles of obesity and alcohol abuse in the etiology of diabetes mellitus are described. Finally, a brief summary of findings is given.

Diabetes Epidemiology Among Native Americans

Many Native American populations surveyed in the past 20 years have shown a prevalence of adult-onset, noninsulin-dependent or type II diabetes much greater than that of the general US population. The range of diabetes prevalence is great, however, with the peak rate occurring among the Pima tribe of Arizona. The epidemic of diabetes is a relatively recent phenomenon, dating to the mid-1940s in onset, and continuing to increase proportionate to the Native American population [1]. The rising diabetes rate is seen in almost all groups of the Native American population. The notable exceptions are the Athabascan Indians and Eskimos of Alaska and the Tarahumara of Mexico. These three groups, although ethnically distinct from one another, share an active outdoor life-style, and largely consume their traditional diets [2, 3]. The wide geographic and climatic range inhabited by the affected tribal groups, and the representation of every major language group among affected tribes, combine to make the diabetes epidemic truly continental in character (table I).

In 1965, 29% of Cherokee surveyed on the Qualla Reservation in North Carolina over 34 years of age were found to have diabetes, with an additional 12% showing borderline glucose tolerance. Within the diabetic group, 17.2% were previously confirmed diabetics and 11.8% were new cases which showed definite abnormal glucose tolerance. Notably, 29.6% of these new cases were 20% or more overweight. Also, 33% of those with more than 50% Indian blood had diabetes, showing a positive correlation of Indian genetic quanta and diabetes rate. The diet on gross appraisal appeared to be high in carbohydrate and total calories [4].

Table I. Diabetes glucose intolerance prevalence in selected Native American populations

Tribe	Area	Year	Prevalence %	Age group years	Reference(s)
Athabascan	Alaska	1969	1.3	adult	2
Cherokee	North Carolina	1965	33.0 12.0 borderline	≥34	4
Choctaw	Oklahoma	1965	5.3	all ages	5, 6
Pawnee	Oklahoma	1966	11.7	all ages	7
Aleuts	New York	1969	2.1	≥20	10
Seneca	New York	1969	13.4	adult	11
Washoe	Nev, Calif.	1973	10.7	≥15	12
N. Paiute	Nev, Calif.	1973	11.5	≥15	12
Mandan	N. Dakota	1978	39	≥35	13
Arickara	N. Dakota	1978	22.8	≥35	13
Hidatsa	N. Dakota	1978	21.1	≥35	13
3 Affil.	N. Dakota	1978	27.1	≥35	13
Zuni	New Mex.	1978 1984	6 23.9 26.5 40.0	25–45 45–64 ≥64 45	14 15
Cocopah	Arizona	1969	17 34	≥5 ≥35	17
Mohave	Arizona	1969	60.0 21.1	adult ≥5	18 18
Pima	Arizona	1971	50	≥35	22
Papago	Arizona	1976	42.3	≥35	25
Apache	Arizona	1976	11.0	≥35	25
White River Apache	Arizona	1976	24.8	≥35	25
San Carlos Apache	Arizona	1976	29.9	≥35	25
Yumas, Navajo	Arizona	1976	12.8	≥35	25
Washoe	Arizona	1976	16.9	≥35	25
Paiute	Arizona	1976	25.9	≥35	25

Also by 1965, a 5-year study of diabetes prevalence among 80% of southeastern Oklahoma's Choctaws had shown a diabetes rate of 53.2 per 1,000 in full-blood Indians, which was six times the national average. Mixed-blood Choctaws, with one eighth or more Choctaw lineage, showed a rate of 18.3 per 1,000. This rate was two times the then-current national average. The Choctaw subjects were screened via a retrospective chart review of all inpatients and outpatients registered at Talihina Indian Hospital between September 1, 1956, and August 31, 1961. The Choctaw diet was high in calories, approximately 4,000 kcal per day, and had a low-protein, high-carbohydrate, high-fat content [5, 6].

In 1966, the clinical records of Oklahoma Indian diabetics attending the Diabetic Clinic at the Pawnee Indian Hospital showed that the incidence for the annual population load was 11.7%. This was higher than the general population's and was predominantly of the adult onset type [7].

By 1969, 19 Native American tribes had been studied since the mid-1950s, and 14 had shown a prevalence of diabetes between 4 and 23%. In addition, a 1969 evaluation of diabetic sequellae among Winnebago and Omaha diabetic patients in Nebraska showed that the disease produced as much vascular and infectious sequellae in Native Americans as in the general US population [8]. The fact that very harmful health consequences were evident was reemphasized when a cross-sectional study of Hopi and Navajo Indians with noninsulin-dependent or type II diabetes was done in 1983. Duration of diabetes was strongly related to vascular complications. Diabetic patients with a problem of 10 years' duration or greater showed rates for retinopathy (57%), nephropathy (40%), peripheral vascular disease (28%), and peripheral neuropathy (21%), similar to those seen in many other populations [9].

One hundred ninety-three Aleuts on the Pribiloff Islands of Alaska, a mixed Native American-European population genetically, showed significantly higher fasting glucose levels than Athabascans or Eskimos, and an incidence of type II diabetes among those 20 years and older of 2.1%. In addition, the percent of glucose intolerance among those Aleuts 39 years of age and older was 13.7, which was as high as that in the Athabascans and more than four times higher than that in Eskimos. Intolerance to glucose was seen in 38.5% of obese Aleuts, which was a much greater intolerance rate than that seen in the nonobese. As a group, the Aleut men were more overweight than Eskimos or Athabascans, but the Aleut women were at the same level of overweight as Athabascan women [10].

In 1969, the first diabetes survey of a northeastern US Native American population was done on a sample of members of the Seneca Nation of Indians residing on the Cattaraugus reservation in western New York State. Eleven and six-tenths percent of men and 14.6% of women were previously known diabetics, for an overall rate of 13.4%, with type II diabetes being the rule. As a group, the Senecas were found to be obese, with 32% of previously diagnosed diabetics being 30% or more overweight, and 30% of new diabetics being equally heavy. Their diet was similar to that of non-Indians, with 42% carbohydrate, 18% protein, and 40% fat contributing to total calories [11].

In 1973, prevalence of hyperglycemia in the Washoe and Paiute of western and central Nevada and eastern California was determined at 10.7 and 11.5%, respectively, in those aged 15 years and older. These individuals included those with a history of treated diabetes. The diets were not closely studied but were thought to be high in carbohydrate content [12].

In 1978, members of the Three Affiliated Indian Tribes of Fort Berthold, North Dakota, who were 35 years and older, were studied via retrospective analysis of clinical records for diabetes prevalence. Overall, full-blood Indians had a prevalence rate of 22.3%, those between half and full-bloodedness showed a 14.9% rate, and those with less than half Indian blood had a 4.1% rate, which was similar to that of Whites on the reservation. Ranked by tribe among full-blood Indians, prevalence was greatest in Mandans at 39%, next highest in mixed Mandan, Arickara and Hidatsa persons at 27.1%, next in Arickara at 22.8%, and next in Hidatsa at 21.2% diabetic [13].

The Zuni Indians of New Mexico, a Pueblo group, showed an overall 1978 prevalence rate for diabetes of 23.9% in those over 45 years of age to 64 years. Also, their prevalence rate was significantly higher than that of the general population, at 6%, in those 25–44 years of age [14]. By 1984 those over 45 years old showed a 40% diabetes prevalence rate [15].

Oklahoma and Arizona have the two largest Native American Indian populations in the USA. Seven of the 8 Native American linguistic groups of North America are represented among the Oklahoma tribes. By 1974, diabetes was a very common problem in all Oklahoma tribes, and it was projected that if then-present rates continued, about half of Oklahoma Indians, or 50,000, would eventually develop diabetes [16]. The other state with a large and varied Native American Indian population, Arizona, had a more complex diabetic prevalence picture. The Pima had the highest rate on record. The Papago, Yumas, Hualapis, Havasupis, Cocopahs, Maricopas, and some Apaches also showed high rates, while those of the Hopi, Navajo, and some Apaches were lower [1].

The Cocopah, a Yuman group living in Arizona's southwest desert area near Mexico, showed a 17% diabetes prevalence in those with at least one-fourth Cocopah blood in those 5 years old and older. This 1969 rate increased to 34% in those 35 years old and older. A high obesity frequency was seen in those 15 years old and older [17]. In 1966, the Mohave Indians of the Colorado River Reservation were studied via clinical observation, charts review, and statistical survey. At least 60% of the people had adult-onset diabetes mellitus. Obesity was seen in 90% of the people. Their diet consisted of 75% fried carbohydrate. Obesity notwithstanding, they carried on an active life with a great deal of physical exercise [18].

Due to their very high diabetes prevalence rate, the Pima have been intensively studied regarding various aspects of diabetes for years [19–27]. In 1971, this prevalence was conservatively estimated at 50% among Pimas aged 35 years and older [22]. The rate from 5 years and older was 21.1%, which was 12.7 times higher than that experienced by a predominantly White population in Rochester, Minnesota, at 1.66% [23]. Diabetes patients were usually obese. The adult-onset, or type II diabetes type was seen, and low-calorie, low-carbohydrate diets could restore β-cell responsiveness to glucose [24]. This suggested that β-cell insensitivity to glucose was involved, rather than nonproduction of insulin. Young Pimas have a high diabetes prevalence rate also, at almost 9.1 per 1,000 between 15 and 24 years of age. Increased glucose intolerance in this age range was also evident, and was associated with obesity [26]. Overall, the Pima diabetes incidence was 26.5 cases per 1,000 person years. The rate increased through adulthood until age 40 in males and 50 in females, and then it declined [23]. Hyperinsulinemia was correlated with obesity in both Pimas and Caucasians, but was significantly higher in Pimas after adjustment for obesity, age, and sex. A greater insulin resistance in obese Pimas than in comparably obese Caucasians was thus indicated [21]. The closely related Papago tribe of Arizona also has a high prevalence at 42.3% in those 35 years and older [25]. One puzzling dichotomy in prevalence rates for diabetes was seen among Apaches, with two closely related Apache tribes of eastern Arizona showing a twofold difference in glucose intolerance. White River Apaches had 11.0% and San Carlos Apaches had 24.8% glucose intolerance prevalences in those 35 years old and older [25]. Perhaps small population size studies may have affected results. Nevertheless, both Apache groups had rates higher than those of the general population.

Genetics and Environment:
Interactional Effects on Obesity and Diabetes

The relative impact of heredity versus the environmental factor of obesity has been explored by several researchers. Lee et al. [28] studied the relationship between type II diabetes, parental diabetes status, and obesity in 2,095 Oklahoma Indians. Both diabetic and nondiabetic subjects were examined via a complete physical examination and a personal interview. The Five Civilized Tribes (Cherokee, Choctaw, Chickasaw, Creek, and Seminole) and the Plains Tribes including Comanches, Kiowas, Caddos, Wichitas, Cheyennes, Osages, Shawnees, Arapahoes, Apaches, and Poncas from 27 contiguous Oklahoma counties were among the 41 tribes represented in the studied population. The results showed a statistically significant association between diabetes and parental diabetes status. Families with affected parents had significantly higher diabetes frequency among siblings than those families without diabetic parents. However, families with one diabetic parent showed no significant difference from those with two diabetic parents [28]. In this study, obesity was defined as percent body mass index more than 120. By this criteria, 77% of all subjects and 84% of diabetic subjects were obese. Fifty-six percent of subjects had at least one diabetic parent. Subjects with diabetes were more obese than nondiabetic subjects both at 18 years of age and at time of interview. In women without diabetic parents, the difference in percent body mass index (PBMI) was significantly higher in diabetics than in nondiabetics. Also among women, a significantly higher PBMI occurred in the diabetic group within both parental diabetes groups. Adjustments for possible age and sex effects were made. Even so, the obese of both sexes had almost twice as much risk for diabetes than did the nonobese. The average ages of maximum weight for male and female diabetic subjects with at least one diabetic parent were 9 and 5.5 years younger, respectively, than male and female diabetic subjects without diabetic parents. Thus, having a diabetic parent was correlated with a younger age of onset of obesity, a higher PBMI, and a higher frequency of diabetes [28]. The researchers also looked at the association of Indian blood with diabetes. Average quantum of Indian blood was 90%, and 73% of subjects were full-blood Indians. Diabetic subjects had a significantly ($p < 0.001$) higher quantum of Indian blood than nondiabetic subjects. As the quantum of Indian blood increased, the proportion of obese subjects increased significantly ($p < 0.001$). Of the subjects with less than or equal to 50% Indian blood, 60%

were obese, whereas 80% of those with greater than 50% Indian blood were obese. Obesity and parental diabetes were uniformly prevalent among all tribes [28].

Since univariate analysis indicated that parental diabetes and obesity were each associated individually with diabetes, the researchers examined the simultaneous effect of these variables. In both men and women, the highest proportion of diabetic individuals occurred among obese subjects with one or two diabetic parents and the lowest proportion occurred among nonobese subjects with nondiabetic parents. A much higher diabetes rate occurred among obese subjects with no diabetic parents (27%) than among nonobese subjects with diabetic parents (18%) [28]. Thus, both genetic and environmental influences were confirmed, with obesity having a greater influence alone than genetic makeup alone.

The proportion of diabetic individuals among siblings of obese and nonobese diabetics was also compared. Diabetic subjects' siblings had a significantly higher diabetic rate than did siblings of nondiabetic subjects. The lowest diabetes rate occurred among siblings of nonobese, nondiabetic subjects (7.2%), followed by siblings of obese, nondiabetic subjects (10%). However, siblings of nonobese, diabetic subjects had a nonsignificant, slightly higher diabetes rate (31.4%) than those of the obese, diabetic subjects (25.2%). The researchers speculated that the difference could have been caused by the relatively small number of nonobese diabetic subjects. After the researchers subdivided the nonobese subjects into two subgroups, those with PBMI equal to or greater than 100 but less than 120 and those with PBMI less than 100, they found that as the subjects' PBMI increased, so did the siblings' diabetes rate. The lowest diabetes rate (6%) occurred in siblings of the nondiabetic subjects with PBMI less than 100 [28]. This correlation between subjects' PBMI and siblings' diabetes rate suggests a hereditary-obesity-diabetes linkage within families.

West [29] has reported that obesity alone is believed to produce diabetes if the degree and duration of obesity are severe and long enough [29]. The fact that diabetes is 10 times more frequent in the obese and 20 times more frequent in the grossly obese supports this contention [30]. Kissebah et al.'s [31] longitudinal studies also support the theory that upper-body obesity is diabetogenic. Also supporting this was Kempner's finding that 63% of 106 very fat patients with an average age of 34 had elevated plasma glucose levels 2 h after a test meal [32]. Obesity may not only be diabetogenic, it may also exacerbate the severity of the diabetic state [18, 19, 33]. Other reserachers have investigated the way in which obesity may interact with diabetes mellitus. Several researchers have noted an association between diabetes and the location of adipose tissue in women [31, 34–37]. Their studies indicated that upper-body obesity resulted in a higher at-risk status for diabetes than did lower-body obesity. A very recent study by Sparrow et al. [38] has shown an association between diabetes and upper-body obesity in men. A significant correlation was seen between body fat distribution, adjusted for overall degree of obesity, and glucose tolerance in both normal and diabetic men unselected for physique. Higher 2-hour serum glucose levels following glucose load after adjustment for age and BMI were correlated with greater ratios of upper-body fat to lower-body fat. Intra-abdominal fat (as opposed to subcutaneous fat) as measured by computed tomography (CT), was particularly correlated with 2-hour glucose [38].

The Oklahoma Indian women studied by Lee et al. [28] usually had upper-body obesity. Trunkal fat deposition was previously recognized as characteristic of the diabetic Plains Indian women by West et al. [39]. They noted in 1974 that the fat distribution of the diabetic Plains Indian women was quite distinctive, with a triceps to subscapular skinfold width ratio of 0.78 as opposed to one of 1.2 in matched Whites [39]. Dogrib adults, both men and women, studied in Canada by Szathmary, exhibited a trunkal or upper-body fat deposition also [40]. These Native American populations exhibit the type of body fat distribution which is most closely associated with diabetes mellitus. One theory used to explain this association suggests that a greater number of large fat cells occur in those with upper-body obesity. These large fat cells have fewer insulin receptors and a greater glucose intake than small fat cells. The theory suggested also purports that a greater number of small fat cells occur in those with lower-body obesity. Small fat cells are less resistive to insulin's effect [35–37]. Therefore, upper-body obesity theoretically results in more insulin-insensitive fat cells proportional to total fat cells than does lower-body obesity.

Obesity is associated with increased fasting insulin level, not only in Native Americans [41, 42] but also in Caucasians [43, 44]. Basal insulin and BMI are important predictors of insulin response to oral glucose [45]. High basal insulin is also evidence of insulin resistance in peripheral tissues. Weight loss can improve tolerance and significantly increase the pancreas' insulin-secreting ability. This suggests that the initial obesity-related defect lies in the sensing mechanism of the beta-cells which tell them to produce insulin as needed [46]. Low calorie, low carbohydrate diets can restore beta-cell responsiveness to glucose [24], indicating that lowered beta-cell sensitivity to glucose rather than inability to produce insulin is involved.

Although conflicting results were obtained in the past concerning relative influences of environment versus heredity on familial fatness in adopted twin studies, the studies done were limited because they lacked information on biologic parents and because they did not explore body weight ranges from lean to obese [47–50]. Very strong evidence for the predominant role of genetics in familial fatness was recently presented by Stunkard et al. [51]. They conducted a study on adopted twins in Denmark, utilizing the records of the Danish Adoption Register, which contains the official records of every nonfamilial adoption granted there between 1924 and 1947. Adoptees' BMI closely correlated with those of biological, but not adoptive, parents across all weight categories. Thus both obesity and leanness were shown to be strongly influenced by genetics [51]. Stunkard's study is notable because it does not have the limitations of the previous adopted twin studies. It confirmed the results of those previous studies which had indicated an important role for genetics in familial fatness. It also refuted the previous studies which had indicated an important role for environment in familial fatness by showing that family environment in non-familial adoptions was of little importance [51]. Poehlman et al. [52] have shown that changes in body fat following a 22-day overfeeding period have a genetic basis, not only in amount but in distribution. Six male monozygotic twin pairs supplemented with 1,000 kcal/day extra showed significant within-pair resemblance for absolute changes in: body weight, percent body fat, fat mass, sum of skinfolds, trunk skinfolds, and extremity skinfolds. The genetic role in sensitivity of response to excess energy was thus suggested. In addition, variation in genotype dependency was suggested for various subcutaneous fat sites as measured by significance of pair resemblance. Biceps, triceps, and thigh measurements were more significant and subscapular, abdomen, suprailiac, calf, auxiliary, and chest sites less significant for within-pair resemblance [52]. The greater influence of genetic makeup in appendage fat deposition than in trunkal fat deposition suggested in this study may have been a function of the small population studied. Only six genotypes were represented in the twelve twin pairs.

Genetically influenced obesity's diabetogenic effect is only one of the etiologic factors in the increasingly alarming rise in type II diabetes mellitus rates seen among Native American populations in the past few decades. West [53, 54] and Lee et al. [28] noted that diabetes was rare in Indian populations in Oklahoma prior to 1940. This was based on Indian hospital records and interviews with knowledgeable Indian elders and with physicians of Indian patients. The traditionally very active life-style contributed to the lean physique of the Indian population prior to the present century. Particularly since the 1940s, a markedly more sedentary life-style has developed, while the traditionally high-fat diets and emphasis on eating to be very full with each meal have remained fairly unchanged in these Oklahoma Indian populations [28, 53]. West [54] showed evidence for the rarity of diabetes mellitus in various Native American populations prior to 1940, the rapid increase in its incidence and prevalence since then, and the simultaneous transformation of these same populations from a lean to an obese state. West [54] noted that some tribes, most particularly the Pima of southern Arizona, showed higher fasting and post-prandial blood glucose than the general population and speculated that this indicated peculiarities in the insulin secretion pattern of these tribes. West et al. [39] noted that regardless of origin, all Oklahoma tribes were fat and suffered from high type II diabetes mellitus rates. Weights averaged 171% of standard in 230 Plains Indians prior to diabetes mellitus onset. This phenomenon is also occurring in Indian tribes in other parts of the country. A 1982 survey of Mississippi Choctaws showed that this 5,000-member band suffered from obesity, with weights from 20 to 50% above ideal weight. A high-fat, high-carbohydrate diet was eaten, with a traditional emphasis on urging people to eat more and more [55]. The survey showed a close association between the Choctaws' obesity and diabetes. Type II diabetes mellitus was their most common disease. Alcoholism was also a factor in the Choctaw life-style, and according to the health records its more overt form of damage was hepatic encephalopathy [55].

The Zuni Indians of western New Mexico have also experienced a rapidly rising diabetes prevalence rate. By 1978, Long [14] reported that 25% of Zuni adults over 45 years of age had diabetes by physician's diagnosis. By 1984 the same age group showed 40% diabetes prevalence rate. This increase is linked to a sudden shift to more sedentary life-style as agriculture, stock-raising, hunting, hand labor, foot transportation, and foot-racing were supplanted by mechanization, motor vehicle transportation, jewelry-making and marketing, and television viewing. The traditional Zuni high-fiber diet based on beans, corn meal foods, and supplemental meat has given way to a highly refined Western-style diet rich in simple carbohydrates, animal fat, and protein. The abundance of food is now perennial, whereas Zuni traditionally coped with feast-and-fast cycles [15].

The Pima tribe resides in southern Arizona, where they have adapted to a feast-and-fast cycle for millenia. Pimas are more obese now than the general US population as measured by mean body mass index for age, but particularly so in young adults. More than 90% of Pima adults from 20 to 34 years of age exceed the US age-specific BMI medians, and more than half of the Pimas exceed the US 90th percentiles [20]. They also have the highest well-documented diabetes rates on record. Between 1967 and 1977, the Pima experienced an overall rate increase in diabetes in adults of 42% (58% for males and 38% for females). They also became more obese in the same time period, with those below 35 years of age gaining the greatest increases in weight and obesity [56]. When Bennett et al. [57] did a follow-up study on 187 Pima women who originally did not have diabetes in 1968, they found that 47% had subsequently developed it. Those who did subsequently develop diabetes had significantly higher baseline carbohydrate and starch intake. Viewed in tertiles of consumption, significantly higher rates of diabetes developed in those who initially consumed more total carbohydrate and starch [57]. Although starch consumption was apparently related to diabetes development, many individual dietary components had high correlations among them. In addition, a nondietary factor could have co-varied with the dietary factors. Thus, the authors could not state with certainty that starch was the primary factor responsible for diabetes development in the Pima [57]. The marked effect of obesity in the Pima is shown by their age-sex adjusted incidence rates as a function of BMI. The range started with the thinnest people who had a rate near zero, and ended with a rate of 72 new cases per 1,000 person-years in the most obese persons [58].

The cultural attitudes of many Indian tribes toward desirable weight are a factor in excessive caloric intake. The Plains Indian idea of women's ideal weight at middle age was reported by West to be 50 pounds greater than that which upper class White women in the USA would consider desirable [53]. He also wrote of Oklahoma Indian women patients worrying 'a little when my diets cause them to fall below 170 pounds' – 'say they don't feel as well when they are so peculiarly "thin". They tell me of concerns of friends and family to whom they may appear dangerously frail at weights under 200' [53].

The diverse genetic, historic, and cultural heritages as well as the varied geographic and climatic environments of the Native American peoples of North America is such that one must be cautious of any generalizations or extrapolations of data from one tribe to the general Native American population. Yet, generalizations have been done concerning Native Americans' susceptibility to obesity, alcohol abuse, and diabetes. The need for caution extends to theoretical explanations of the mechanism(s) underlying the complex interrelationships among modern Westernization, obesity, and type II diabetes mellitus. Lee et al. [28] suggested that the positive correlation of both degree of obesity and diabetes rate with increasing 'Indianness' was directly related to the cultural concept of ideal weight, the Indian diet, and the metabolic system adapted to the former feast-and-famine, high-activity life-style. This is similar to Neel's 'thrifty gene' hypothesis except that it emphasizes the culturally and environmentally influenced state of metabolism whereas Neel's theory emphasizes the genetically influenced 'quick insulin trigger' and resulting state of metabolism under modern conditions.

Neel's 'thrifty gene' hypothesis describes Native American propensity to become obese with modern Western diet and life-style as having been an evolutionary advantage developed through millenia of feast-famine cycles [59, 60]. The mechanism Neel originally based his theory on was a 'quick insulin trigger'. His later mechanism was differential cellular response to insulin action. Knowler et al. [58] suggested that differences in sensitivity to insulin in metabolic paths consisting of greater insulin resistance in glucose utilization than in fat metabolism was the mechanism producing obesity under modern conditions. An over-responsive β-cell, and a down-regulation of insulin receptor response to given insulin levels have also been proposed as mechanisms [60]. All these mechanisms focused on the pancreas or peripheral tissue response to insulin. The advent of a steady food supply in Neel's scenario was the precipitator of obesity, which in turn precipitated noninsulin-dependent diabetes mellitus.

A study of Australian aborigines who were obese and diabetic supports the Neel hypothesis [61]. When these aborigines began consuming their traditional diet they experienced a marked improvement in glucose tolerance and a steady loss in weight [61]. Another study supportive of Neel's hypothesis is of the Tarahumara Indians of Mexico. They live a physically active life and eat a traditional diet, and data shows that this unacculturated tribe has almost a complete lack of obesity [3]. They have no problems with alcoholism and diabetes either. Their diet is high in carbohydrates, high in fiber, adequate in protein, and low in fat [3]. They are perfectly adapted to their environment with a cultural milieu which is largely unchanged from ancient times. The Pima tribe also fits the pattern of Neel's hypothesis. Pimas exhibit hyperinsulinemia, which would be expected in insulin-resistant people or in those with a 'quick insulin trigger'. Nondiabetic Pimas were significantly more hyperinsulinemic than Caucasians even after adjustment for obesity, age, and sex when fasting insulin concentrations were measured [21]. Since Pimas have the highest well-documented type II diabetes mellitus rate on record, however, they may represent a unique population in this respect [22, 23]. A great deal has been extrapolated from the Pima to the general Native American population, but the Pima are not necessarily representative of other tribes. The Pimas' dietary environment, predominantly that of dry-land farmers for the past several centuries, is not representative of that of far-North hunting-fishing nomads. The Pimas' traditional diet did not significantly differ from the Western diet in fat, carbohydrate, and protein proportions [40]. In addition, the Pima were introduced to Western dietary and other cultural elements much earlier than some of the tribes of the far North. Some far-North Native American groups are only partially and recently acculturated or remain unacculturated to modern Western diets and life-styles to date.

One tribe which lives a predominantly traditional life-style is the Dogrib of the Canadian Northwest Territories [62]. Adult-onset diabetes was unknown among them as recently as 1979. Dogribs are not obese by Caucasian skinfold standards. In 1979, a study of adult Dogribs in three villages showed a significant age-adjusted association of hyperglycemia with locality/season and with trunkal deposition of body fat. Increased centripetality of fat, as opposed to long-term obesity per se, was thought to be the more important risk factor for Dogrib hyperglycemia [62].

Szathmary [40] has noted that only Pima and Navajo nondiabetics have shown elevated serum insulin levels. This is expected where Neel's hypothesis is appropriate. Szathmary [40] pointed out that Eskimos, normal Senecas, and unacculturated South American Indians have not shown elevated serum insulin levels compared to Whites. She has focussed on adaptation at the gastrointestinal, peripheral tissue, and pancreas levels, and has suggested several alternative possibilities for mechanisms of diabetogenesis in a series of papers [40, 63–66].

Szathmary [40, 63–66] studied the Dogrib, a tribe belonging to the Athapascan language family. This tribe has had a relatively recent exposure to Western diet and life-style, and the degree of acculturation varies within its territory. Szathmary conducted a series of studies on the Dogrib in her search for a mechanism of diabetes etiology more appropriate for peoples traditionally accustomed to a no-carbohydrate diet.

The Northern hunter-fisher tribes' traditional diets were predominantly protein and fat, with virtually no carbohydrate content except during the very short end-of-summer berry season. The nature of the dietary transition for the Dogrib was the addition of new, carbohydrate-rich foods to a stable traditional diet with a net increase in carbohydrate intake and in total calories ingested [49]. Recent information on 149 adult Dogrib shows that consumption of a nontraditional diet was associated with significantly higher glucose levels and significantly higher insulin levels. Thus insulin resistance was seen in those Dogrib consuming the nontraditional diet [66]. Age affected food consumption, with Dogrib over 65 years old consuming almost totally traditional foods, middle-aged Dogrib consuming some nontraditional foods, and Dogrib adults less than 45 years old consuming the largest amount of nontraditional foods [40]. However, Szathmary's study of age-adjusted Dogrib glucose levels in different categories of first-degree relatives showed significant association among adult siblings but not between intergenerational adults [63]. She has suggested that complex and polygenic inheritance was involved, including additive and dominant effect genes and an unspecified intragenerational effect. In the Dogrib, the degree of fatness per se as measured by BMI was not significantly associated with hyperglycemia [63]. Increased BMI was, however, significantly associated with increased insulin level [64]. Greater upper body obesity pattern was associated with hyperglycemia in the Dogrib. This type of obesity is the same as that seen in Oklahoma tribes. As noted before, it is this trunkal fat pattern which is considered diabetogenic.

The increase in obesity accompanying increased caloric intakes and sedentary life-styles among Native Americans has been recognized as a public health threat, particularly where diabetes mellitus and cardiovascular disease are concerned. As a result, health practitioners are focusing on tailoring local programs to assist affected people to shift back toward more healthful life-styles. One notable program is the Zuni Diabetes project, which is a model of an exercise-education program for Zuni diabetics [15]. The Zuni community suffers from a high obesity prevalence. Type II diabetes is the most prevalent disease among Zunis [15]. The Zuni Diabetes Project is based on the theory of genetic predisposition brought to phenotypic expression by the sudden dietary and exercise shifts experienced in recent decades. It has focused its resources on promoting life-style changes in physical activity and diet. Criteria for participation in the program, which has been ongoing since July of 1983, includes a high projected compliance likelihood. A 20-week behavior-modification program with a 0.5-pound/week weight loss goal is combined with exercise classes, health and fitness lectures, and written and exercise homework. Rewards are given to complying participants consisting of exercise-oriented clothing and equipment [15]. Participation by the community has increased so that 30–50 people participate in each exercise class. Reported successes include an average weight loss of 21 pounds for 61 individuals, and improvement in fasting serum glucoses for most of 35 diabetic participants despite reduction of dosage or discontinuance of diabetes medications [15].

Environmental interaction with genetic makeup may be crucial in the etiology and expression of diabetes not only after birth, but also in the womb. In addition, the relationship may not simply be a one-way case of obesity causing diabetes, but a two-way case whereby both cause each other in a certain cyclical circumstance. Pettitt et al. [67] have reported that among children of Pima Indian women, those whose mothers had diabetes during pregnancy had a higher prevalence of obesity than children of women who had diabetes subsequent to pregnancy or than children of women who remained nondiabetic [67]. The researchers differentiated their subjects by age groups. Three were used; 5–9, 10–14 and 15–19 years old. Obesity was defined as 140% or more than the desirable weight. Using this criteria, in all age groups there were considerably larger percentages of obese people among children of diabetics than among children of subsequent diabetics or nondiabetics. For instance in the 15- to 19-year age group 58, 25, and 17% of children of diabetics, subsequent diabetics, and nondiabetics, respectively, were obese. The implication was that the mother's diabetes per se produced a prenatal environment conducive to development of childhood and early adulthood obesity.

The large birth weights of offspring of diabetic mothers also indicate that fetal over-nutrition is a prime factor in their environment. As discussed in Freinkel's review, even mildly altered carbohydrate tolerance can result in excessive fetal nutrition [68]. Freinkel [68] has suggested that some fetal changes may be permanent. This seems to be borne out by Pettitt et al.'s [68] findings. The early and long-range obesity seen in children of mothers who were diabetic during their pregnancy may have occurred partly through the abnormal uterine nutriture, and partly through postnatal environmental factors, however. Pettitt et al. [68] therefore looked at the relative importance of heredity and the extrauterine environment in the development of obesity. They found that maternal and childhood obesity were not correlated among the children of diabetics, although they were among the older children of nondiabetics and subsequent diabetics. The diabetic fetal environment's effect was strong enough to submerge hereditary and extrauterine environmental effects. Thus, it seems to be of prime importance in the early and long-range obesity of the diabetic mothers' offspring.

Pettitt's results indicate that a vicious cycle may exist whereby a pregnant diabetic mother gives birth to a child at high risk for obesity which in turn can then produce diabetes in the offspring. This, coupled with a cultural milieu which is conducive to overeating relative to energy expenditure, may be an important component in the phenomenon of familial diabetes among Native Americans. Control of diabetes during pregnancy may be of the utmost importance in altering the lifelong and intergenerational ramifications of maternal diabetes to the offspring [67].

The early-onset obesity seen with children of diabetic mothers at pregnancy may be implicated in the strong relationship shown between diabetes incidence and preceding obesity reported among Gila River Pimas by Knowler et al. [94] in a 15-year follow-up study [69]. By contrast, concurrent obesity had little relationship to diabetes prevalence [69]. The relationship of preceding obesity with diabetic prevalence increased from 0.8 $\pm$ 0.8 cases/1,000 person-years in subjects with less than 20 kg/m^2 to 72.2 $\pm$ 14.5 cases/1,000 person-years in subjects with more than or equal to 40 kg/m^2 BMI, as age and sex adjusted to the 1980 US White population. The association persisted regardless of the subjects' parental diabetes status. However, the hereditary component was reflected in highly significant variance in relative diabetes incidence from one parental group to another. Subjects with two or one diabetic parents had age- and obesity-adjusted diabetes rates 3.9 and 2.3 times higher, respectively, than subjects with no diabetic parents [69]. As is true for many other Native American tribes, the Pimas' obesity and diabetes rates have concurrently and rapidly risen in the past few decades [20]. Viewing familial obesity-diabetes-obesity-diabetes as an intergenerational vicious cycle may help to visualize the familial type II diabetes in Pimas and other Native American populations as resulting at least partly from maternal diabetes during fetal life as a starting point.

Overall, the Mexican American community has a 30–40% Native American contribution to their genetic admixture [70, 71], with the rest primarily composed of European genes. Since the US Mexican American population is of mixed European and Native American ancestry, both genetic and cultural factors transmitted as part of their Native American heritage could influence the prevalence rates of diabetes among them. In the past few years, several reports based on epidemiologic studies done among Texas Mexican Americans have presented evidence of both cultural and genetic influences on the diabetes rates seen among various socioeconomic levels of Mexican Americans compared to Texas Anglo-Americans [72–78]. These reports also showed the influence of obesity on diabetes rates of the communities studied. Stern et al. [72] studied the prevalence of overweight and diabetes in 40- to 74-year-old Mexican Americans in Laredo, Texas. They found that Mexican Americans had rates of overweight and fasting hyperglycemia intermediate between those of the predominantly Caucasian general US population and the Pima Indians [72]. Stern et al. detected no lowering of medical control level of diabetes in the Laredo Mexican Americans, and concluded that a true excess of diabetes prevalence was indicated among them. They also suggested that the overweight seen reflected adult adipose deposition and not accretion to lean body mass, since it occurred after the age of 20 years [72]. The authors refrained from assigning cause of the intermediary Mexican American measures to genetic admixture. Rather, they noted it as a possibility while noting that differential cultural environments could also be implicated [72].

Reports based on the San Antonio Heart Study found both cultural and physical correlations with diabetes rates among Mexican Americans [73–79]. The San Antonio Heart Study was a comprehensive epidemiologic study of life-styles as they related to obesity, diabetes, and other cardiovascular risk factors in Mexican Americans and Anglo-Americans resident in San Antonio. The term Anglo was defined as Caucasians of non-Hispanic descent. The study's purpose was to clarify the life-style versus the genetic background components of ethnic differences in these health variables [73–79]. Three levels of social class and acculturation of Mexican Americans and two levels of social class of Anglos were measured for knowledge, attitudes, and behavior related to obesity and dieting, for degree of obesity (lean, average, and obese) using the Anglo-American distribution of the sum of the triceps and subscapular skinfold, and for hypertriglyceridemia, high-density lipoprotein cholesterol levels, and diabetes rates [73–75]. The study population was comprised of 25- to 65-year-old men and nonpregnant women. In a preliminary report of two socioeconomic levels of subjects, from a middle income transitional area and from a high-income suburban area, Mexican Americans of both levels were found to be more overweight than their Anglo counterparts [73]. This was true of both men and women. In both ethnic groups, suburbanites were leaner than those in the transitional neighborhood. Mexican Americans of both sexes and areas were more skeptical about the importance of losing weight, and transitional Mexican Americans scored lower on sugar avoidance and dieting behavior scales than their Anglo counterparts [73]. This indicated to the authors that they had not fully accepted the Anglo cultural emphasis on the importance and desirability of being lean. The researchers noted that the attitudinal differences between Mexican Americans and Anglos within each socioeconomic status level could be either a culturally based contributing cause to obesity or a rationalization for preexisting, genetically based obesity. They suggested, however, that the behavioral differences were strongly supportive of an environmental basis for obesity among Mexican Americans [73]. The suburban Mexican American and Anglo groups showed no ethnic behavioral differences in dietary and sugar avoidance, yet the Mexican Americans maintained a greater overweight than the Anglos. This meant to the authors that some unexplained residual noncultural obesity-generating factor was also operative in the suburbs among the Mexican Americans [73].

Mexican American men and women were respectively two to four times as likely to fall into the obese category as Anglo-American counterparts [74]. Within each weight category, both ethnic groups' skinfold measurements closely matched [74]. However, even within each obesity category, the prevalence of type II diabetes was significantly greater in Mexican Americans than in Anglo-Americans. After controlling for obesity, the summary diabetes prevalence ratios of Mexican American to Anglo-American groups were 2.54 and 1.70 for men and women, respectively. In addition, within each obesity category, Mexican Americans had significantly higher plasma glucose than Anglo-Americans [74]. In both groups, fasting and post-glucose plasma glucose rose with increasing degrees of obesity. Thus, although obesity was shown to contribute to type II diabetes in both ethnic groups, it did not explain the entire Mexican American excess prevalence rate [74].

Researchers also studied Native American genetic admixture among San Antonio Mexican Americans and showed that type II diabetes prevalence did parallel the degree of Native American genetic admixture [76, 77]. This was clearly shown in their study of Mexican Americans in the three different socioeconomic status neighborhoods in San Antonio [76, 77]. A genetic admixture study determined that the Native American contribution to the heritages of the three areas' residents decreased with increasing socioeconomic status. Determined on the basis of skin color, these percentages were: 46% for the low-income barrio, 27% for the middle-income transitional neighborhood, and 18% for the high-income suburb [76, 77]. Thus, there was a correlation of native American genetic background with lower socioeconomic status and with lower acculturation to the mainstream Anglo society. The percentage of Native American contribution to the gene pool also clearly correlated positively with age-adjusted noninsulin or type II diabetes prevalence rates. Prevalences of 14.5, 10, and 5% were seen in neighborhoods having 46, 27, and 18% Native American genes in their admixtures, respectively [76, 77]. Compared with these rates, the predominantly Anglo-American HANES (Health and Nutrition Examination Survey) rate was 3.1%, and the San Antonio Anglo American population rate was 3.0% [76, 77]. Since the dose-to-pure Native American genetic background in the Pimas is associated with a 49.4% diabetes rate, the Mexican American rates represent intermediate rates between those of full-blooded Native Americans of the Southwest and non-Native Americans of the Southwest [77]. Such is expected if the genetic contribution of Native American genetic background is related to susceptibility to diabetes. The fact that cultural differences occurred along with genetic differences between the neighborhoods could mean that both cultural and genetic factors were operative. Since the obesity rate also correlated negatively with increasing socioeconomic states and positively with increasing Native American genetic contribution, the link between susceptibility to type II diabetes and obesity in Native Americans was also supported by the data. Again, both genetic and cultural factors could be impinging on the obesity according to this data.

The hypothesis that as Mexican Americans became more acculturated to mainstream US life-style and/or more affluent, they would progressively lose their obesity-related pattern of cardiovascular risk factors including obesity and diabetes, was tested [75]. They found that this did occur in Mexican American women. However, Mexican American men lost the pattern much less so. The difference in diabetes prevalence from barrio to suburbs was twofold in Mexican American men as opposed to fourfold in Mexican American women [75]. Within each socioeconomic status category, both sexes of Mexican Americans had higher obesity-related risk factors than their Anglo-American counterparts [76]. The authors concluded that the data suggested that a stronger influence of cultural factors than purely socioeconomic factors was operative on obesity and diabetes rates in Mexican Americans [75].

Another group of researchers conducted the Diabetes Alert Study, a multidisciplinary, genetic and epidemiological study of Mexican Americans in Texas [78, 79]. The first phase was a random screening of about 14% of the Mexican American population of Starr County in southern Texas to determine the prevalence and morbidity of type II diabetes among this population [78]. Age-specific prevalences in males were: 0% from 15 to 24 years, 2.6% from 25 to 34 years, 3.3% from 35 to 44 years, 12.6% from 45 to 54 years, 16.5% from 55 to 64 years, 16.7% from 65 to 74 years, and 17.6% in those above 75 years. In females, age-specific prevalences were: 0.4% from 15 to 24 years and from 25 to 34 years, 5.7% from 35 to 44 years, 10.8% from 45 to 54 years, 19% from 55 to 64 years, 17% from 65 to 74 years, and 8% in those over 75 years. The overall prevalence was 6.8%. Both sexes had high increases from 45 to 54 years of age and high rates after that. Starr County subjects had a 2- to 5-times greater risk of diabetes than the general US population. Researchers noted that the results implied that more than 50% of this Mexican American community either suffered from diabetes personally or had a first-degree relative who suffered from it. Thus, they found diabetes to constitute a major public health problem in Starr County's Mexican American community [78].

The second phase of the Diabetes Alert Study examined the diabetic probands identified in the first phase together with their extended families for their social, demographic, medical, genetic, and physical characteristics [79]. The anthropometric results with particular reference to overweight, fatness, and anatomical fat patterning were reported. The children of both sexes from 10 to 18 years of age were growing at the 50th percentile of reference HANES-1 data for height, weight/height^2 (Wt/Ht^2), and triceps and subscapular skinfolds [79]. The adults were well above median Wt/Ht^2, and skinfolds but well below median height. Thirty percent or more of adults were obese by age 30. Fat patterning results showed that in both sexes the ratio of lower to upper body fat decreased over the life cycle, with the highest ratio at adolescence and the lowest at ages 40–50. Diabetics had shorter sitting heights, more upper body fat by subscapular skinfold, less lower body fat by lateral calf skinfold, and had heavier age 18 and maximum weights than age/sex-matched nondiabetics [79]. Thus, greater upper body to lower body fat patterning ratio was associated with presence of diabetes. The authors did not characterize whether genetic or ecological influences were responsible for the age-related changes in fat patterning [79]. The precipitous weight gain after maturity was ascribed to obesity, not muscle accretion. Recent improvement in environmental circumstances was suggested as the basis for the secular increase in children's height median scores compared to those of adults. The authors felt the evidence that diabetics were shorter than nondiabetics of similar age supported the hypothesis that poverty followed by improved environmental circumstances may predispose small-framed adults to glucose intolerance [79]. They noted that diabetics were already heavier than nondiabetics by age 18, and that it seemed to point to overweight early in life as a correlate of upper body obesity [79].

Overall, the Laredo, San Antonio, and Starr County studies showed both genetic and cultural influences on obesity and diabetes rates. Cultural influences included attitudes, behaviors, and differences in socioeconomic status. The genetic component was ascribed to Native American background since the rates seen paralleled percents of Native American genetic contribution to the gene pool. The importance of upper body fat patterning as well as obesity per se in diabetes rate increases was underlined. The role of early poverty and the presence of Native American genes were both implicated in the upper body fat patterning. Similarly, the prevalences of obesity and diabetes were both seen to be influenced by socioeconomic status and other cultural factors as well as by Native American genetic heritage. Thus, the complexity of interaction between nature and nurture was again confirmed, with Native American genetic heritage interacting with the environment to produce obesity, and a certain type of fat patterning, which were themselves associated with excess diabetes rates. There does seem to be a susceptibility to diabetes conferred with Native American genes through the development of obesity in certain environmental circumstances among the Mexican American populations examined in these studies.

Genetics and Diabetes

Researchers have long differentiated type I (juvenile onset) from type II (adult onset) diabetes in terms of heritability or genetic influence. Studies done through the 1970s propounded autosomal dominant, autosomal recessive, X-linked, and multifactorial modes of diabetes inheritance [69, 80, 81]. However, heterogeneity, or two or more distinct entities with similar phenotypes, is now generally recognized as most likely [82, 83]. None of the various modes is proven, and objections have been raised to all of them. In addition, the various types of studies devised to separate genetic from environmental influences all fell short of their goal to a certain extent and have also been criticized. However, valuable information has come from these studies.

In 1967, Falconer [84], who studied familial aggregation via heritability index, or HI, suggested that juvenile and maturity onset diabetes were genetically different. The HI assesses the relative effects of genetic and environmental etiologic factors of a disease, with a 100% HI being theoretically totally genetically based, and 0% HI being wholly environmental in origin [84]. Falconer [84] based her theory on the finding that the HI decreased with age from 70–80% among young diabetics to 30–40% in those more than 55 years of age.

In addition to the HI, twin studies have been used to assess heredity versus environmental effects of diseases with familial aggregation [85]. An index of the relative effects of each is obtained by comparing the degree of similarity, or concordance, of identical or monozygotic twins with that of fraternal or dizygotic twins. Theoretically, a 100% concordance rate for monozygotic twins only would indicate genetic factors were responsible for a given trait, whereas similar concordance in mono- and dizygotic twins would indicate the prime importance of environmental factors [86].

Rimoin [86] discussed how twin studies conducted up to 1971 on clinical, glucose tolerance, and combined data almost invariably found monozygotic twins' concordances ranged from 3 to 37%. In addition, as age increased, and as more sensitive markers were used, the monozygotic twins' concordance rate approached 100%. The greater concordance of monozygotic versus dizygotic twins' diabetes mellitus indicated a role for genetic makeup in diabetes etiology. However, the phenotypic expression of the diabetic genotype was thought to be greatly influenced by environment, as shown by lower concordance among young monozygotic twins. Now it is recognized that this reflects much greater concordance for type II versus type I diabetes. Rimoin [86] noted that two diabetic parents produce offspring of whom only about 50% are affected by diabetes. Possible explanations for this had focused on 'lack of penetrance' due to remoteness of studied parameters from the mutant gene's basic action, on the mode of inheritance being anything other than simple autosomal recessive, and on the possibility that diabetes mellitus was heterogenous – a group of distinct disorders caused by different gene mutations at different loci, each of which produced carbohydrate intolerance. Well-documented clinical variability in prevalence and clinical features of diabetes involve both environmental and genetic factors. In addition, more than 30 distinct genetic disorders occur with all types of abnormal carbohydrate metabolism, in some cases leading to both type I and type II diabetes mellitus as part of the syndromes. Finally, Rimoin [86] enumerated several problems that genetic studies on diabetes mellitus were limited by, including variability in the disease's age of onset, lack of uniformity in defining affected subjects, lack of knowledge concerning the basic defect in diabetes, and the extent of the environmental influence on variable expression of the diabetic genotype [86].

Some researchers have examined genetic heterogeneity between type I and type II diabetes. In 1979, Zavala et al. [87] reported the results of their complex segregation analysis on data from 1,293 Mexico City nuclear families having at least one diabetic patient. Two treatment groups, insulin-dependent and insulin-independent, were studied. Families were divided into different mating types for the heterogeneity analyses. A significantly higher recurrence risk was seen within the insulin-independent groups in those with affected mothers. No such difference was found within the insulin-dependent group or between insulin-dependent and insulin-independent groups. When testing for a major locus, strong evidence in favor was found in the insulin-independent group but no evidence was found in the insulin-dependent group. Thus heterogeneity between insulin-independent and insulin-dependent groups was seen [87].

Focusing on weight and diabetes, twin studies have shown that despite significant differences in body weight, the majority (almost 100%) of monozygosity twin pairs are concordant for type II diabetes [88]. This is not true for type I diabetes [88]. Cahill [89] has cited this as supportive of inherited heterogeneity in diabetes mellitus [56]. Cahill [89] reviewed the evidence for heterogeneity, and described type II diabetes mellitus as a component of a spectrum ranging from pure β-cell deficiency to severe degree of insulin resistance due to obesity and other factors. Clinical heterogeneity in β-cell capacity to handle the insulin resistance associated with over-consumption, obesity, and physical inactivity was suggested to be the genetic component to type II diabetes. Alternatively, an age-related heterogenous distribution of β-cell function, survival, and/or capacity to divide with challenge within the normal population was also purported to be a possible heterogenous genetic factor. This proposed senescence of β-cells was described as the endocrinological Achilles heel pierced by the triad of obesity-overnutrition-physical inactivity [89].

That insulin resistance is a factor in type II diabetes mellitus when obesity is not a factor was indicated when 16 nonobese Asian Indian patients in South Africa showed evidence for insulin resistance via fasting hyperinsulinemia and hyperglycemia, as well as significantly lower index of insulin resistance, K_1, than controls showed [90]. A significant inverse correlation was seen between the K_1 and fasting plasma glucose level, and the authors concluded this showed that insulin resistance was a significant contributor to fasting hyperglycemia [90].

Genetic research has shown that certain histocompatability antigens (HLA antigens) are particularly common in children suffering from type I diabetes. The HLA known as DR3 and DR4 are possessed by 90% of all diabetic children. In the US general population, at least one in three people have either or both of these two HLA. Such people have about 2.5 times more likelihood to develop type I or insulin-dependent diabetes than those who do not possess either [91]. Since diabetes mellitus is really a group of diseases in which different pathogenetic processes result in impaired glucose metabolism, the etiopathology of various types of diabetes differs with respect to the relative contribution by genetic and environmental factors [92]. A great deal of research is needed to shed more light on the role of such genetic factors as HLA antigens in etiology of type II diabetes, but some interesting findings have already been seen.

Focusing on genetic susceptibility to type II diabetes, King et al. [93] found evidence of increased genetic susceptibility in Nauruans, an urbanized Micronesian population. Nauruans suffer from a very high prevalence of type II diabetes mellitus. They were compared with Gilbertese residents of Betio islet, another urbanized Micronesian population. Both groups chosen led physically inactive life-styles. Nauruans had three times the probability of contracting type II diabetes mellitus compared with Gilbertese after controlling for age and obesity. Dietary fat was a weak but significant predictor of diabetes in females after controlling for age, but was not a significant predictor after controlling for body mass or for ethnicity also. Ethnicity was the prime predictor for both males and females, even after controlling for age and body mass [93].

Eight blood genetic markers were compared for frequency between the Gilbertese and Nauruans. Red cell enzyme ACP1*A's gene frequencies were 25.4% in Nauru and 2.6% in Betio. In contrast, red cell enzyme PGD*C's gene frequencies were 2.8% in Nauru and 15.4% in Betio. Serum component BF*F's gene frequencies were 8.4% in Nauru and 1.5% in Betio. Finally, a rare variant of complement component C6, C6*NAURU, was completely absent in Betio and had a frequency of 6.7% in Nauru [94]. Several genetic differences thus exist between these two populations whose significantly different type II diabetes rates are related primarily to ethnicity rather than to obesity. The researchers concluded, however, that although ethnicity was the prime predictor, unknown environmental influences could not be discounted [93].

The character and site of possible genetic sources of increased diabetes susceptibility in Native Americans were explored by Knowler et al. [94]. They looked at variation in DNA sequences flanking the insulin gene in a study on type II diabetes mellitus in 87 unrelated Pima Indians at least 35 years old [94]. The Pimas studied showed less allele variation in this region than other previously studied racial groups had shown. Two classes of alleles, classes 1 and 3, were found, with no within-class variation. Allele frequency was 0.77 and 0.23 for classes 1 and 3, respectively, in the diabetic subjects. This distribution was almost identical with that of a larger sample of 115 Pimas which included nondiabetics as well as the 87 diabetics. For class 3 alleles, homozygosity was found only in diabetics, although 47% of nondiabetics and 37% of the diabetics had at least one class 3 allele [94].

No genotype differences occurred with varying obesity, fasting or post-load glucose or insulin levels, or interrelationships of glucose and insulin levels. The authors concluded that the insulin gene polymorphism was thus probably not important in the Pimas' noninsulin-dependent diabetes mellitus genesis. However, they found that 61% of the diabetics with a class 3 allele were receiving drug treatment for diabetes whereas that was true of only 26% of diabetics without a class 3 allele. Knowler et al. [94] suggested that the class 3 allele, particularly when homozygous, may have influenced the disease's severity in the Pimas and therefore their need for drug therapy. The HLA-A2 antigen has also been found in the Pimas and is thought to confer susceptibility to type II diabetes [58].

Szathmary [63] found an association between plasma glucose elevation and the Serum Group Specific Complement subtype Gc^1s in Dogribs. This complement binds vitamin D [95]. As noted later in the section on alcohol and diabetes, vitamin D has an important role in insulin metabolism [96–101]. Kirk et al. [102, 103] had previously reported an association between Gc^1 with type II diabetes mellitus in Pacific populations. Eighty four percent of Gc protein variation is under genetic control, with 19% of the variation explained by the Gc structural locus [104].

Szathmary [64] examined the distribution of fasting insulin by Gc genotype by assessing fasting insulin levels and determining Gc genotypes, including subtypes of Gc, for 144 adult Dogrib. She showed that differences in basal insulin levels were associated with Gc genotype. Two parameters, BMI and Gc genotype, explained 23% of the $\log_{10}$ fasting insulin variation [64]. After BMI was adjusted for, Gc genotype was the only variable that had a significant effect on $\log_{10}$ fasting insulin by sex [65]. This was true also for a subset of people who had never shown an abnormal response to oral glucose challenge on any occasion. The lowest fasting insulin levels were shown by homozygotes for Gc^{1F} [64]. Gc^{1s} possession was associated with increased fasting insulin. Finally, Dogrib GC^2 heterozygotes had higher fasting insulin levels than the Gc^1 homozygotes [64]. Szathmary [64] suggested that Gc polymorphism maintenance as connected to the insulin effects of the active form of vitamin D may provide valuable leads as to differential genotype risk for diabetes.

Genetics and Environment: Interactional Effects on Alcohol Use and Alcoholism

Cultural Influences on Alcohol Consumption

Philosophers have contemplated the collective nature of drinking behavior within and between cultures and have developed more than one theory to explain the distribution and magnitude thereof. Ledermann [105] proposed a single-distribution theory which postulated that the population distribution along the consumption scale could be mathematically described via a variant of a log-normal distribution function. He postulated that there was an exact relation between the average and the variance in distributions [105]. His theory has been criticized on both theoretical and evidential grounds [106].

Skog [106] proposed two hypotheses in 1985 to explain the distribution of alcohol consumption within and between cultures. First is that drinking behavior is determined by a large number of factors which tend to combine multiplicatively. Second is that the individual drinker is to a large extent influenced by the habits in his personal social network. Skog [106] analyzed data from several countries and showed that alcohol consumption distribution is skewed, and that populations behave like collectives, moving in concert up and down the consumption scale. Skog [106] noted that changes in drinking behavior will typically be a group phenomenon, for as mean consumption increases, the consumption level of all kinds of drinkers increases. He also noted that the notion of a qualitative distinction between normal drinkers and alcoholics has been increasingly questioned in the past 10 years. He supported the supplanting of the rigid concept of alcoholism as a distinct abnormal entity with the more flexible concept of alcohol-dependence syndrome, which can come in varying degrees within any culture since it has a pluralistic causal base and which allows definitional variation between cultures. Skog [106] used data on 1956–57 Finnish and 1959 French alcohol consumption, per capita and for alcoholics, as an example which clearly depicted cultural definitional differences. Finnish per capita alcohol consumption was cited at 1.8 liters per year, and Finnish alcoholics consumed 3,650 cl pure alcohol annually. By contrast, French per capita consumption was almost 19 liters per year, and French alcoholics consumed 12,410 cl pure alcohol per year. Whereas the French alcoholics consumed more than 3 times more alcohol than Finnish alcoholics, the French per capita consumption was more than 10 times greater than that of Finns. Finally, Skog [106] noted that the data base in hand represents only the recent history of the industrialized world and as such is a view of a free consumers' society only. It thus does not indicate what the distribution characteristics of consumption behavior would be in a strict or controlled society. In a rationed society or in one in which religious beliefs proscribed alcohol consumption, the distribution would most likely be different due to different social interaction dynamics.

Skog's theory, supported by much data, leads one to expect that as alcohol consumption increases in a given culture, it also increases in all parts of that culture. Any thorough examination of the characteristics and trends of alcohol consumption among Native Americans must therefore take into account the fact that Native American individuals and communities are surrounded by and interact continuously with the larger American community, and that Native American cultures are similarly surrounded and influenced by the greater American culture. In view of this, and in view of the collective character of cultural trends up and down the scale in terms of alcohol-consuming behavior, it behoves us to understand what has happened to alcohol consumption in the greater American culture in this century.

To this end, Room [107] has researched the history of 20th century American drinking norms and mores. She has shown how American middle-class drinking norms shifted in the late 1920s, particularly among American youth, away from abstinence and carefully moderated drinking toward drinking heavily to become drunk. Room [107] noted that this shift was greatly influenced by the literary works, and films based on them, of a cotery of famous American expatriate authors known as the 'lost generation'. These authors, many of whom were heavy drinkers in their college years, spent time in Paris after World War I. They were themselves greatly influenced by the French drinking style, which used heavy drinking as an individual and group symbol of defiance against the state's laws and official morality. The lost generation used drunkenness as a symbol of liberation from the moral hegemony of traditional America. The lost generation's writings exposed American culture to new drinking values, and their expatriate Paris community supported heavy drinking among the middle-class American tourists who flooded to Paris in the late 1920s. This flood was partly a result of Americans' exposure to the expatriates' literary works. Drinking and drunkenness were widely portrayed as attractive to the public, and this new image ultimately changed cultural mores so that heavy drinking was no longer perceived as undesirable but became progressive, cosmopolitan, and eventually respectable.

The shift in cultural perception and increased alcohol usage have continued to this day, and increased particularly during World War II and in the 1960s. As a result the USA currently ranks high among nations for per drinker alcohol consumption [107]. Two thirds of the US adult population is currently believed to use alcohol [108]. Seven percent of the adult population can be classified as alcoholics [109]. Alcohol abuse is the third leading cause of death in the nation [108]. It accounts for 1 in 10 deaths, 1 in 3 hospital admissions, and costs $60 billion annually in the USA [110]. Alcoholism's costs nationally include medical problems, accidents, family problems, suicide, social isolation, economic problems, employment problems, and incalculable human suffering. In 1978, the Nationwide Food Consumption Survey listed alcohol intake per person 15 years old and older at an average of 2.7 gallons of ethanol. This equals about 1 oz of ethanol per person 14 years and older per day [111].

One would expect that Native American communities would show heavier alcohol consumption today than early in the century, with a steady trend toward higher consumption in the intervening years, if only because they are a part of the greater American culture. In addition, subcultural influences affect the drinking patterns and habits of people. Within the general US population, Hispanic Americans and Native Americans, groups which reflect significant social disruption, particularly in vocational and economic areas, were found to have a greater tendency than Anglo-Americans to drink in happy social settings such as in bars and in groups [112]. Since, as Skog [106] pointed out, alcohol consumption moves in concert collectively along the scale, permissive group-drinking practices would be particularly effective in producing heavy drinkers. That this may occur among both of these groups will be discussed in more detail later.

That there are other environmental effects on the etiology of alcoholism and on its course and the prospects of successfully treating it have long been purported. Among the environmental factors which were long ago reported to affect the onset of alcoholism and abusive alcohol intake were stressful life events [113–115]. This was more true for women than men in some studies [114, 116]. Higher social status was reported to diminish the correlation between stressful life events and onset of abusive alcohol intake [117–122]. This was thought to be related to the higher stress level and lower health services available in the lives of lower social class women [121, 122]. Most of the early reported connections were obtained through interviews, and the question arose as to whether subjective patients' reports were reliable. To answer this question, Morrissey and Schuckit [123] examined the temporal relationship between some potentially stressful life events and the occurrence of alcohol-related problems in 293 women entering a county detoxication center. Women were categorized as primary alcoholics, secondary alcoholics, or problem drinkers. Of specific events, gynecological events and deaths of family members were most closely related to onset of alcohol-related problems for any age of women studied. Some significant differences between groups were seen.

Primary alcoholics showed the lowest level of association between stressful life events and alcohol problems, whereas the nonalcoholic problem drinkers showed the closest relationship between the two. The investigators noted that the latter may have been exhibiting transient alcohol-related problems in time of severe stress rather than the 'disease' of alcoholism [123]. Primary alcoholics had greatest likelihood of experiencing an alcohol-related problem in a year with a potentially stressful gynecological event, such as miscarriages and hysterectomy, whereas the same was true for problem drinkers and secondary alcoholics subsequent to an abortion [123]. Family members' deaths were most closely related to alcohol-related problems occurring among secondary alcoholics. A depression episode or serious suicide attempt was more likely to be related to that year's alcohol-related problems in problem drinkers than in either category of alcoholic. Lower class women were most likely to experience their first alcohol-related problem in a year with any one of the potentially stressful life events examined, and for them it was most often an abortion or birth of a first child. When death-in-family events were examined, higher social class women were most likely to begin having an alcohol-related problem in the same year as the death of a parent whereas lower class women did so with the death of a child or a parent equally often.

Despite the group differences in the temporal correlation between specific potentially stressful life events and onset of alcohol-related problems, the investigators concluded that their study failed to demonstrate a convincing level of association between stressful life events and the onset of alcoholism, and that the results were not greatly influenced by the social class of the women. Only 22% of the subjects reported events in the same year as onset of alcohol-related problems, and 27% more reported events within the subsequent three years, with all events combined [123]. Thus, although life circumstances affected what events correlated most closely with onset of alcohol-related problems, the alcoholics were not precipitated into alcoholism by stressful life events per se.

Another area with some environmental influence is that of successful alcoholism therapy. Moos et al. [124] found that the efficacy of a Salvation Army's alcoholism treatment program for skid row alcoholic men was good, and compared favorably with that of four other treatment programs they studied. They noted that two unique, integral Salvation Army program characteristics were social climate and treatment approach. The social climate emphasized overall functioning of the patient rather than lowering or stopping the drinking per se. Two unique treatment experiences which impressed the authors were Sunday worship and spot jobs. These and vocational counseling were thought to contribute to significant occupational, behavioral, and psychological function improvement [124]. A program which spiritually nurtures and occupationally stimulates and rewards one in a cohesive social climate, as the Salvation Army program did, may help the minority of Native American problem drinkers who are chronic overimbibers. Such a program would need to be tailored to the specific local group's cultural milieu and needs to be accepted by those it would seek to help. The success of treatment programs for alcoholism is also influenced by post-treatment environmental aspects. This is particularly true of the family setting [125–128]. Moos et al. [128] studied this aspect and found that families which had higher cohesion, active-recreational orientation, and organization and lower conflict and control produced alcoholics who had better treatment outcome, more positive and fewer negative life events, and fewer reported physical and emotional symptoms and disagreements.

Pedersen [129] examined the relative influences of familial versus nonfamilial factors on common legal drug usage (tobacco, coffee, beer, wine, and spirits) in 238 Swedish families using multivariate behavioral analysis. Familial correlation was generally greater among alcohol-related measures than was nonfamilial correlation. This was also true between smoking and wine and spirits consumption. Familial and nonfamilial correlation was the same for beer consumption and smoking use patterns, but nonfamilial correlation was significantly larger between heavy drinking and smoking than was familial correlation [129]. The author noted that her results needed to be replicated. Thus, she only stated that the results suggested that the phenotypic structure reflected familial factors more than nonfamilial influences [129].

The question of the need for culturally determined differential personality norms for alcoholic patients of minority groups, including Native Americans, was addressed by Page and Bozlee [130]. They compared Caucasian, Hispanic American, and Native American veterans in treatment for alcoholism at a small VA Medical Center in Walla Walla, Washington, for responses on the Minnesota Multiphasic Personality Inventory (MMPI) [130]. All subjects had similar secondary diagnoses, similar acculturation through military service, and similar ages, situational and educational levels. Differences between ethnic groups were only modestly seen, with the three groups more similar than dissimilar in clinical diagnoses and composite MMPI profiles [130]. The authors noted that their results were similar to those obtained in previous studies which also had controlled rigorously for age-related, socioeconomic, and educational differences [130–133].

Other cultural factors within the patient can affect the success of treatment programs by influencing the dropout rate [134]. When Black and White male voluntary admissions to a VA Hospital Inpatient Substance Abuse Unit were compared on functioning, motivation, attitudes, symptoms, and mood using reliable and valid scales and on a 12-factor scale measuring perception of the treatment milieu, different cultural factors influenced attrition between the two groups. This was true even though the attrition rate was the same for both groups. Higher motivation and poorer adjustment influenced Whites to stay whereas environmental factors, particularly a more 'therapeutic' approach in terms of insightfulness, spontaneity, autonomy, and practicality on the ward influenced Blacks to stay [134]. These types of cultural differences could prove crucial in the efficacy of a given treatment program, not only for Whites and Blacks, but also for Native Americans. Internalized attitudes, responses, and adjustments to the cultural milieu, whether positive or negative, can also affect the development, course, and successful treatment of alcoholism both in terms of overall personality and coping mechanisms produced in response to environmental reality and in terms of how the patient is perceived in an interaction between him and professionals in the course of treatment [135, 136].

In addressing the first type of interaction, Townsley and Goldstein [135] described the longstanding 'parent-child' dependency relationship between the Federal government and Native Americans and charged it with being responsible for reducing Native Americans to passively dependent people lacking important decision-making opportunities and having a lifelong negative self-evaluation. These authors noted that studies on the Ojibwa showed personality regression with progressive acculturation which produced apathetic personality without inner resources [135]. The adverse environmental milieu of many Native Americans includes high community unemployment and low education levels, factors which depress people and make them amenable to the temporarily comforting effects of substances like alcohol [135]. The lack of control over one's daily life, future planning, and expectations which dependency produces causes personality disruption and poor adjustment in Oglala Sioux eighth graders [135]. These children were found to be poorer than White eighth graders on 20 of 28 personality variables, despite academic excellence at younger ages [135]. Finally, Townsley and Goldstein [135] noted two causes for hope on the horizon; the Indian Self-Determination Act and the increasing recognition and acceptance of the Christian pan-Indian, Native American Church. They expressed the hope that these two developments will enable Native Americans to regain control over important aspects of their own lives and thereby regain self-respect and inner strength. This would be expected to diminish any need they may have developed to replace missing inner strength with the temporary, false strength of the bottle.

Leland [136] analyzed a first interview between a caseworker and a northeastern Algonkian alcoholic woman patient which had originally been characterized by Popham as evidence that five cultural traits common to Algonkians hindered the treatment process for alcoholism. These traits were all described by Popham as attributable to emotional inhibition which was common among Algonkians. Leland [136] showed that there were indeed cultural traits which were inhibiting the treatment process, but that they were the interviewer's and not the patient's. Four of the five traits: lack of affect, lack of spontaneity, never contradicting anyone, and no perception of drinking problem, purported to have been present in the patient at time of interview, were shown on examination of the transcript of the interview to have been untrue of this patient [137]. Leland [136] showed that the barriers to successful treatment were rudeness, preoccupation, judgmental attitude, lack of courtesy, warmth, and caring, and resultant cultural mislabeling and mischaracterization of the patient on the part of the interviewer. The professional's bias and misjudgment inhibited the patient's chances for successful recovery even though she perceived her problem as undesirable and sought to obtain treatment. Thus, interactions between two people of different cultures when the one in a helping capacity fails to understand and empathize with the one seeking help can be a barrier to recovery.

Native Americans and Alcohol Use

Alcohol consumption among Native American populations is not only affected by constant cultural interaction with the larger American environment, but is also affected by the local population's own historical cultural foundation, by the relative acculturation history it has experienced, and by the acculturation stage it currently has attained. Interindividual differences are also produced with varying social status, education, occupation, urbanization, and psychiatric status [137, 138]. Clearly, numerous differences in each of these factors exist from tribe to tribe and individual to individual. Thus, one would expect that these differences would produce differences in drinking behavior, level, and consummatory patterns from one local population to another, and within a given population. Wide variation is seen in percentages of heavy drinkers reported from one Native American community to another [139–143]. The same is true of alcohol-related problems. Levy and Kunitz [144] showed that tribal level of social organization affected both. Tribes with band-level, loose social organization generally had a higher incidence of alcohol-related problems compared with tribes having strict, highly structured organization. These paralleled the higher level of drinking in these tribes.

Throughout the USA, the extent of Indian drinking is less among women than men [137]. This is particularly so in some Southwest tribes [137]. Nevertheless, drinking among Indian women greatly varies from tribe to tribe, as reflected by the distribution of fetal alcohol syndrome damage [143]. The pattern follows the overall tribal pattern discussed by Levy and Kunitz [144], with strict, highly structured tribes having the fewest drinking mothers and lowest fetal alcohol-syndrome-damaged children [143]. Several surveys have looked at the magnitude of consumption and the usage patterns of various Native American populations for alcohol and other drugs in the past 24 years. We will focus on a few more recent ones. Some of the Native American populations studied have been compared for usage level and pattern with other ethnic US groups [140, 145, 146]. These same studies focused exclusively on youth [140, 145, 146], as did one other [142]. Some selected relatively isolated communities [141, 142, 146, 147]. Few examined the reasons for drinking, drinking attitudes, or environmental correlates predictive of drinking behavior [140, 142, 147].

In a recent review, Beauvais and La Boueff [148] have noted that little generalization is possible concerning Native American alcohol and drug use rates because most available information is anecdotal, or if quantitative, is limited to one or two locations, or is from a skewed sample of subjects. However, they cited a 9-year series of studies conducted by Oetting and colleagues which used a nationwide sample of several thousand Native American youths in schools to provide a comprehensive epidemiological record, and to examine many antecedents and consequences of drug and alcohol use [148]. Unfortunately, Oetting et al.'s [146] work does not include school dropouts or adults, so it provides only a partial picture, for school-attending youth only. Beauvais and La Boueff [148] cited literature estimating that from 30 to 80% of reservation adults drank at least once a year compared to 68% for all US adults. They noted that the variability reflected true differences among studied tribes as well as variations in methodology [148]. In their review, Beauvais and La Boueff [148] cited an earlier, very complete review of Indian alcoholism literature done in 1980 by Mail and McDonald [149] to substantiate their statement that heavy drinking is a more serious problem for Indian populations. The 1982 mortality data of the US Public Health Service reports and of May and Broudy's [150] 1980 study of age-adjusted death rates for related causes for Indians and other US populations was used to highlight some of the disastrous sequellae of alcohol abuse [150]. Alcohol use at young ages (7th to 12th graders) was significantly greater among reservation Indians than among non-Indian youths, with use reported at 82 versus 66%, respectively [148, 151] in a study done by Beauvais et al. [151]. A sample of 9 to 12 year old Indian reservation children studied by Oetting and Beauvais [148, 152] reported that over 1/3 had 'ever used' alcohol, with 58% reporting recent usage, compared to 27% recent usage among comparable US non-Indian youngsters.

A plethora of environmentally related factors are used to explain drug use among Native Americans. These 'nurture' factors include family cohesiveness and strength, poor socioeconomic conditions in general, peer

Table II. Environmentally related reasons for drug use among Native Americans

'Nurture' factors	Reference(s)
Few restraining forces	152
Poverty-related conditions	153
Stressful living conditions	153
Family cohesiveness and strength	154–158
Peer influence	158, 159
School adjustment	158–160
Perception as nondeviant behavior	159
Personal coping mechanism	159
Cultural base	159

influence particularly among the young, adjustment at school, cultural base (i.e. traditional, acculturated, or bicultural), perception of alcohol use among Indian youth as nondeviant behavior, and use of alcohol as a coping mechanism for stress [147, 148, 152–160] (table II).

May [137] in 1982 cited four studies on different Native American adult populations with reputations as 'hard drinking' groups to substantiate his view that the overall incidence of Indian alcohol use is probably similar to that of the general US population. Of the 'hard drinking' tribes studied, the Southwest's Navajo had 30%, Standing-Rock Sioux of South Dakota had 69%, the Ute of Igacio Colorado had 80%, and the Ojibwa of Brokenhead Reserve in Canada had 84% adult drinkers [141, 144, 147, 161]. May [137] also noted that although reasons for drinking were similar for Indian and non-Indian US youth, most groups of Indian youth have higher drinking incidence than do youth in general (56–89% vs 53–73%, respectively, for 7th to 12th graders). May [137] noted that both recreational drinkers and anxiety drinkers in most tribes abused alcohol. The difference in the two drinking styles was that recreational drinkers, who predominated, abused alcohol infrequently, whereas anxiety drinkers, of whom there were few in most tribes, did so constantly. It was only the latter who fitted the classic description of 'alcoholic', but both groups suffered from alcohol-related problems. May [137] concluded that it was the drinking style of heavy, forced drinking for social recreational purposes that resulted in alcohol-related problems for most Indian alcohol abusers. The Fourth Special Report to the US Congress on Alcohol and Health, 1981, cited a study by Wanberg and associates in which the Alcohol Use

Inventory (AUI) was used to measure drinking patterns in Native American, Black, Hispanic, and White groups treated in a single State hospital program [138]. The AUI found significant differences in drinking style in all four groups, with Native American and Hispanic subjects having a greater tendency to drink in convivial, gregarious settings. No differences were found between groups for affective association, drinking benefits, or symptoms of alcohol use [138]. These findings corroborate those reported by May [137, 138] that the predominant Native American drinking style is a recreational drinking pattern in a social group setting.

Flores studied Native American volunteer admissions and Anglo staff subjects in a southwestern community mental health center for a 9-month period [162]. He addressed the issue of whether the specific cultural values of Native Americans versus those of Anglos were important in the pathology of Native American's alcoholism [162]. This was an important question to determine because Native Americans have poorer prognosis rates of alcoholism recovery than Anglos [162]. Significantly different cultural values were measured between Native Americans and Anglos [162]. However, individual pathology and personality differences overrode cultural influences and differences. Native American and Anglo alcoholics were more similar to each other than they were to their respective nonalcoholic cultural peers [162]. Thus, alcoholism itself was seen as the strongest influence on personality and pathology [162].

In a brief review, Longclaws et al. [147] noted that studies on alcohol use among Native Americans as compared to the general American population using arrest rates, social indicators, cirrhosis statistics, and survey findings have been criticized for their lack of control on extraneous variables which are highly correlated with ethnicity. These authors also noted that despite this, four major types of theories had been postulated to explain the basis of Native American drinking problems. They listed these theory types as: biological predetermination based on racial differences in metabolism; lack of social control; assuagement, and positive functions of alcohol use [147].

It is useful to examine the results of a 1971 survey of high school students in Anchorage Alaska which was administered by means of a questionnaire [145]. This survey sought to determine the past and then-current rates of drug usage in relation to sex, grade, age, and race [145]. Of the 15,634 students who completed questionnaires, 5.7% were native Aleut, Eskimo, or Indian. Results showed that 43.5% of Natives, a higher percentage than that of any other racial group, responded that they had used at least one drug other than alcohol or tobacco. They were followed by Whites at 35.7%, Blacks at 32.2%, and Orientals at 26.0% [145]. Natives also showed a lower percentage (21.8%) of nonusers of any type of drug including alcohol and tobacco than did Whites (26.8%), Blacks (32.7%) and Orientals (22.0%). Unfortunately, the questionnaire did not elucidate the reasons for these differences in drug usage, so it was not useful in enlightening one on the impact of specific cultural and attitudinal differences. Thus, there is no way to separate, even in a gross way, any biological predisposition from cultural and attitudinal predispositions. In addition, the authors did not separate alcohol and tobacco usage in their report, but lumped them together so that the actual consumption rates for alcohol per se were not examined.

Oetting et al. [146] compared Native American adolescents from 5 Southwestern tribes for drug use with a large predominantly urban national sample. The survey on the Native Americans, who were students attending junior through senior high school, was done in 1979, whereas the national sample was surveyed in 1973 [146]. The questionnaires of a final sample of 1,744 male and female adolescents between 12 and 18 years of age were used to compile the data on past and then-current drug usage. Comparisons of data were performed on three different grade groups; 7th and 8th graders, 9th and 10th graders, and 11th and 12th graders. Results showed a significantly greater use of alcohol, marijuana, and inhalants, and significantly lesser use of barbiturates by Native American youth at all 3 grade levels compared to the national sample [146]. Alcohol prohibition, which the authors noted was in force by tribal codes in most of the Native American communities involved in this survey, failed to prevent the youth from engaging in a high level of alcohol experimentation. This, despite the relative isolation of the surveyed communities, the least remote of which was 40 miles from an urban community. The fact that 17.3% of the Native American respondents reported blackouts on more than one occasion indicated according to the authors, that they engaged in a guzzling drinking pattern to get drunk. Again, the sociocultural factors causing the reported levels of drug use were not addressed in the survey questionnaire [146]. Thus, its usefulness in indicating relative importance to nature versus nurture components in this higher reported usage remained nil.

More recently, Oklahoma college students were assessed by questionnaire on drinking behavior [140]. The data from 181 White men and 250 White women were compared with that of 34 culturally active Native American men and 24 culturally active Native American women [140].

The Native Americans represented mainly the central Oklahoma tribes, particularly Pawnee, Ponca, Kaw, Tonkawa, and Otoe-Missouria. They were at least one quarter Indian, with most being half or more Indian. While 96.7% of Native Americans and 86.2% of White students were classified as drinkers, Native American students had started drinking at 17.5 years of age compared to 16 years of age for White students [140]. Whites reported drinking more alcohol and drinking it more often than did Native Americans, except for beer consumption. More Native Americans reported high beer consumption than did Whites. Differences in reasons for drinking between the two groups were indicated, with Native Americans tending to report social and escapist reasons and drinking for effect (to get high), and Whites tending to cite hedonistic reasons [140]. Native Americans, particularly women, reported more drinking-related problems, and they were considered suggestive of future alcoholism. These problems were the more serious ones of arrest, blackouts, impaired school and work performance, and human relationship problems. The authors noted that possible police bias could have been involved in the disproportionately higher Native American arrest report rate, for the Native Americans as a whole tended to drink less often, less heavily, and more in private homes rather than in public places and parked cars like Whites. However, the increased reporting of the other serious alcohol-related problems, especially by Native American women, caused concern among the researchers as to the likelihood of future alcoholism. The higher blackout report rate of Native Americans, given their lower drinking frequency and volume, was considered suggestive of a biological predisposition, in terms of metabolism of alcohol, for later alcoholism. Clearly, cultural differences between Whites and Native Americans were indicated by the differences in reasons for drinking and in drinking styles and locations.

Longclaws et al. [147] conducted a study to examine characteristics within a Native American population which might be predictive of alcohol or drug use. The population studied consisted of 123 persons, aged 6 and over, living on the Brokenhead Indian Reservation, an Ojibwa community located about 45 miles from Winnipeg, Manitoba, Canada [147]. The population was divided into 4 age groups: students 6–12 and 13–17, and adults under 35 and over 35 years of age. Alcohol use was very uncommon in younger students, 29 of 34 not having used alcohol in the previous 6-month period. However, 10 of 18 older students had used alcohol in that time period, with 7 drinking 2 or more times per month. Among younger adults, alcohol use was very common, with 34–38 having used alcohol within 6 months, and 21 reporting frequent alcohol use (more than 2 times per week). In older adults, 22 of 29 used some alcohol. Observations of drinking pattern indicated that heavy weekend drinking during group gatherings, with an 'avid drinking' pattern was common. Among adults, 11% were reported to be abstainers. Also among adults, 27 drank 2–5 times per week, and 3 drank about daily. Thus, 42% of adult respondents were considered to be heavy drinkers.

Criterion-variables which had no significant predictive value for alcohol use were social assets, acculturation, sex, traditional upbringing, sports participation, and mother's and father's drug use. Among students, predictors of all types of drug use were older age, poorer family relationships, and less involvement in hobbies. These predictors accounted for 49% of variance in alcohol use. Among adults, only 26% of alcohol use variance was accounted for by these predictors, with only one, less participation in hobbies, emerging as a significant predictor of alcohol use [147]. Unfortunately, the researchers did not ask questions to determine quantity of alcohol consumed. This study was useful for showing that almost half of the variance in alcohol use in youth was attributable to essentially cultural factors, the same being true for over one quarter of the adults' alcohol use variance. This leaves a substantial amount of alcohol use variance still to be accounted for. Other cultural predictors not used in this study, and variance in biological predisposition, are only two possible salient factors which could also have been involved.

The Hispanic American population is a mixed-descent US minority group of 7.2 million people, with the Mexican American population the largest subgroup within this population [163]. Since Native American genetic and cultural contributions in Hispanic Americans may each impinge on their alcohol consumption patterns and consequences, it is germaine to briefly review the epidemiology of alcoholism among Hispanics compared to the general US population. Nace [163] reviewed current drinking patterns and prevalence of alcohol-related problems in five subgroups in the USA, including Hispanics. He noted that available data indicated a greater prevalence of heavy drinking and alcohol-related problems among the Hispanic population than in the general US population [163]. He also noted greater sex-related differences in drinking patterns among Hispanics, with 33% of women abstaining. This is three times the rate for men. Avoidance of treatment facilities and turning to alternatives to alcoholism treatment services, such as the church, curanderos (medicine men), and the extended family, were seen as obstacles to treatment.

Caetano [164] also reviewed the literature on drinking patterns and alcohol problems among Hispanic Americans, and suggested that the literature was sparse, contradictory, largely based on small numbers of respondents, and had methodological limitations. Epidemiological studies based on alcohol-related indicators of mortality, traffic accidents, arrests, and treatment for alcohol-related psychiatric conditions indicated a sharper increase in Mexican American alcohol-related deaths between 1950 and 1970 compared to Whites and Blacks [164]. Higher arrest rates for drunk driving and public drunkenness than expected for Hispanics, and over representation of Hispanics in private, state, and county mental hospitals, and alcohol treatment programs were also seen. Two community surveys, one national and one in San Francisco, which assessed drinking patterns and alcohol-related problems, were reviewed, and their different results were ascribed to one having used a small number of subjects and the other having had a possibly biased sample [164]. Both were criticized. Another study, done in Colorado, showed that Hispanics drank twice as much as Anglo-Americans but with the same drunkenness frequency and rate of drinking problems. Native Americans in this study drank seven times as much alcohol as Anglos and three times as much as Hispanics. They also had seven times higher intoxication rates and six times as many alcohol-related problems [165]. Reported lifetime abstinences in this study were: Anglo – 25%, Hispanic – 17%, and Native American – 3%. The rates for reported 'usually heavy' drinkers were: Anglos – 2%, Hispanics – 9%, and Native Americans – 26%. Reports of morning drinking and 5 or more drinking-related deviance occurrences were lowest for Anglos, intermediate for Hispanics, and highest for Native American [165]. Ethnic differences in drinking habits between Mexican Americans and Anglo-Americans were investigated in two other studies which found Anglos of both sexes to have more restrictive views on drunkenness than Mexican Americans [164]. Mexican Americans preferred drinking with friends whereas Anglos preferred drinking with the family [157]. As to alcohol use in general, 44% of Mexican American men agreed that it was all right for a person to get drunk at a party, whereas only 25% of Mexican American women and 16 and 12% of Anglo men and women, respectively, thought so [164]. Caetano [164] concluded that given the survey research limitations, a tentative picture of US Hispanic drinking showed concentrations of Hispanics at both ends of the drinking scale distribution – either heavy drinkers or light drinkers/abstainers. He also noted there were permissive norms for men and more restrictive norms for women, a sharp contrast between male and female drinking patterns, and a higher general rate of alcohol problems than the overall US population has [164].

Munoz [166], a Hispanic American psychotherapist with Hispanic American clients, cautioned against Hispanic American professionals viewing some traits which were tendencies among many Hispanic Americans as if they were culturally typical, unique, unavoidable, and/or benign when they were signs of psychopathology. Among the tendencies often perceived as cultural and sometimes excused on cultural or sociopolitical grounds which he cited was the tendency that encouraged many Hispanic Americans toward alcoholism as a response to stress. Munoz [166] pointed out that the response of alcohol overconsumption was more related to stress than culture and was shared by many other groups, particularly in those with similar socioeconomic situations. That this Hispanic American professional felt it necessary to clarify this point indicated that among Hispanics themselves the tendency to overindulge in alcohol was accepted as culturally normal.

Nature versus Nurture: Varying Viewpoints on Alcoholism

Alcoholism's environmental and genetic etiologic aspects have been the subjects of much study and the influences of both nurture and nature factors have been at least partially demonstrated [167–169]. The relative importance of each type of factor has attracted widely differing points of view. Miller and Fagan [167] characterized alcoholism as a polygenic, multifactorial disease in a review. Based on the reviewed literature, they stated that the disease phenotype is caused by multiple genetic and exogenous factors interacting in a complex way [167]. They cited several studies showing that various genetic markers had been identified and that biochemical evidence of genetic influence had been produced [167]. One example given was the higher blood acetaldehyde seen in first-degree relatives of alcoholics versus first-degree relatives of nonalcoholics. Another example was the possibility that alcoholics may metabolize alcohol by a pathway additional to those seen in nonalcoholics [167]. They acknowledged that intermediary metabolism of alcohol was incompletely understood, and that future investigation of intermediary metabolism and its genetic control in alcoholics was a necessary next step [167].

Goodwin [168] approached the nature-nurture problem differently. He noted a number of problems with family studies of alcoholism, including the 'nature-nurture' type studies. Goodwin [168] listed eight categories of problems with family studies in general. They were: retrospective, unsystematic, hard-to-evaluate and validate sources of information; conflicting stories which were probably only reconciled by investigator's bias; definitional chaos concerning alcoholism; sample bias due to generalization; observer bias; the paucity of knowing which relatives had entered the age-at-risk for alcoholism in any given study; the problem of which came first, the sociopathy and depression or the alcoholism when they all appeared in patients and their families; and assortative mating of alcoholics with other alcoholics, manic depressives, and schizophrenics. Goodwin [168] also noted problems specific to classic 'nature-nurture' studies. He questioned the assumption of equally similar environments for identical versus fraternal twins in twin studies (1974). He noted that identical twins lived together a longer number of years, married at the same age more, and had a more similar social and physical environment than did fraternal twins [168]. In addition, Goodwin [168] noted several characteristics of twins which showed that generalization from them to the general population may not be valid. Similarly, adoption studies were criticized on several lines. Intrauterine environmental differences between adopted babies of alcoholics versus those of nonalcoholics could greatly influence a differential propensity to later development of alcoholism [168]. In addition, the unreliability of reported paternal parentage in the largely illegitimate adopted babies was cited as a problem with genetic certainty in adoption studies [168]. Goodwin [168] noted that given all these problems, the consistency across studies definitely shows alcoholism to be familial in nature, but that it may not necessarily be genetic. To put the question in perspective, Goodwin [168] noted that speaking a given language, such as French, is also definitely familial, but not genetic.

Goodwin [169] pointed out that there are two chemical theories on why alcohol makes some feel better quicker than others, and that they are probably influenced by genetic differences [163, 169]. The first is the theory that alcohol brings the brain serotonin level of pre-alcoholics with too little serotonin up to a normal level or above, thus making alcoholic beverages highly reinforcing until the overstimulated brain cells run out of serotonin. This would prompt the alcoholic to futiley drink more and more alcohol. The other chemical theory is an overproduction hypothesis that assumes alcohol produces morphine-like substances in the brain, more in some than in other individuals. This theory purports that alcohol causes physiological changes yielding overproduction of morphine-like substances (endorphins) in the pre-alcoholic and results in a habit-forming addictive, unusually rewarding drinking behavior [163, 169]. Goodwin

[169] reduced the complex question to a root cause of one of two possible chemical mechanisms influenced by genetic makeup.

Although almost all of the papers cited in this review are studies involving human subjects only, one elegant little animal study neatly pointed out that even in highly specialized genetically isolated populations of laboratory mice the environmental influence of early experience could alter a well-characterized, genetically based preference for alcohol [170]. For this reason, it is included in this paper [163]. Male mice from three inbred strains were given either control conditions or infantile handling. When they were 60 days old, all were tested in a 2-choice situation for selection of water versus 10% ethanol, and for 15 days selection ratios for alcohol per total fluid volume and consumption from both drinking tubes were measured. C57 mice, known for a high preference for alcohol, and BALB mice, known for a low preference for alcohol, both showed increased preference for alcohol as a result of early handling. C3H mice, who have an intermediate preference for alcohol, showed a biphasic response to early handling, with greater initial acceptance followed by decreased selection compared to controls [170]. These results very neatly showed clear influence of early environmental experience regardless of the specialized genetic disposition for appetite for alcohol [170]. Thus, even in highly purified genetic strains selected specifically for alcohol appetite an environmental effect is evident.

Alcohol and Diabetes

Alcoholism is a chronic behavioral disorder manifested by repeated drinking of alcohol-containing beverages in excess of the dietary and social uses of the community. Thus, it interferes with the drinker's health or his social or economic functioning producing physical, mental, or biochemical derangements in the body [171]. The complex illness of alcoholism has physical, emotional, genetic, and sociological aspects [172].

In examining the ways by which abusive alcohol intake and alcoholism may relate to type II diabetes mellitus rates, it is necessary to differentiate between direct and indirect relationships. Direct relationships would include direct organ damage, particularly to the pancreas and liver, and disturbances of glucose metabolism leading to glucose intolerance. Indirect relationships would include production of obesity, and micronutrient depletions which could in turn be implicated in the diabetogenic process or in exacerbation of diabetic symptoms. Since the possible indirect relationships are nutritionally mediated they will be discussed separately from the direct effects on organs and glucose metabolism.

Effects of Alcohol on Organs and Glucose Metabolism

Alcoholism can produce glucose intolerance, pancreatitis, and cirrhosis of the liver. Since each has been implicated in diabetogenic processes, study and prevention of diabetes problems should consider these possible effects of alcohol. Although there is a pronounced familial tendency towards alcoholism, the proportion due to sociocultural environments versus genetic endowment is unknown. Native Americans overall show two to seven times as many alcohol-related health problems as the general US population, but there are large differences between groups. Generalizations are therefore inaccurate and unfair if made from one tribe to the next.

Alcohol affects pancreatic function by increasing the secretion of water and bicarbonate and by causing morphological changes. Only a small number of alcoholics develop clinically evident pancreatitis. However, three stages of progressive alcoholic pancreatitis exist. They are the latent, acute, and chronic stages. During the long, silent latent stage, continuous toxic metabolic alcohol pancreatic injury occurs subclinically, accompanied by pancreatic hypersecretion [173]. By some unknown mechanism, in some individuals acute alcoholic pancreatitis develops, characterized by acute acinar cellular necrosis [173]. Acute pancreatitis associated with abusive alcohol intake has been seen accompanied by type IV and V hyperlipoproteinemia [174]. What this means is unknown. One longstanding belief existed in a nutritional cause of differential development of either pancreatitis or liver damage in alcoholics. This was laid to rest when Wilson et al. [175] found no nutritional differences in intakes of alcoholic liver cirrhosis patients compared to alcoholic pancreatitis patients.

When complications of the inflammatory process develop from recurrent acute and subacute inflammations, chronic pancreatitis with exocrine and endocrine insufficiency results [173]. Endocrine deficiency or diabetes occurs in 30% of chronic pancreatitis cases [173]. Testoni et al. [176] showed via pancreatogram that asymptomatic pancreatitis is frequent in chronic alcoholics, being present in 48.6% of 35 patients with alcoholic chronic liver disease who had no clinical evidence of pancreatitis. The pancreatic lesions showed no correlation with length of alcoholism history or with hepatic lesions, but were significantly more frequent in those who ingested more than 200 g of alcohol per day [176]. Evidence of parallel toxic metabolic processes has also been seen in other studies of the pancreases and livers of alcoholics [175, 177].

Acute or chronic pancreatitis may decrease the functional islet cell mass and can lead to atrophy and fibrosis of the pancreatic tissue, impaired β-cell function, decreased insulin production, and resultant diabetes [178, 179]. The glucose intolerance associated with acute pancreatitis exhibits hypoinsulinemia due to delayed insulin response, and hyperglucagonemia. This results in an alteration in the handling of an intravenous glucose load. In one study by Duckworth et al. [180], 30% of participants who had only one acute attack of pancreatitis still had glucose intolerance one year later.

The liver is the primary site for alcohol metabolism. It is also the major source of glucose to the body in the post-absorptive state [181]. Cirrhosis is the most common clinical problem associated with alcohol consumption [182]. Impaired glucose tolerance is present in about 80% of patients with liver cirrhosis and about 10–15% develop frank diabetes [183–186]. Cirrhotic glucose intolerance is characterized by insulin resistance, hyperinsulinemia, decreased hepatic clearance, peripheral underutilization of glucose, hepatic overproduction of glucose, hyperglucagonemia with decreased suppressibility, and a decreased number of insulin receptors on monocytes [187–190].

Impaired insulin secretion may also combine with insulin resistance in patients with liver cirrhosis due to concurrent pancreatitis. Peak C-peptide levels and total C-peptide response to glucagon were low normal in cirrhotics and significantly reduced in patients with cirrhosis and diabetes. Plasma glucose response to glucagon was reduced in cirrhotics [191]. Insulin resistance occurs when normal concentrations of insulin produce a less than normal biologic response, which can be due to decreased sensitivity to the hormone, or decrease in maximal response to the hormone, or a combination of decreased sensitivity and decreased responsiveness [192]. As Kahn [192] has noted, molecular mechanisms are likely to differ among them, for decreased responsiveness is more likely to result from alterations in intracellular insulin interactions whereas decreased sensitivity may be due to changes in extracellular or pre-receptor insulin interactions, and insulin receptor affinity or number changes may produce either, with changed sensitivity more frequently occurring.

The abnormal glucose metabolism seen in cirrhotics is also due to the altered pancreatic-hepatic-peripheral interrelationship [182, 190, 191]. The hyperinsulinemia is in part due to a decreased hepatic removal of insulin as indicated by a decreased peripheral C-peptide/insulin ratio. Cirrhotic hyperinsulinemia is also caused by increased release of insulin [190]. The hyperinsulinemia in time causes a decreased number of insulin receptors on monocytes. The increase in insulin going to peripheral tissue due to decreased hepatic removal and increased pancreatic secretion down-regulates peripheral tissue receptors [190, 193]. This results in insulin resistance via decreased insulin sensitivity. The altered liver function and decreased number of receptors lengthens the clearance rate of exogenous insulin [182, 183]. In addition to decreased insulin sensitivity, alcoholic cirrhosis patients have shown insulin resistance marked by decreased maximum insulin effect [194]. This indicates that a combined receptor-postreceptor defect underlies the insulin resistance [194]. Hepatic damage can also alter drug metabolism, including that of alcohol, and lead to a vicious spiral of increasing alcohol-induced damage.

Alcohol affects glucose metabolism even when alcohol abuse is not a factor. Alcohol intakes can induce symptomatic hyperglycemia. This type of alcohol-induced diabetes can be reversed in insulin-dependent diabetics by abstention from alcohol. Abstention has resulted in the normalization of fasting glucose levels and no future clinical symptoms [195]. Nonalcoholic, nondiabetic subjects who consumed alcohol followed by glucose loading initially showed increased peak insulin levels and accelerated plasma glucose clearance. Upon repeated trials decreased insulin release occurred, indicating that insulin reserves became depleted, rendering further stimulation incapable of inducing a quick-release response. Thus, chronic drinkers who consume high-carbohydrate meals repeatedly stimulate insulin release, exhausting insulin reserves and resulting in glucose intolerance [196].

Large amounts of alcohol in nondiabetic drinkers can cause a transitory rise in blood glucose. This may result from a release of hormones which induce hepatic glycogen mobilization, and it has unknown consequences [197]. Alcohol's induction of reversible symptomatic hyperglycemia in diabetics and transient hyperglycemia in normal nonalcoholics, its production of pancreatitis, and the higher incidence of diabetes in cirrhotic alcoholics are all suggestive of the harmful effects of both short- and long-term heavy alcohol use and alcoholism on carbohydrate metabolism.

The true toll of alcoholism goes far beyond this physiological damage. A New Mexico study in 1975 showed alcohol abuse to be directly related to five of the ten major causes of death among Native Americans. These causes were accidents, cirrhosis of the liver, alcoholism, suicide, and homicide [198].

Diabetes and obesity can cause differential metabolism of glucose in response to alcohol ingestion. Whether this may affect development of alcoholism is unknown. Nikkila and Taskinen [199] compared nonalcoholic normal, obese, and diabetic subjects for insulin and blood glucose metabolic responses to a 1-mg/ml ethanol blood concentration. Both oral and intravenous routes of ethanol administration were employed to define more closely the glucose tolerance and insulin secretion in relation to acute or prolonged intake of moderate amounts of alcohol. In nonfasting normal subjects the intravenous ethanol dose enhanced the immediate and prolonged insulin response, increased the glucose disposal rate, accentuated the post-glucose disposal rate, and accentuated the post-glucose hypoglycemia. Thirty-minute blood glucose and plasma insulin values increased but oral glucose tolerance was not changed by ethanol administration. Alcohol was administered for one week at a dose equal to 25% of daily caloric intake and substituting for fat. The insulin response remained unchanged even though both the oral and intravenous glucose tolerances were impaired in each subject [199]. Thus, even after only one week of heavy alcohol ingestion, normal subjects experienced impaired glucose tolerances without a compensating increased insulin response.

In obese, nondiabetic subjects ethanol increased the prolonged but not the immediate insulin response to intravenous glucose, and did not increase glucose disposal rate and post-glucose hypoglycemia. In diabetic patients, the ethanol did not improve glucose utilization. Neither did it restore the absent early insulin response in insulin-deficient diabetic subjects, and intravenous alcohol increased prolonged insulin release only a little [199]. The authors concluded that either the β-cells of obese subjects were less sensitive to ethanol's primary action or that the pool of immediately releasable insulin had been depleted by the obese person's basic hyperresponse of insulin to acute glucose loading. The decreased glucose tolerance seen after one week of ethanol at 25% of total calorie intake caused some decreased liver function expressed as a lowered removal of glucose from the blood. Thus, the decrease in glucose tolerance must have been caused by peripheral insulin resistance because the plasma insulin response did not change with alcohol treatment [199].

Bordy et al. [200] have found an association between chronic alcoholism and type I, or insulin-dependent diabetes mellitus. They took family histories of 100 type I diabetes mellitus patients and 100 nondiabetic controls, and their siblings, parents, grandparents, aunts, and uncles. A highly significant difference in incidence of chronic alcoholism in one or more family members was found between families of diabetes mellitus patients and families of nondiabetic controls (54 families versus 28 families, respectively). When parents only were considered, there were 20 versus 4 alcoholics in diabetes mellitus patients' families and controls' families, respectively. Bordy et al. [200] concluded that first-degree relatives of the type I diabetes mellitus patients studied had a significantly higher chronic alcoholism incidence than did those of nondiabetic patients. What this finding means in terms of etiology has yet to be determined. This is true both for alcoholism possibly increasing diabetes and the diabetes possibly increasing alcoholism in these families. Also, since type I diabetes patients are insulin-dependent, the effect of the insulin therapy on alcoholism must be considered and explored. The concurrence of alcoholism and type II diabetes needs to be determined in similar studies.

Nutritionally Mediated Effects

Alcoholism frequently produces nutritional deficiencies when coupled with a borderline or inadequate diet. Chronic alcoholism is the major cause of malnutrition in countries with adequate food supplies [201, 202]. Alcohol's effects on nutrient sufficiency depend on several factors. Most notable are the frequency and levels of ingestion and length of time of habitual ingestion, the socioeconomic status of the imbiber, dietary quality, and whether or not the imbiber supplements with vitamins and minerals [203–213]. A great dichotomy in prevalence of malnutrition in alcoholics exists according to socioeconomic status. Goldsmith et al. [204] used anthropometric measures and epilation force to measure malnutrition in lower- and middle-income alcoholics. They found 8% of middle-income alcoholics to be moderately malnourished, but 24% of low-income alcoholics to be moderately malnourished and an additional 8% to be severely malnourished [204]. Thus, it is important to distinguish among subgroups of alcoholics when assessing alcoholism's adverse impacts on nutrition.

Alcohol ingestion need not be done to the extent one associates with alcoholism in order for nutrient density of drinkers' diets to significantly decrease. The nutrient density of nonalcoholic drinkers has been found to be lower than that of nondrinkers in several studies [111, 214, 215]. Protein, carbohydrate, fat, iron, phosphorus, calcium, thiamine, and vitamin A were significantly lower in drinkers according to data from the 1977–78 Nationwide Food Consumption Survey [111].

Reports on micronutrient effects accompanying abusive alcohol ingestion indicate that alcoholics have been found in at least one study to be deficient in each of the fat- and water-soluble vitamins [210, 211, 216–219]. The balance and status of several electrolyte and nonelectrolyte minerals are also affected by excessive alcohol intake [220–223]. In the case of alcoholics, decreased intake, absorption, and utilization, and increased loss through diarrhea and vomiting contribute to lowered levels of the affected minerals [222]. Micronutrients of interest in relation to diabetes etiology are magnesium, zinc, and vitamin D.

Low serum magnesium concentrations are often seen in chronic alcoholics [224, 225]. Total body magnesium deficiency and a need for magnesium repletion have been indicated by the markedly positive magnesium balances seen in chronic alcoholic patients during 6- to 10-day repletion periods [225]. Both magnesium and zinc deficiencies have been found in alcoholic patients with Wernicke Korsakoff's syndrome [226]. Magnesium deficiency in alcoholics may be a contributory factor in the peripheral insulin insensitivity seen with alcoholism [224, 227]. Magnesium is thought to be important determinant of insulin sensitivity in noninsulin-dependent diabetes mellitus, acting to improve insulin sensitivity of tissues. Plasma magnesium levels inversely correlate with both plasma glucose and plasma insulin in noninsulin-treated adult-onset diabetics [224, 227]. A direct relationship has also been seen between fasting plasma magnesium levels and the rate of glucose disposal during glucose tolerance test [224, 227].

Zinc deficiency is a common finding in chronic alcoholics [228–230]. Plasma zinc has decreased to 60% of normal levels in chronic alcohol abusers, especially cirrhotics, due to zincuria [231]. Common symptoms of zinc deficiency as seen in alcoholics include impaired retinal function and night vision, immune dysfunction, and characteristic skin lesions known as acrodermatitis [228]. Zinc has a role in storage and mobilization of vitamin A, and optic atrophy has been seen with zinc deficiency [232–234]. Primary biliary cirrhosis patients' impaired dark adaptation has been reversed with zinc and vitamin A therapy [235].

Nephropathy and retinopathy are common complications of diabetes. Among the factors predisposing an individual to these complications are the level of hyperglycemia and the duration of diabetes [236]. Retinopathy is also related to heavy alcohol consumption [237]. In cases where a diabetic individual develops alcohol-induced zinc and/or vitamin A deficiencies, these conditions can exacerbate the process leading to retinopathy.

Zinc is found associated with insulin in the β-cells of the pancreas, and zinc concentration in β-cells decreases after glucose administration [232]. Zinc is thought to be involved in storage, synthesis, and/or release of insulin, and alcohol-induced zinc deficiency may contribute to impaired insulin metabolism. This in turn can lead to impaired glucose tolerance. Zinc is necessary for wound healing. It is also essential for maintenance of an adequate humoral and cellular immune defense [238–240]. The chronic pancreatitis of alcoholism may be partly precipitated by decreased pancreatic tissue healing during zinc deficiency. The increase in infections due to decreased immune function with alcohol-induced zinc deficiency could exacerbate the pancreatitis.

Vitamin D has been found deficient in alcoholics with lowered blood levels and reduced bone mass [241]. Deficiency in this vitamin has adverse effects on calcium absorption and mobilization which can contribute to the low calcium levels seen in some alcoholics [242]. Vitamin D has a vital role in glucose metabolism via a direct regulatory role in maintaining insulin levels [96–101]. The B cells of the pancreas have receptors for the active form of vitamin D which is 1,25-$(OH)_2D_3$ [96]. Vitamin D deficiency in humans causes reduced pancreatic insulin secretion but does not affect glucagon secretion by pancreatic A cells [97, 100]. In vitamin-D-deficient rats, 1,25-$(OH)_2D_3$ administration results in a significant insulin level increase [98]. Long-term (6 months), but not short-term (2 weeks) of vitamin D supplementation to deficient human subjects resulted in significant increases in insulin levels [97, 100]. Nyomba et al. [99] and Kadawaki and Norman [101] have shown in rabbits and rats, respectively, that it is the 1,25-$(OH)_2D_3$ rather than calcium which is the agent directly influencing insulin. Vitamin D deficiency has resulted in reduced insulin secretion and delayed insulin response to glucose [99, 101]. In cases where alcohol abuse has resulted in vitamin D deficiency, insulin response could be impaired thereby.

For years alcohol was thought to cause weight gain in heavy imbibers. This belief was based on the fact that alcohol is second only to fat as concentrated energy source, yielding 7 kcal/g combusted in the laboratory. In addition, beer, wine, and mixed drinks contain not only alcohol but also carbohydrates, thus providing substantial calories in some instances. Heavy and chronic ingestion of these alcoholic beverages does increase total caloric intake prior to the onset of appetite-depressive effects. However, clinical observations suggest that alcohol's energy value is minimized by the changes in other factors accompanying alcohol intake [243, 244]. Several studies conducted in the past few years have produced results which consistently indicate that alcohol ingestion, particularly abusive ingestion, leads to weight loss, not gain [214, 215, 243, 245–251].

Habitual intake of alcoholic beverages by nonalcoholic men and women ranging from 27 to 62 years of age over 6-month to 1-year periods resulted in 88% showing no significant difference in diet between drinking and nondrinking days, and the remaining 12% showing no pattern relative to the change in nutrients on drinking and nondrinking days [245]. In this type drinker then, calories from nonalcoholic beverage sources did not significantly vary between drinking and nondrinking days. However, alcohol calories added to the basic daily diet on drinking days did not produce weight increases. The authors noted that the failure of added alcohol calories to produce weight gain in nonalcoholic drinkers could be explained by invalid data, increased caloric expenditure on drinking days, or short-term and long-term mechanisms to regulate caloric intake based on caloric need [245]. A recent study by Hillers and Massey [252] on relationships of habitual alcohol consumption with diet and nutritional status was done using 179 middle-class US males with a wide range of alcohol consumption. Similar results were obtained, with nonsignificant trends toward increased energy intake with increased alcohol consumption and a simultaneous significant decrease in percent of energy derived from proteins, fat, and carbohydrates from the lowest to the highest tertile of alcohol intake [252].

Barboriak et al. [214] conducted a study in 1978 on 51 elderly residents of the VA Domicilary who were nonalcoholics. Of the subjects, 26 were abstainers and 25 regularly consumed alcohol. Unfortunately, only 9 of the 25 imbibers volunteered information on daily amounts of alcoholic beverages consumed. The imbibers in this study ate fewer food calories, the decrease extending to protein, fat, and carbohydrate calories, and they had lower serum albumin levels than did the abstainers. This occurred despite availability of ample food. The average daily energy intake of the abstainers was 2,415 kcal, and the imbibers had an average nonalcohol energy intake of 2,140 kcal. For the 9 imbibers who gave alcohol consumption information, an average of 473 kcal of alcohol energy was ingested per day, bringing their total caloric intake to 2,613 per day, almost 200 kcal more than that of the abstainers. The imbibers in this study were on average 3 pounds heavier than the abstainers, and were on average 3 years younger than abstainers. Although intakes of several micronutrients were decreased along with food energy intake, total energy intake and weight was maintained in these elderly nonalcoholic imbibers [214]. Analysis of nutrient intakes based on amount of alcohol consumed was done on data from the first National Health and Nutrition Examination Survey [215]. Intakes of food calories decreased with increasing alcohol intakes, drinkers had significantly higher total caloric intakes than abstainers only due to alcohol calorie intakes, and drinkers nonetheless were not more obese than abstainers. Nutrient intakes were decreased in drinkers compared to abstainers, particularly in the case of carbohydrates [215].

The data concerning alcoholics' weight change is consistent in pointing to weight loss as the likely result of alcohol abuse. In a 1982 review, Morgan [246] noted that most alcoholics reported a weight loss history over a period of years, and that weight gain was commonly seen in alcoholics following abstinence from alcohol. Evidence indicates that the improved diet is responsible for weight gain in alcoholics on hospital admission, as opposed to alcohol abstinence per se [247]. Weight loss in alcoholics is accounted for mainly by reductions in both muscle tissue and fat tissue [248, 249]. Causes for muscle mass losses in chronic alcoholics include deficient protein and calorie intake due to dietary neglect, anorexia, vomiting, impaired gastrointestinal absorption, and partial starvation, and direct promotion of muscle catabolism by alcohol [250].

Body weight loss in alcoholics has been so well established as a concomitant of alcohol abuse that it has been suggested and used as a simple indicator of continuing alcohol abuse for alcoholics attending outpatient clinics [250, 251]. It was the best indicator of apparently continuing alcohol abuse in a 1984 6-month outpatient study of chronic alcoholics with undercompensated liver disease [251]. World et al. [251], who conducted this study, also conducted a rat study in which the epididymal fat pad weights of rats following 28 days of alcohol administration as 37% of total calories in a nutritionally adequate liquid diet were compared with those of initially weight-matched pair-fed controls. Although both groups had the same body weight gain, the mean weight of fat pads of alcohol-fed animals was a significant ($p < 0.025$) 29% greater than that of pair-fed controls. In summary, the adipose tissue loss in chronic alcoholics was probably the result of inadequate nutrient intake, and the alcohol itself did not prevent increased body weight or fat deposition even when hepatic steatosis was present [251].

To summarize, the endemic obesity seen in the USA including in many Native American communities is not a result, even partially, of alcoholism, for weight loss, not weight gain, attends this condition. Even moderate to heavy imbibers who are nonalcoholics do not as a group experience weight gain due to their alcohol ingestion. The evidence is overwhelming at this point that alcohol intake, including alcoholism, even when endemic in local Native American populations, is not related to their diabetes rates by way of obesity.

Genetics and Alcoholism

Despite the problems with genetics studies cited by Goodwin and others, there is a good deal of evidence that suggests there are genetic components which affect metabolization of alcohol and effects of it on the individual. Researchers have looked for genetic differences predisposing to alcoholism by studying adopted-away children, and monozygotic versus dizygotic twins [253]. Both subjective and objective components comprise predictors of increased risk for alcoholism. Metabolic markers, such as prolactin response to ethanol ingestion [254] and high circulating acetaldehyde response to alcohol, as well as lowered subjective response of feeling 'high' with alcohol ingestion, increased reduction in electromyograph levels at rest in response to alcohol [255] and alcohol-related flushing [256] have been found in those at high risk due to familial alcoholism. A decreased P_3 component of event-related brain potentials has also been recently found in boys at high risk for alcoholism due to parental alcoholism [257]. Nonalcoholic young male drinkers who had an alcoholic first-degree relative (family history positive, FHP) showed significantly less static ataxia or body-sway increase following a measured alcohol dose compared to matched young men with no known first-degree alcoholic relative (family history negative, FHN) [258]. Similar were previous findings of lowered cortisol and prolactin blood levels and less deterioration on 7 of 7 cognitive tests and neuropsychomotor tests in FHP men following 7.5 ml/kg of ethanol ingestion compared to FHN men [254, 257, 259]. The consistently decreased intensity of reaction to alcohol in FHP men in the above areas may be seen as possible genetic trait marker of a predisposition to increased vulnerability to alcoholism.

Significantly increased phenotype frequency of HLA antigen CW3 has also been found in chronic alcoholics with positive family history compared to controls (58.5 versus 30% respectively) [260]. Even more pronounced was this distinction in alcoholics with liver disease, in whom the phenotype frequency was 64% in those with alcoholic hepatitis and 59% in those with alcoholic liver cirrhosis [260].

Three recent reviews of alcoholism and heredity literature all uncritically cited results of twin studies, adoption studies, and studies of populations at high risk for future alcoholism development (sons of alcoholics) [261–263]. Two failed to differentiate specifically between the familial nature of alcoholism and heredity per se [261, 262]. Schuckit [261] reviewed the twin and high-risk population studies and noted tentative results from the latter such as possible decreased amplitude of the P300 wave of the event-related potential, a possible decreased α-wave activity amount on the background cortical electroencephalogram (CAT scan), and a probable decreased intensity of reaction to modest alcohol doses. He also noted that some, but not all, studies of acetaldehyde level after drinking showed higher levels in sons of alcoholics than in controls [261]. Personality test results were divergent, and Schuckit [261] concluded they did not justify solid conclusions in connection with alcoholism. He also noted no relatively obvious neurological or intellectual problems correlated with later development of alcoholism. Given the tentative nature of the results cited, Schuckit [261] surprisingly stated that the studies indicated important genetic influences in alcoholism. He concluded that multiple genes interacted with environment to produce a final risk level.

An editorial review emphasized predisposition to alcoholism by genetically transmitted factors, but acknowledged that alcoholism most likely was a heterogenous condition [262]. Metabolic factors cited included differential liver alcohol dehydrogenase activity affecting preference for dilute alcohol over water in laboratory rodents or producing the flushing response in Japanese via high acetaldehyde levels [262]. The latter is purported to be 'protective' by some. However, conflicting evidence, such as production of high acetaldehyde by relatives of alcoholics, raises questions as to the usefulness of high acetaldehyde levels as a protective agent [262]. This review also mentioned the electroencephalographic differences found in a twin study and the lessened subjective feeling of intoxication and lessened ethanol-induced body sway in healthy young FHP men [262].

Boyd's [263] review was more well-balanced in perspective, acknowledging the not-necessarily-genetic familial transmission of alcoholism and the importance of environmental factors. However, he too was relatively nonquestioning of the strictly genetic meaning of results from twin and adoption studies. Boyd [263] noted that the differential alcohol dehydrogenase response in some Orientals was the only inherited enzymatic defect affecting resistance to alcoholism found to date. Childhood conduct disorder in adopted biological children of alcoholics was cited as possibly inherited from alcoholic parents. Boyd [263] noted that in polygenic disorders, as alcoholism is thought to be, one cannot know with certainty who has genetic or nongenetic alcoholism. In addition, one can carry a dozen potentially lethal genes without harm due to their lack of expression. Thus, even a person in a family with no alcoholism history could theoretically be genetically predisposed [263]. This could be particularly true in teetotaling populations, where the environment would not be conducive to the expression of the harmful gene. Boyd [263] listed socioeconomic status and availability of alcohol as two environmental factors which have a large influence on drinking habits and alcoholism incidence even in adoption studies. Finally, he noted that the disorder itself was not inherited, only the risk or vulnerability was thought to be.

A 1984 editorial urged the scientific community to address the questions of relative contribution of genetic factors, cultural influences, and level of liquor supply to prevalences of drinking problems without bias toward the extremes of genetic and social determinism [264]. Based on the literature and reviews seen to date, this remonstration is timely and relevant. Sometimes the advice is taken. The correlation between diabetes mellitus and alcoholic liver disease among a group of Piman-speaking people in south central Arizona was studied via a check on automated records. The overall occurrence of concurrent diabetes and cirrhosis did not significantly exceed expected levels. However, actual versus expected prevalence was higher in males and lower in females. Researchers concluded that the male drinking behavior accounted for the increments in concurrent cirrhosis and diabetes as well as cirrhosis per se among them compared to females [265]. This same population was seen to have about the same clinically detected cirrhosis prevalence as the general US population, but a much higher rate of death associated with alcoholic cirrhosis. The researchers noted that there appeared to be few social restraints upon alcohol abuse, and that social traditions might even have favored excessive alcohol use [266].

Goodwin [267] urged the use of the term 'familial' alcoholism in a 1981 paper based on his review of the four then-completed twin studies, the then-contradictory findings of genetic marker studies, his own series of adoption studies in Denmark, and the four other adoption studies then extant. Following are his criteria for familial alcoholism: (1) a family history of alcoholism; (2) early onset of alcoholism; (3) severe symptoms requiring treatment at an early age, and (4) absence of other conspicuous psychopathology [267]. Goodwin [268] has more recently speculated about physiologic reactions possibly protective against development of alcoholism. Specifically he mentioned the unpleasant side reactions of many women (dizziness, nausea, somnolence) to alcohol ingestion and the flushing reaction of many Orientals. He cited the finding that in most studies of hospitalized alcoholics, half are FHP and half are not. He differentiated between the two, characterizing familial alcoholics as consistently showing first signs of dependence at a younger age and consistently having a more severe form of dependence with a more rapid, fulminating course [268]. He noted that familial and primary alcoholics were similar except that familial alcoholics often had more antisocial personality [268]. A differential treatment outcome was seen between familial and nonfamilial alcoholics, with the latter more often returning to controlled drinking after treatment [268]. Familial alcoholism has repeatedly been shown to be the strongest predictor of future alcoholism in adolescents, but occupational choice also predicts it. Other predictors include hyperactivity in childhood, poorer performance on a categories test, a modest elevation of blood acetaldehyde, greater muscular relaxation, and more behavioral tolerance of alcohol in those at high risk for alcoholism [268]. All of these predictors can be influenced by environment as well as by genetics.

Knop [269] conducted a study of 19-year-old sons of alcoholics compared to sons of nonalcoholics and found several pre-morbid differences between the two groups. The most striking differences in those at high risk were: (a) significantly worse performance on the Halstead category test, the vocabulary test, and the Porteus maze; (b) a significant decrease in the fast α-energy in resting EEG and significant reduction of the P1 latencies in evoked post-alcohol visual potential, and (c) significantly higher scores on impulsivity and restlessness tests [269]. The boys' teachers also reported high risk boys to be significantly more impulsive and less verbally proficient. Knop will conduct a follow-up study in 6–7 years to determine which if any of these variables may prove to have been predictive of alcoholism.

Cook and Winokur [270] conducted a family study on 259 alcoholic probands and 507 first-degree relative. They suggested that their results showed separate genetic transmission of alcoholism and psychotic symptoms [270]. Their conclusion was based on results showing that alcoholic relatives of probands with psychotic symptoms were significantly more likely to have psychotic symptoms than those related to probands without psychotic symptoms [270]. However, neither socioeconomic status nor nutritional status of probands and relatives was characterized. Thus, at least two important environmental variables which could be operative were not measured. Since the possible affect of even the major potential environmental factors is not known, the purported separate heritability could just as well be separate sets of conditionally produced symptoms [270].

Only 18% of children of alcoholics will eventually develop alcoholism [271]. This means sporadic alcoholism occurs in history-positive families and that some do and some do not have a predisposition to develop alcoholism within the same history-positive family. Volicer et al. [272] explored the intergenerational aspects of familial alcoholism. They found that a history of alcoholism in parents, grandparents, and siblings of parents was associated with accelerated rate of alcoholism development in male probands. There was also a positive association between the number of generations within the proband's family in which alcoholism occurred and their rate of alcoholism development. However, the history of alcoholism in the proband's siblings and children was not associated with their rate of alcoholism development [272]. The results were similar for both paternal and maternal family histories. The authors claimed that the results indicated that alcoholism in first-degree relatives other than parents and grandparents could be used as indicators of a genetic predisposition to alcoholism. This conclusion is unjustified and premature on the basis of this study's results because the environmental effects were not even considered. It is just as likely that alcoholism in parents, grandparents, and siblings of parents is an environmental predisposition to alcoholism due to the utter misery imposed upon the proband from early childhood on. The lack of association between accelerated development of alcoholism in probands and their siblings' and children's alcoholism history could mean that the misery impact of their alcoholism was greatly decreased compared to the misery impact of the older generation's alcoholism. Of course, one could go to obviously ridiculous extremes here too by claiming a genetic predisposition to desire to obliterate misery, but genetic extremist determinism is already too evident in the focus and conclusion of this study.

Several researchers have focused on susceptibility to increased organ damage from abusive alcohol ingestion as a route to study accelerated rate of damage from alcoholism. Saunders et al. [273] examined the link between presence of HLA-B8 and rate of development of liver cirrhosis in those drinking potentially hepatotoxic amounts of alcohol. They found that both men and women with the antigen had developed cirrhosis a significantly shorter number of years after onset of drinking greater than

40 g alcohol/day than did men and women without the antigen (16.6 ± 1.4 and 9.4 ± 2.6 versus 23.7 ± 1.7 and 15.8 ± 2.0 years, respectively) [273]. Thus, HLA-B8 may be a marker for increased susceptibility to early liver damage with high alcohol intake.

In 1981, Jenkins and Thomas [274] reviewed the literature on variations in alcohol- and acetaldehyde dehydrogenases and HLA-B loci associated with increased susceptibility to alcohol-induced liver damage. They cited studies showing that HLA-B8, HLA-B-13, and HLA-BW40 were associated with alcohol-induced cirrhosis in British, Chilean, and Scandinavian patients, respectively [274]. They also cited literature whose findings indicated that Japanese populations had approximately an 85% incidence of atypical liver alcohol dehydrogenase as well as a 52% incidence of atypical liver acetaldehyde dehydrogenase, whereas German livers did not have the unusual acetaldehyde dehydrogenase and only 13% had atypcial alcohol dehydrogenase. The original researchers had speculated that the flushing response of Japanese might be due to delayed oxidation of acetaldehyde by the unusual acetaldehyde dehydrogenase [275]. This led to speculation by the reviewers that the possibly protective flushing effect might be caused by either faster acetaldehyde production or delayed oxidation of acetaldehyde, or both [274]. The reviewers also noted that a much higher rate of concordance in alcohol drinking behavior was seen in monozygotic twins than in dizygotic twins. They speculated that a genetic basis for inherited drinking patterns could be related to alcohol metabolism variations, such as ethanol elimination rates and levels of blood acetaldehyde [274].

In connection with this speculation, Zeiner and Paredes [276] noted Reed et al.'s [277] 1976 study which compared clearance rate of ethanol in Native Americans, Orientals, and Caucasians. Caucasians had the slowest rate, Orientals were intermediate, and Native Americans the fastest in clearance rate of ethanol [277]. Reed et al. [277] found that as ethanol clearance rate rose, so did acetaldehyde levels [268, 269]. Farris and Jones [278, 279] also found Native Americans to metabolize ethanol faster than Caucasians, and to reach higher peak blood alcohol concentrations and sooner than did Caucasians [276]. However, Ijiri's [280] finding that flusher Japanese developed a twofold higher acetaldehyde level than did nonflushers hindered any attempt to connect Farris and Jones' [279] finding with increased susceptibility to alcoholism in Native Americans [276, 280]. In addition, other studies have been reviewed which found comparable rates of ethanol metabolization for Native Americans, Caucasians, and Orientals [275]. One study, Fenna's, found the opposite results, with Canadian Eskimos and Canadians Indians clearing an intravenously infused ethanol slower than Canadian Caucasians [275, 276]. However, this study was criticized for several reasons [276].

The 1979 Conference on Genetic and Biochemical Variability in Response to Alcohol held at The Johns Hopkins University School of Medicine featured much of the data then extant on the genetic aspects of alcoholism, including genetic variation in metabolism of alcohol and genetic variation in organ-specific pathology response to alcohol [281]. Wolff cautioned against ascribing a relationship to the flushing response with development and course of alcoholism and cited the results of studies which contradicted each other concerning a possible protective effect. He noted that in Orientals the flushing response was associated with low alcoholism incidence whereas in some Native American groups the same response was associated with high rates of alcoholism [281].

Veech reported at the same conference that two thirds of 100 admitted to a detoxication center showed 2,3-butanediol in the blood compared to 16 normal controls and 4 normals fed ethanol who did not show or produce it [281]. In addition, 90% of normals showed no more than 0.01m*M* of 1,2-propanediol and 10% showed 0.01–0.15 m*M* of it after ethanol ingestion. All the alcoholics showed much higher blood concentration, in a range from 0.05 to 0.95 m*M*, and it persisted in their blood for up to 10 days after cessation of drinking [281]. As of the time of the conference the genetic significance of the compound was not known. Several other topics were reported on which have already been discussed in this paper.

In 1974, Bert P. Eder, as chief of the Indian Desk of the National Institute on Alcohol Abuse and Alcoholism, noted that 'no proof exists that the physiological reaction of Indians to alcohol is any more severe than that of other racial groups' [282]. A few studies have been done, however, which have shown faster ethanol metabolization by individual Indians compared to people of other ethnic groups [137, 283, 284]. May [137] cited these but made the point that biological differences, even if found, had only a remote link to behavior and that factors for susceptibility and drinking behavior are more probably to be found in historical, social, cultural, and psychological variables. In addition, one should keep in mind that the whole concept of biological predetermination tends to differentiate a single group, perhaps falsely, from other peoples. To use an analogy carried to its logical extreme, one could say that the human race has a biological predetermination to die, but that does not mean that other mammals, indeed all other living creatures, do not have the same biological predetermination. Similarly, if anyone abuses alcohol consumption enough, he or she will become an alcoholic and suffer the physical, psychological, social, and other sequellae of alcoholism. This is true for all races and both sexes.

Now that the necessary cautionary note has been sounded, an examination of some more of the literature dealing with differential metabolism of alcohol involving Native Americans follows. Paredes reported for himself, Zeiner, and Cowden in the 1979 conference that US Native Americans and the Tarahumara Indians of Mexico metabolized alcohol faster than Caucasian controls [278, 281, 283]. This was noteworthy particularly in the Tarahumara, who are still successfully maintaining their traditional, pre-Columbian way of life and diet and among whom such Western-associated health problems as obesity, diabetes, and alcoholism are unknown [281]. The researchers noted that interpreting this difference in rate of metabolization was difficult because there is great genetic variability among Indians, even intratribally. Paredes compared this variability with that found in great modern urban centers [281]. He also noted that the effect could be attributable to a combined effect of multiple genes, and that ascribing metabolization differences according to race was poor practice since only 6% of human genetic diversities are due to between-race variation whereas 85% is attributable to intra-individual variation within race [281]. He also cited the highly variable pattern of intensity of alcohol problems from tribe to tribe, which in some cases were more variable than in Caucasian-Native American comparisons [281].

Underscoring the intertribal variation was Stratton and Zeiner's [285] work. They found differences between eastern and western Oklahoma Indian tribal areas for the highly intercorrelated data on arrests for public drunkenness, driving under the influence, and alcohol-related deaths [286]. The Native Americans from the 5 Eastern civilized tribal areas had much lower-than-expected mortality from alcohol-related deaths. However, the Native Americans from the Western tribal areas had much higher-than-expected mortality from such deaths [286]. Since east-west Caucasian mortality rates from alcohol-related deaths were similar, the Native American east-west tribal area differences were noteworthy evidence of a much higher intraracial variability among Oklahoma Native Americans than there was among Oklahoma Caucasians [286].

The prevalence of alcohol abuse varies not only from tribe to tribe, but also within a given tribe. A case in point is the Papago tribe of Arizona. Based on a survey by the Papago Alcoholism Program, an estimation of the percentage of Papagos in ten districts who were problem drinkers was obtained in 1981. The overall rate was 54.7%, with an estimated weighted overall mean of 53.9%. However, within this overall mean was a more than twofold variation between the highest and lowest local means. Problem drinker weighted mean percents ranged from a low of 32.8 at San Xavier to a high of 73.2 at Hickiwan [287]. Clearly, local conditions were affecting the problem drinking rates within this tribe.

The hypothesis of biological sensitivity to alcohol on a racial basis was given a blow from the results of the studies on the Tarahumara Indians [283, 286]. This tribe cleared ethanol faster than Caucasians, and had less physiological reactivity to alcohol than Caucasians, both effects which some researchers have noted in the sons of alcoholics, yet alcoholism is unknown among them [283, 286]. The Tarahumara had lower post-ingestion blood alcohol at 40 min than Caucasians [283, 286]. The unacculturated life-style of the Tarahumara could be an important factor in their freedom from Western-associated health problems, including alcoholism. Nevertheless, here is a population of Native Americans who showed two characteristics of alcohol metabolism and response to alcohol ingestion – purported to be predictors to heightened susceptibility to alcoholism in certain high-risk populations and interracial studies, respectively, in whom they are associated with lack of alcoholism. Clearly, whatever predisposition toward alcoholism may be genetically endowed, it was accompanied by massive cultural and social disruption with attendant misery before such predisposition was expressed among Native American populations.

Conclusion

The documented, rapid, widespread rise in type II diabetes mellitus rates among Native Americans in the USA has been accompanied by a similarly rapid and widespread rise in obesity rates. The upper-body or trunkal type of fat patterning has been associated with diabetes prevalence among Native Americans. The influence of maternal diabetes on fetal nutritional environment and subsequent predilection of offspring to develop early and lifelong obesity has been shown to be related with the offspring's subsequent higher diabetes rates. Both cultural factors, including higher ideal body weight concepts, and genetic factors are implicated in the obesity rates seen in Native American communities. Environmental factors such as the advent of a steady food supply with development of a high carbohydrate, high total calorie diet, and the advent of a sedentary life-style are also implicated. Communities of mixed European-Native American background, such as the Mexican American community, show intermediate rates of diabetes mellitus, and studies among them have shown both environmental and genetic influences on both diabetes mellitus and obesity. Genetic studies have found some link between allele class and diabetes frequency, and between serum group-specific complement subtype and plasma glucose elevations in Pimas and Dogribs, respectively.

A multitude of cultural, socioeconomic, and other environmental factors affect collective and individual drinking behavior and pathology among Native Americans. Widely varying rates of alcohol abuse are seen intratribally, intertribally, and interregionally. The intertribal and interregional variation is related to level of social organization, with more highly structured tribes having lower rates of alcoholism and alcohol-related problems. Permissive attitudes toward male heavy drinking on social occasions and in social groups are implicated in heavy incidence of alcohol-related problems both in Native American communities and in mixed-heritage Mexican American and other Hispanic American communities. Genetic studies on alcoholism in Native American communities are sparse. However, one study done has shown higher than expected cirrhosis rates in men but lower rates in women. This finding implicated the heavy social drinking pattern seen among males in their cirrhosis incidence rate. Genetic studies on alcohol metabolism rate among Native Americans have been equivocal in results, with some genetic studies connecting alcoholism with faster metabolism rates, one showing slower metabolism rates with alcoholism, and one showing an absence of alcoholism with faster metabolism rates.

Some of the physiological effects of alcohol abuse are clearly diabetogenic. These are production of pancreatitis and liver cirrhosis, both of which can produce glucose intolerance. Glucose intolerance in the absence of clinical organ damage is also seen via stimulation of insulin release and exhaustion of insulin reserves. Alcohol adversely affects zinc, magnesium, and vitamin D nutriture and status, which also adversely affects insulin response and glucose metabolism. One physiological effect long thought to be related to alcohol abuse was obesity. This has now been shown not to be the case. Several studies have consistently shown that alcohol abuse produces weight loss, not weight gain. In fact, weight loss has actually been used to diagnose continuing clandestine alcohol ingestion in alcoholics undergoing a treatment regimen.

The interrelationships of alcohol abuse, obesity, and diabetes have yet to be studied in depth. However, one study showed that diabetes and obesity each caused differential glucose metabolism following alcohol ingestion. The implications of this finding in terms of etiology and exacerbation of alcoholism are unknown. Genetic studies on non-Native American subjects have supported the hypothesis that susceptibility to increased organ damage from abusive alcohol ingestion is related to certain HLA antigens. However, no studies of this kind have been done on Native American populations.

Overall, the extreme complexity of the etiologic picture for type II diabetes mellitus has been confirmed. Much work remains to be done, particularly in the area of genetic studies. The effects of obesity and diabetes on development of alcoholism also need to be investigated. The findings of the studies reviewed have great import for many American citizens, for many millions have some Native American inheritance in their background. The combination of interactions between environmental factors of diet and life-style with genetic heritage may impact on these Americans as well as on identifiable Native American communities. Thus, it behoves researchers to continue their thrust to identify and describe the etiologic entities and interrelationships among the genetically and environmentally affected conditions of diabetes mellitus, obesity, and alcoholism.

Acknowledgements

Encouragement and support for initial writing from a grant to P. Skinner from the National Institute on Disability and Rehabilitation Research, Cop. Ag. No. G0083C0094.

References

1 West, K.M.: Diabetes in American Indians. Adv. metab. Disord. *9:* 29–48 (1978).
2 Mouratoff, G.J.; Berkeley, M.D.; Carroll, N.V.; Scott, E.M.: Diabetes mellitus in Athabascan Indians in Alaska. Diabetes *18:* 29–32 (1969).
3 Connor, W.E.; Cerqueira, M.T.; Connor, R.W.; Wallace, R.B.; Malinow, M.R.; Casdorph, H.R.: The plasma lipids, lipoproteins, and diet of the Tarahumara Indians of Mexico. Am. J. clin. Nutr. *31:* 1131–1142 (1978).
4 Stein, J.H.; West, K.M.; Robey, J.M.; Tirador, D.F.; McDonald, G.W.: The high prevalence of abnormal glucose tolerance in the Cherokee Indians of North Carolina. Archs intern. Med. *116:* 842–847 (1965).

5 Drevets, C.C.: Diabetes mellitus in Choctaw Indians. Diabetes Forecast *5:* 322–329 (1977).

6 Kalb, W.: Diabetes stalks state Choctaw Indians. Daily Oklahoman *July 26:* 2 (1965).

7 White, W.D.: Diabetes in the Oklahoma Indian. Abstr. Proc. 1st Joint Meet. Clin. Soc. Commissioned Officers Ass., 1966, p. 31.

8 Waring, G.O.: The sequellae of diabetes mellitus in midwestern American Indians. Am. J. Diabetes *19:* suppl., pp. 403–404 (1968–69).

9 Rate, R.G.; Knowler, W.C.; Morse, H.G.; Bonnell, M.D.; McVey, J.; Chervenak, C.L.; Smith, M.G.; Pavanich, G.: Diabetes mellitus in Hopi and Navajo Indians. Diabetes *32:* 894–899 (1983).

10 Mouratoff, G.J.; Scott, E.M.: Diabetes mellitus in the Aleutians of Alaska. Diabetes *25:* 227 (1976).

11 Doeblin, T.D.; Evans, K.; Ingall, G.B.; Dawling, K.; Chilcote, M.E.; Elsea, W.; Bannerman, R.M.: Diabetes and hyperglycemia in Seneca Indians. Hum. Hered. *19:* 613–627 (1969).

12 Bartha, G.W.; Burch, T.A.; Bennett, P.H.: Hyperglycemia in Washoe and Northern Paiute Indians. Diabetes *22:* 58–62 (1973).

13 Brosseau, J.D.; Eelkema, R.C.; Crawford, A.C.; Abe, T.A.: Diabetes among the three affiliated tribes: correlation with degree of Indian inheritance. Am. J. publ. Hlth *69:* 1277–1278 (1979).

14 Long, T.P.: The prevalence of clinically treated diabetes among Zuni Reservation residents. Public Health Briefs. Am. J. publ. Hlth *68:* 901–903 (1978).

15 Leonard, B.; Leonard, C.; Wilson, R.: Zuni diabetes project. Publ. Hlth Rep. *101:* 282–288 (1986).

16 West, K.M.: Letter on diabetes problems in Oklahoma Indians (University of Oklahoma Health Sciences Center, Norman 1974).

17 Henry, R.E.; Burch, T.A.; Bennett, P.H.; Miller, M.: Diabetes in the Cocopah Indians. Diabetes *18:* 33–37 (1969).

18 Richey, D.F.: Observations of an obese population. Abstr. Proc. 1st Joint Meet. Clin. Soc. Commissioned Officers Ass., 1966, p. 22.

19 Knowler, W.C.; Savage, M.; Nagulesparan, M.; Howar, B.V.; Bennett, P.H.: Obesity, insulin resistance and Diabetes mellitus in the Pima Indians; in Kobberling, Tattersall, The genetics of diabetes mellitus. Serono Symp. 47, pp. 243–250 (Academic Press, New York 1982).

20 Knowler, W.C.; Pettitt, D.J.; Savage, P.J.; Bennett, P.H.: Diabetes incidence in Pima Indians: contributions of obesity and parental diabetes. Am. J. Epidem. *113:* 144–156 (1981).

21 Nagulesparan, M.; Savage, P.J.; Knowler, W.C.; Johnson, G.C.; Bennett, P.H.: Increased in vivo insulin resistance in non-diabetic Pima Indians compared with Caucasians. Diabetes *31:* 952–956 (1982).

22 Bennett, P.H.; Burch, T.A.: Diabetes mellitus in American (Pima) Indians. Lancet *ii:* 125–128 (1971).

23 Knowler, W.C.; Bennett, P.H.; Hamman, R.F.; Miller, M.: Diabetes incidence and prevalence in Pima Indians: a 19-fold greater incidence than in Rochester, Minnesota. Am. J. Epidem. *108:* 497–505 (1978).

24 Bennett, P.H.; Savage, P.J.: Natural history of Diabetes mellitus in the Pima. Diabetes *26:* 355 (1977).
25 Bennett, P,H,; Rushforth, N.B.; Miller, M.; Le Compte, P.M.: Epidemiologic studies of diabetes in the Pima Indians. Recent Prog. Horm. Res. *32:* 333–376 (1976).
26 Savage, P.J.; Bennett, P.H.; Senter, R.G.; Miller, M.: High prevalence of diabetes in young Pima Indians. Diabetes *28:* 937–942 (1979).
27 Howard, B.U.; Lisse, J.R.; Knowler, W.C.; Davis, M.P.; Pettitt, D.J.; Bennett, P.H.: Diabetes and atherosclerosis in the Pima Indians. Mount Sinai J. Med. *49:* 169–175 (1982).
28 Lee, E.T.; Anderson, P.S.; Bayan, J.; Bahr, C.; Coniglione, T.; Cleves, M.: Diabetes, parental diabetes, and obesity in Oklahoma Indians. Diabetes Care *8:* 107–113 (1985).
29 West, K.M.: Epidemiology of diabetes and its vascular lesions (Elsevier, New York 1978).
30 West, K.M.: Report to the Indian people on the diabetes problem (Oklahoma Indian Health Service, Oklahoma City, Okla. 1976).
31 Kissebah, A.H.; Vydelingun, N.; Murray, R.; Evans, D.J.; Hartz, A.Z.; Kalkhoff, R.K.; Adams, P.W.: Relation of body fat distribution to metabolic complications of obesity. J. clin. Endocr. Metab. *54:* 254–260 (1982).
32 Kempner, W.; Newberg, B.D.; Peschel, R.L.; et al.: Treatment of massive obesity with rice-reduction diet program. An analysis of 106 patients with at least a 45-kg weight loss. Archs intern. Med. *135:* 1575–1584 (1975).
33 Pettitt, D.G.; Lisse, J.R.; Knowler, W.C.; Bennett, P.H.: Mortality as a function of obesity and diabetes mellitus. Am. J. Epidem. *115:* 359–366 (1982).
34 Vague, J.: The degree of masculine differentiation of obesity: a factor determining predisposition to diabetes, atherosclerosis, gout, and uric-calculous disease. Am. J. clin. Nutr. *4:* 20–34 (1956).
35 Kalkhoff, R.K.; Hartz, A.H.; Rupley, D.; Kissebah, A.H.; Kelber, S.: Relationship of body fat distribution to blood pressure, carbohydrate tolerance, and plasma lipids in healthy obese women. J. Lab. clin. Med. *102:* 621–627 (1983).
36 Kissebah, A.H.; Vydelingum, N.; Adams, P.W.; et al.: Morphology and metabolism of fat cells in females with gynoid and android obesity; in Vague, Vague, Diabetes and obesity, pp. 148–152 (Excerpta Medica, Amsterdam 1979).
37 Hatz, A.J.; Rupley, D.C.; Remm, A.A.: The association of girth measurements with disease in 32,856 women. Am. J. Epidem. *119:* 71–80 (1984).
38 Sparrow, D.; Borkan, G.A.; Gerzof, S.G.; Wisniewski, C.; Silbert, C.K.: Relationship of fat distribution to glucose tolerance: results of computed tomography in male participants of the normative aging study. Diabetes *35:* 411–415 (1986).
39 West, K.M.; Bailey, C.P.; Coniglione, T.C.; Smith, W.O., Jr.; Scroggins, K.R.; Ellison, M.G.; Maxwell, E.L.; Sanders, M.L.; Whayne, T.F.: Diabetes in nineteen Oklahoma Indian tribes (Abstract). Diabetes *23:* suppl., p. 385 (1974).
40 Szathmary, E.J.E.: Diabetes in Amer-Indian populations: the Dogrib studies; in Armelagos, Swedlund, Health and diseases of populations in transition (Bergin & Garvey, New York, in press).
41 Genuth, S.M.; Bennett, P.H.; Miller, M.; Burch, T.A.: Hyperinsulinism in obese diabetic Pima Indians. Metabolism *16:* 1010–1015 (1967).

42 Savage, P.J.; Dippe, S.E.; Bennett, P.H.; Gorden, P.; Roth, J.; Rushforth, N.B.; Miller, M.: Hyperinsulinemia and hypoinsulinemia. Insulin responses to oral carbohydrate over a wide spectrum of glucose tolerance. Diabetes *24:* 362–368 (1975).
43 Kreisberg, R.A.; Boshell, B.R.; Di Placido, J.; Roddam, R.F.: Insulin secretion in obesity. New Engl. J. Med. *276:* 314–319 (1967).
44 Bagdade, J.D.; Bierman, E.L.; Porte, D., Jr.: The significance of basal insulin levels in the evaluation of the insulin response to glucose in diabetic and non-diabetic subejcts. J. clin. Invest *46:* 1549–1557 (1967).
45 Mohan, V.; Sharp, P.S.; Cloke, H.R.; Burris, J.M.; Schumer, B.; Kohner, E.M.: Serum immunoreactive insulin responses to a glucose load in Asian-Indian and European type 2 (non-insulin-dependent) diabetic patients and control subjects. Diabetologia *29:* 235–237 (1986).
46 Bennett, P.H.: The Pima Indians: Do they hold the key? Diabetes Forecast *58:* 318–319 (1977).
47 Withers, R.F.J.: Problems in the genetics of human obesity. Eugen. Rev. *56:* 81–90 (1964).
48 Hartz, A.; Giefer, E.; Rimm, A.A.: Relative importance of the effect of family environment and heredity on obesity. Ann. hum. Genet. *41:* 185–193 (1977).
49 Garn, S.M.; Cole, P.E.; Bailey, S.M.: Effect of parental fatness levels on the fatness of biological and adoptive children. Ecol. Food. Nutr. *7:* 91–93 (1977).
50 Annest, J.L.; Sing, C.F.; Biron, P.; Mongeau, J.G.: Familial aggregation of blood pressure and weight in adoptive families. III. Analysis of the role of shared genes and shared household environment in explaining family resemblance for height, weight, and selected weight/height indices. Am. J. Epidem. *117:* 492–506 (1983).
51 Stunkard, A.J.; Sorensen, T.I.A.; Hanis, C.; Teasdale, T.W.; Chakraborty, R.; Schull, W.J.; Schulsinger, F.: An adoption study of human obesity. New Engl. J. Med. *314:* 193–198 (1986).
52 Poehlman, E.T.; Tremblay, A.; Despres, J.-P.; Fontaine, E.; Perusse, L.; Theriault, G.; Bauchard, C.: Genotype-controlled changes in body composition and fat morphology following over-feeding in twins. Am. J. clin. Nutr. *43:* 723–731 (1986).
53 West, K.M.: Culture, history, and adiposity, or should Santa Claus reduce? Obesity bariatr. Med. *2:* 48–52 (1974).
54 West, K.M.: Diabetes in American Indians and other native populations of the new world. Diabetes *23:* 841–855 (1974).
55 Thomas, P.: Choctaws control 40-bed hospital and treat ills of poverty, isolation. Med. Tribune *Nov. 7:* 18 (1984).
56 Bennett, P.H.; Knowler, W.C.: Increasing prevalence of diabetes in the Pima American Indians over a ten-year period. Diabetes *32:* 507–511 (1979).
57 Bennett, P.H.; Knowler, W.C.; Baird, H.R.; Butler, W.J.; Pettitt, D.J.; Reid, J.M.: Diet and development of non-insulin-dependent diabetes mellitus: an epidemiological perspective; in Pozza et al., Diet, diabetes, and atherosclerosis, pp. 109–119 (Raven Press, New York 1984).
58 Knowler, W.C.; Pettitt, D.J.; Bennett, P.H.; Williams, R.C.: Diabetes mellitus in the Pima Indians: genetic and evolutionary considerations. Am. J. phys. Anthrop. *62:* 107–114 (1983).
59 Neel, J.V.: Diabetes mellitus: a 'thrifty' genotype rendered detrimental by 'progress'? Am. J. hum. Genet. *14:* 353–362 (1962).

60 Neel, J.V.: The thrifty genotype revisited; in Kobberling, Tattersall, The genetics of diabetes mellitus. Serono Symp. 47, pp. 283–293 (Academic Press, New York 1982).

61 O'Dea, K.: Marked improvement in carbohydrate and lipid metabolism in diabetic Australian Aborigines after temporary reversion to traditional lifestyle. Diabetes *33:* 596–603 (1984).

62 Szathmary, E.J.E.; Holt, N.: Hyperglycemia in Dogrib Indians of the Northwest Territories, Canada: association with age and a centripetal distribution of body fat. Hum. Biol. *55:* 493–515 (1983).

63 Szathmary, E.J.E.: The search for genetic factors controlling plasma glucose levels in Dogrib Indians; in Chakraborty, Szathmary, Diseases of complex etiology in small populations: ethnic differences and research approaches, pp. 199–226 (Liss, New York 1985).

64 Szathmary, E.J.E.: The effect of Gc genotype on fasting insulin level in Dogrib Indians (unpublished manuscript, 1986).

65 Szathmary, E.J.E.: Diabetes in arctic and subarctic populations undergoing acculturation (submitted to Collegium Anthropologicum, Zagreb 1986).

66 Szathmary, E.J.E.; Ritenbaugh, C.; Goodby C.S.M.: Dietary change and plasma glucose levels in an Amerindian population undergoing cultural transition. Soc. Sci. Med. *24:* 791–804 (1987).

67 Pettitt, D.J.; Baird, H.R.; Aleck, K.A.; Bennett, P.H.; Knowler, W.C.: Excessive obesity in offspring of Pima Indian women with diabetes during pregnancy. New Engl. J. Med. *308:* 242–245 (1983).

68 Freinkel, N.: Of pregnancy and progeny. Diabetes *29:* 1023–1025 (1980).

69 Rimoin, D.L.; Schinke, R.N.: Endocrine pancreas; in Remoin, Schinke, Genetic disorders of endocrine glands, pp. 150–194 (Mosby, St Louis 1971).

70 Reed, T.E.: Ethnic classification of Mexican Americans. Science *285:* 283 (1974).

71 Gottlieb, K.; Kimberling, W.J.: Admixture estimates for the gene pool of Mexican Americans in Colorado (Abstract) Am. J. phys. Anthrop. *50:* 44 (1979).

72 Stern, M.P.; Gaskill, S.P.; Allen, C.R.; Garza, N.; Gonzales, J.L.; Waldrop, R.H.: Cardiovascular risk factors in Mexican Americans in Laredo, Texas. I. Prevalence of overweight and diabetes and distributions of serum lipids. Am. J. Epidem. *113:* 546–555 (1981).

73 Stern, M.P.; Pugh, J.A.; Gaskill, S.P.; Hazuda, H.P.: Knowledge, attitudes, and behavior related to obesity and dieting in Mexican Americans and Anglos. The San Antonio Heart Study. Am. J. Epidem. *115:* 917–928 (1982).

74 Stern, M.P.; Gaskill, S.P.; Hazuda, H.P.; Gardner, L.I.; Haffner, S.M.: Does obesity explain excess prevalence of diabetes among Mexican Americans? Results of the San Antonio Heart Study. Diabetologia *24:* 272–277 (1983).

75 Stern, M.P.; Rosenthal, M.; Haffner, S.M.; Hazuda, H.P.; Franco, L.J.: Sex differences in the effects of sociocultural status on diabetes and cardiovascular risk factors in Mexican Americans. The San Antonio Heart Study. Am. J. Epidem. *120:* 834–851 (1984).

76 Gardner, L.I.; Stern, M.P.; Haffner, S.M.; Gaskill, S.P.; Hazuda, H.P.; Relethford, J.H.; Eifler, C.W.: Prevalence of diabetes in Mexican Americans. Relationship to percent of gene pool derived from Native American sources. Diabetes *33:* 86–92 (1984).

77 Stern, M.P.; Relethford, J.H.; Ferrell, R.E.; Gaskill, S.P.; Hazuda, H.P.; Haffner, S.M.; Gardner, L.I.: Diabetes and genetic admixture in Mexican Americans. The San Antonio Heart Study. Diabetes *31:* suppl. 2, p. 45A (1982).

78 Hanis, C.L.; Ferrell, R.E.; Barton, S.A.; Aguilar, L.; Garza-Ibarra, A.; Tulloch, B.R.; Garcia, C.A.; Schull, W.J.: Diabetes among Mexican Americans in Starr County, Texas. Am. J. Epidem. *118:* 659–672 (1983).

79 Mueller, W.H.; Joos, S.K.; Hanis, C.L.; Zanaleta, A.N.; Eichner, J.; Schull, W.J.: The diabetes alert study: growth, fatness, and fat patterning, adolescence through adulthood in Mexican Americans. Am. J. phys. Anthrop. *64:* 389–399 (1984).

80 Neel, J.V.: Diabetes mellitus: a geneticist's nightmare; in Creutzfeldt, Kobberling, Neel, The genetics of diabetes mellitus, pp. 1–11 (Springer, Berlin 1976).

81 Simpson, N.E.: The genetics of diabetes mellitus: a review of family data; in Creutzfeldt, Kobberling, Neel, The genetics of diabetes mellitus, pp. 12–20 (Springer, Berlin 1976).

82 Report on the work group on genetics of the Committee on Scope and Impact to the National Commission on Diabetes. Report of the National Commission on Diabetes to the Congress of US vol. 3, part 2, DHEW publ. No. (NIH) 76-1022, pp. 163–170 (Government Printing Office, Washington 1976).

83 Rotter, J.E.; Rimoin, D.L.; Samloff, I.M.: Genetic heterogeneity in diabetes mellitus and peptic ulcer; in Morton, Chung, Genetic epidemiology, pp. 381–412 (Academic Press, New York 1978).

84 Falconer, D.S.: The inheritance of liability to diseases with variable age of onset with particular reference to diabetes mellitus. Ann. hum. Genet. *31:* 1–20 (1967).

85 Neel, J.V.: The genetics of diabetes mellitus. Adv. metab. Dis. *1:* suppl. 3, pp. 3–10 (1970).

86 Rimoin, D.L.: Inheritance in diabetes mellitus. Med. Clins N. Am. *55:* 807–819 (1971).

87 Zavala, C.; Morton, N.E.; Rao, D.C.; Lalouel, J.M.; Gamboa, I.A.; Tejeda, A.; Lisker, R.: Complex segregation analysis of diabetes mellitus. Hum. Hered. *29:* 325–333 (1979).

88 Barnett, A.H.; Eff, C.; Leslie, R.D.G.; Pyke, D.: Diabetes in identical twins: a study of 200 pairs. Diabetologia *20:* 87–93 (1981).

89 Cahill, G.F.: Heterogeneity in type II diabetes (Editorial). West. J. Med. *142:* 249–250 (1985).

90 Jialal, I.; Nadoo, C.; Rajput, M.; Joubert, S.M.: Evidence for insulin resistance in Indian patients with non-insulin-dependent diabetes in the young. Hormone metabol. Res. *16:* 377–378 (1984).

91 Ginsberg-Fellner, F.: In the genes. Diabetes Forecast *34:* 31–33 (1981).

92 Jenson, A.B.; Doberson, M.J.: Etiopathology of diabetes mellitus. Perspect. pediatr. Pathol. *7:* 167–184 (1982).

93 King, H.; Zimmet, P.; Pargeter, K.; Raper, L.R.; Collins, V.: Ethnic difference in susceptibility to non-insulin-dependent diabetes. A comparative study of two urbanized Micronesian populations. Diabetes *33:* 1002–1007 (1984).

94 Knowler, W.C.; Pettitt, D.J.; Vasquez, B.; Rotwein, P.S.; Andreone, T.L.; Permutt, M.A.: Polymorphism in the 5' flanking region of the human insulin gene. J. clin. Invest. *74:* 2129–2135 (1984).

95 Daiger, S.P.; Schanfield, M.S.; Cavalli-Sforza, L.L.: Group-specific component (Gc) proteins bind vitamin D and vitamin D metabolites. Proc. natn. Acad. Sci. USA *72:* 2076–2080 (1975).
96 Christakos, S.; Norman, A.W.: Studies on the mode of action of calciferol. XXXIII. Biochemical characterization of 1,25-dihydroxy vitamin D receptors in chick pancreas and kidney cortosol. Endocrinology *108:* 140–149 (1981).
97 Gedik, O.; Akalin, S.: Effects of vitamin D deficiency and repletion on insulin and glucagon secretion in man. Diabetologia *29:* 142–145 (1986).
98 Clark, S.A.; Stumpf, W.E.; Sar, M.: Effect of 1,25-dihydroxyvitamin D_3 on insulin secretion. Diabetes *30:* 382–386 (1981).
99 Nyomba, B.L.; Bouillon, R.; De Moor, P.: Influence of vitamin D status on insulin secretion and glucose tolerance in the rabbit. Endocrinology *115:* 191–197 (1984).
100 Nyomba, B.L.; Auwerx, J.; Bormans, V.; Peeters, T.L.; Pelemans, W.; Reynaert, J.; Bouillon, R.; Vontrappen, G.; De Moor, P.: Pancreatic secretion in man with subclinical vitamin D deficiency. Diabetologia *29:* 34–38 (1986).
101 Kadawaki, S.; Norman, A.W.: Demonstration that the vitamin D metabolite $1,25(OH)_2$-vitamin D_3 and not $24R,25(OH)_2$-vitamin D_3 is essential for normal insulin secretion in the perfused rat pancreas. Diabetes *34:* 315–320 (1985).
102 Kirk, R.L.; Serjeantson, S.W.; Zimmet, P.: Genes and diabetes in the Pacific; in Mimura, Baba, Goto, Kobberling, Clinicogenetic genesis of diabetes mellitus, pp. 34–41 (Excerpta Medica, Amsterdam 1982).
103 Kirk, R.L.; Serjeantson, S.W.; King, H.; Zimmet, P.: The genetic epidemiology of diabetes mellitus; in Chakraborty, Szathmary, Diseases of complex etiology in small populations, pp. 105–118 (Liss, New York 1985).
104 Daiger, S.P.; Miller, M.; Chakraborty, R.: Heritability of quantitative variation at the group-specific component (Gc) locus. Am. J. hum. Genet. *36:* 663–676 (1984).
105 Ledermann, S.: Alcohol, alcoholism, alcoholization, vol. 1 (Presses Universitaires de France, Paris 1956).
106 Skog, O.-J.: The collectivity of drinking cultures: a theory of the distribution of alcohol consumption. Br. J. Addict. *80:* 83–99 (1985).
107 Room, R.: A 'reverence for strong drink': the lost generation and the elevation of alcohol in American culture. J. Stud. Alc. *45:* 540–546 (1984).
108 Friedman, H.: Alcohol and heart disease. Primary Cardiol. *Dec.:* 44–49 (1984).
109 Clark, L.: Alcohol use and hypertension. Postgrad. Med. *75:* 273–276 (1984).
110 Eastman, P.: Forgetting the alcohol-HBP link? Med. Tribune *June:* 9–11 (1985).
111 Windham, C.T.; Wyse, B.W.; Hansen, R.G.: Alcohol consumption and nutrient density of diets in the nationwide food consumption survey. J. Am. diet. Ass. *82:* 364–371 (1983).
112 Wanberg, K.; Lewis, R.; Foster, F.M.: Alcoholism and ethnicity: a comparative study of alcohol use patterns across ethnic groups. Int. J. Addict. *13:* 1245–1262 (1978).
113 Wall, J.H.: A study of alcoholism in women. Am. J. Psychiat. *93:* 943–955 (1937).
114 Curlee, J.: Alcoholism and the 'empty nest'. Bull. Menninger Clin. *33:* 165–171 (1969).
115 Lisansky, E.S.: Alcoholism in women; social and psychological concomitants. I. Social history data. Q. Jl Stud. Alcohol *18:* 588–623 (1968).
116 Curlee, J.: Women alcoholics. Fed. Probation *32:* 16–20 (1968).
117 Schuckit, M.A.; Morrissey, E.R.: Alcoholism in women; some clinical and social

perspectives; in Greenblatt, Schuckit, Alcoholism problems in women and children, pp. 5–35 (Grune & Stratton, New York 1976).
118 Cramer, M.J.; Blacker, E.: Social class and drinking experience of female drunkeness offenders. J. Hlth hum. Behav. *7:* 276–283 (1966).
119 Fort, T.; Porterfield, A.L.: Some background and types of alcoholism among women. J. Hlth hum. Behav. *2:* 283–292 (1961).
120 Wood, H.P.; Duffy, E.L.: Psychological factors in alcoholic women. Am. J. Psychiat. *123:* 341–345 (1966).
121 Dohrenwend, B.S.: Events as stressors; a methodological inquiry. J. Hlth Soc. Behav. *14:* 167–175 (1973).
122 Richardson, W.C.: Poverty, illness and use of health services in the United States. Hospitals *43:* 34–40 (1969).
123 Morrissey, E.R.; Schuckit, M.A.: Stressful life events and alcohol problems among women seen at a detoxication center. J. Stud. Alcohol *39:* 1559–1576 (1978).
124 Moos, R.H.; Mehren, B.; Moos, B.S.: Evaluation of a Salvation Army alcoholism treatment program. J. Stud. Alcohol *39:* 1267–1275 (1978).
125 Cadogan, D.A.: Marital group therapy in the treatment of alcoholism. Q. Jl Stud. Alcohol *34:* 1187–1194 (1973).
126 Van Dijk, W.K.; Van Dijk-Koffeman, A.: A follow-up study of 211 treated male alcoholic addicts. Br. J. Addict. *68:* 3–24 (1973).
127 Orford, J.; Guthrie, S.; Nicholls, P.; Oppenheimer, E.; Egert, S.; Hansman, C.: Self-reported coping behavior of wives of alcoholics and its association with drinking outcome. J. Stud. Alcohol *36:* 1254–1257 (1975).
128 Moos, R.H.; Bromet, E.; Tsu, V.; Moos, B.: Family characteristics and the outcome of treatment for alcoholism. J. Stud. Alcohol *40:* 78–88 (1979).
129 Pedersen, N.L.: Multivariate analysis of familial and non-familial influences for commonality in drug use. Drug Alc. Depend. *14:* 67–74 (1984).
130 Page, R.D.; Bozlee, S.: A cross-cultural MMPI comparison of alcoholics. Psychiat. Rep. *50:* 639–646 (1982).
131 Davis, W.E.: Race and the differential 'power' of the MMPI. J. Personal. Assess. *39:* 138–139 (1975).
132 Miller, C.; Mertz, C.; Counts, S.: Racial differences on the MMPI. J. clin. Psychol. *17:* 159–160 (1961).
133 Adams, B.L.; Horovitz, J.H.: Psychopathology and fatherlessness in poor boys. Child Psychiat. hum. Devel. *10:* 135–143 (1980).
134 Linn, M.W.; Shane, R.; Webb, N.L.; Pratt, T.C.: Cultural factors and attrition in drug abuse treatment. Int. J. Addict. *14:* 259–280 (1979).
135 Townsley, H.C.; Goldstein, G.S.: One view of the etiology of depression in the American Indian. Publ. Hlth Rep. *92:* 458–461 (1977).
136 Leland, J.: Comment on 'psychocultural barrier to successful alcoholism therapy in an American Indian patient'. J. Stud. Alcohol *40:* 737–742 (1979).
137 May, P.A.: Substance abuse and American Indians: prevalence and susceptibility. Int. J. Addict. *17:* 1185–1209 (1982).
138 De Luca, J.R. (ed.): Fourth Special Report to the United States Congress on Alcohol and Health for the Secretary of Health and Human Services. US Department for Health and Human Services, Public Health Service, p. 161 (National Institute on Alcohol Abuse and Alcoholism, Rockville 1981).

139 Sievers, M.L.: Cigarette and alcohol usage by southwestern American Indians. Am. J. publ. Hlth *58:* 77–82 (1968).
140 Hughes, S.P.; Dodder, R.A.: Alcohol consumption patterns among American Indian and White college students. J. Stud. Alcohol *45:* 433–439 (1984).
141 Whittaker, J.O.: Alcohol and the Standing Rock Sioux tribe. I. The pattern of drinking. Q. Jl Stud. Alcohol *23:* 468–479 (1962).
142 Cockerham, W.C.: Drinking attitudes and practices among Wind River reservation Indian youth. J. Stud. Alcohol *36:* 321–326 (1975).
143 May, P.A.; Hymbaugh, K.J.: A pilot project on fetal alcohol syndrome among American Indians. Alcohol Hlth Res. Wld *7:* 3–9 (1982–83).
144 Levy, J.E.; Kunitz, S.J.: Indian drinking: Navajo practices and Anglo-American theories (Wiley, New York 1974).
145 Porter, M.R.; Vieira, T.A.; Kaplan, G.J.; Heesch, J.R.; Colyer, A.B.: Drug use in anchorage, Alaska. A survey of 15,634 students in grades 6 through 12, 1971. J. Am. med. Ass. *223:* 657–664 (1973).
146 Oetting, E.R.; Edwards, R.; Goldstein, G.S.; Garcia-Mason, V.: Drug use among adolescents of five southwest Native American tribes. Int. J. Addict. *15:* 439–445 (1980).
147 Longclaws, L.; Barnes, G.E.; Grieve, L.; Dumoff, R.: Alcohol and drug use among the Brokenhead Ojibwa. J. Stud. Alcohol *41:* 21–36 (1980).
148 Beauvais, F.; La Boueff, S.: Drug and alcohol abuse intervention in American Indian communities. Int. J. Addict. *20:* 139–171 (1985).
149 Mail, P.; McDonald, D.: Tulapai to Tokay (HRAF Press, New Haven 1980).
150 May, P.A.; Broudy, D.W.: Health problems of the Navajo area and suggested interventions; 2nd ed. (Navajo Health Authority, Window Rock 1980).
151 Beauvais, F.; Oetting, E.R.; Edwards, R.: Trends in drug use of Indian adolescents living on reservations 1975–1983. Am. J. Drug Alc. Abuse *11:* 209–229 (1985).
152 Oetting, E.R.; Beauvais, F.: Drug use among Native American youth: summary of findings (1975–1981). NIDA Project Report, 5R01-DA-1853 (Colorado State University, Fort Collins 1982).
153 Pinto, L.: Alcohol and drug abuse among Native American youth on reservations: a growing crisis; in Drug use in America: problem in perspective. The Technical Papers of the Second Report of the National Commission on Marijuana and Drug Abuse, appendix vol. 1 (United States Government Printing Office, Washington 1973).
154 Delk, J.; Urbancik, G.; Williams, C.; Berg, G.; Kahn, M.: Dropouts from an American Indian reservation school: a possible prevention program. J. Community Psychol. *2:* 15–17 (1974).
155 Leighton, D.; Kluckhohn, C.: Children of the people (Octagon Books, New York 1947).
156 Mesteth, L.: Gas and glue sniffing among the school age population. Pine Ridge Research Bulletin No. 4 (United States Government Printing Office, Washington 1968).
157 Mendill, C.: Some psychological aspects of normal Indian adolescents and two groups of non-Indian adolescents. Pine Ridge Research Bulletin, No. 4 (United States Government Printing Office, Washington 1968).

158 Oetting, E.R.; Goldstein, G.: Drug use among Native American adolescents; in Beschner, Friedman, Youth drug abuse: problems, issues and treatment (Lexington Books, Lexington 1979).
159 Oetting, E.R.; Goldstein, G.; Beauvais, F.; Edwards, R.: Drug abuse among Indian children. Interim Report, NIDA Grant 1 R01-DA01853 (Colorado State University, Fort Collins 1980).
160 Beauvais, F.: Preventing drug abuse among American Indian young people. NSF final report (Colorado State University, Fort Collins 1980).
161 Jessor, R.; Graves, T.; Hanson, R.; Jessor, S.: Society, personality, and deviant behavior: a study of tri-ethnic-community (Holt, Rinehart, & Winston, New York 1968).
162 Flores, P.J.: Alcoholism treatment and the relationship of Native American cultural values to recovery; PhD diss. Tucson. Diss. Abst. Int. *44:* 306–B (1983).
163 Nace, E.P.: Epidemiology of alcoholism and prospects for treatment. A. Rev. Med. *35:* 293–309 (1984).
164 Caetano, R.: Drinking patterns and alcohol problems among Hispanics in the US: a review. Drug Alc. Depend. *12:* 37–59 (1983).
165 Jessor, R.; et al.: Society, personality, and deviant behavior (Holt, Rinehart, & Winston, New York 1968).
166 Munoz, J.A.: Difficulties of a Hispanic-American psychotherapist in the treatment of Hispanic-American patients. Am. J. Orthopsychiat. *51:* 646–653 (1981).
167 Miller, G.; Fagan, P.: Alcoholism: a polygenic, multifactorial disease. Compreh. Ther. *11:* 72–75 (1985).
168 Goodwin, D.S.: Family studies of alcoholism. J. Stud. Alcohol *42:* 156–162 (1981).
169 Goodwin, D.S.: Speculations on the cause(s) of alcoholism. J. clin. Psychiat. *45:* 491–493 (1984).
170 Jones, B.; Goldstein, R.; Gurley, M.: Appetite for alcohol: influence of genetics and early experience. Neurobehav. Toxicol. Teratol. *7:* 125–127 (1985).
171 Dorlands Illustrated Medical Dictionary; 25th ed., pp. 744–745 (Saunders, Philadelphia 1974).
172 Brock, P. (ed): The alcoholism report. The authoritative newsletter for professionals in the field of alcoholism. *12:* 1–5 (The Johnson Institute, Washington, D.C. 1984).
173 Dreiling, D.A.; Koller, M.: The natural history of alcoholic pancreatitis: update of 1985. Mount Sinai J. Med. *52:* 340–342 (1985).
174 Dickson, A.P.; O'Neill, J.; Imrie, C.W.: Hyperlipidemia, alcohol abuse and acute pancreatitis. Br. J. Surg. *71:* 685–688 (1984).
175 Wilson, J.S.; Bernstein, L.; McDonald, C.; Tait, A.; McNeil, D.; Pirola, R.C.: Diet and drinking habits in relation to the development of alcoholic pancreatitis. Gut *26:* 882–887 (1985).
176 Testoni, P.A.; Masci, E.; Passaretti, S.; Guslandi, M.; Tittobello, A.: Early detection of pancreatic lesions in chronic alcoholism: diagnostic accuracy of ERP. J. clin. Gastroenterol. *6:* 519–523 (1984).
177 Kreel, L.: Diagnostic images: pancreatic and liver disease in an alcoholic. Post-grad. med. J. *61:* 37–38 (1984).

178 Seligson, U.; Cho, J.W.; Nygren, A.; Rachard, P.: Is glucose intolerance after pancreatitis related to pancreatic tissue damage? Acta med. scand. *312:* 119–122 (1983).
179 Longnecker, D.S.: Pathology and pathogenesis of diseases of the pancreas. Am. J. Path. *107:* 115–118 (1982).
180 Duckworth, W.C.; Solomon, S.S.; Jallepalli, P.; Iyer, R.; Bobal, M.A.: Hormonal responses to intravenous glucose and arginine in patients with pancreatitis. Hormone Res. *17:* 65–73 (1983).
181 Myers, J.D.: Net splanchnic glucose production in normal man and in various disease states. J. clin. Invest. *29:* 1421–1429 (1950).
182 Shaw, S.; Lieber, C.: Nutritional support of the medical practice; in Schneider, Anderson, Corsin (Harper & Rowe, London 1977).
183 Megyesi, C.; Samols, E.; Marks, V.: Glucose tolerance and diabetes in chronic liver disease. Lancet *ii:* 1051–1056 (1967).
184 De Moura, M.C.; Cruz, A.G.: Carbohydrate metabolism studies in cirrhosis of the liver. Am. J. dig. Dis. *13:* 891–899 (1968).
185 Conn, H.O.; Schreiber, W.; Elkington, S.G.: Cirrhosis and diabetes. II. Association of impaired glucose tolerance with portal-systemic shunting in Laennec's cirrhosis. Am. J. dig. Dis. *16:* 227–239 (1971).
186 Creutzfeldt, W.; Fredrichs, H.; Kraft, W.: The intravenous tolbutamide test in liver disease. Acta diab. latina *4:* 205–222 (1967).
187 Iverson, J.; Vilstrup, H.; Tygstrup, N.: Insulin sensitivity in alcoholic cirrhosis. Scand. J. clin. Lab. Invest. *43:* 65–73 (1983).
188 Salmela, P.I.; Sartaniemi, E.A.; Pelkonen, R.P.: The evaluation of the drug-metabolizing capacity in patients with diabetes mellitus. Diabetes *29:* 788–794 (1980).
189 Shankar, T.P.; Solomon, S.S.; Duckworth, W.C.; et al.: Studies of glucose intolerance in cirrhosis of the liver. J. Lab. clin. Med. *102:* 459–464 (1983).
190 Iversen, J.; Vilstrup, H.; Tygstrup, N.: Insulin sensitivity in alcoholic cirrhosis. Scand. J. clin. Lab. Invest. *43:* 565–573 (1983).
191 Marchesini, G.; Melli, A.; Checchia, G.A.; Mattioli, L.; Capelli, M.; Cassarani, S.; Zoli, M.; Pisi, E.: Pancreatic B-cell function in cirrhotic patients with and without overt diabetes. C-Peptide response to glucagon and to meal. Metabolism *34:* 695–701 (1985).
192 Kahn, C.R.: Insulin resistance, insulin insensitivity, and insulin unresponsiveness: a necessary distinction. Metabolism *27:* suppl. 2, pp. 1893–1902 (1978).
193 Blei, A.T.; Robbins, D.C.; Drobny, E.; Baumann, G.; Rubenstein, A.H.: Insulin resistance and insulin receptors in hepatic cirrhosis. Gastroenterology *83:* 1191–1199 (1982).
194 Iversen, J.; Vilstrup, H.; Tygstrup, N.: Kinetics of glucose metabolism in relation to insulin concentrations in patients with alcoholic cirrhosis and in healthy persons. Gastroenterology *87:* 1138–1143 (1984).
195 Feingold, K.B.; Siperstein, M.D.: Normalization of fasting blood glucose levels in insulin-requiring diabetes: the role of ethanol abstention. Diabetes Care *6:* 186–188 (1983).
196 Sereny, G.; Endrenyi, L.: Mechanisms and significance of carbohydrate intolerance in chronic alcoholism. Metabolism *27:* 1041–1046 (1978).
197 Arkey, R.A.: Alcohol use and the diabetic patient. Alcohol Hlth Res. Wld *8:* 8–13 (1984).

198 Andre, J.M.; Ghachu, S.: Suicide occurrences in an American Indian community of the southwest (Albuquerque Indian Health Service, Albuquerque 1975).
199 Nikkila, E.A.; Taskinen, M.D.: Ethanol-induced alterations of glucose tolerance, postglucose hypoglycemia, and insulin secretion in normal, obese, and diabetic subjects. Diabetes *24:* 933–943 (1975).
200 Bordy, M.D.; Harris, D.J.; Howard, C.P.; Grunt, J.A.: The relationship of chronic alcoholism and type I diabetes mellitus. Missouri Med. *82:* 84–86 (1985).
201 Lieber, C.S.: Alcohol-nutrition interaction. J. med. Soc. New Jers. *76:* 379–380 (1979).
202 Ryle, P.R.; Thomson, A.D.: Nutrition and vitamins in alcoholism; in Rosalki, Clinical biochemistry of alcoholism, pp. 188–224 (Churchill-Livingstone, New York 1984).
203 Hurt, R.D.; Higgins, J.A.; Nelson, R.A.; Morse, R.M.; Dickson, E.R.: Nutritional status of a group of alcoholics before and after admission to an alcoholism treatment unit. Am. J. clin. Nutr. *34:* 386–392 (1981).
204 Goldsmith, R.H.; Iber, F.L.; Miller, P.A.: Nutritional status of alcoholics of different socioeconomic class. J. Am. Coll. Nutr. *2:* 215–220 (1983).
205 Tomaiolo, P.O.; Kraus, V.: Nutritional status of hospitalized patients. JPEN *4:* 1–3 (1980).
206 Herbert, V.; Zalusky, R.; Davidson, C.S.: Correlation of folate deficiency with alcoholism and associated macrocytosis, anemia and liver disease. Ann. intern. Med. *58:* 977–988 (1963).
207 Leevy, C.M.; Cardi, L.; Frank, O.; Gellene, R.; Baker, H.: Incidence and significance of hypovitaminemia in a randomly selected municipal hospital population. Am. J. clin. Nutr. *17:* 259–271 (1965).
208 Leevy, C.M.; Baker, H.; Ten Hove, W.; Frank, O.; Cherrick, G.R.: B-Complex vitamins in liver disease of the alcoholic. Am. J. clin. Nutr. *16:* 339–346 (1965).
209 Ashley, M.J.; Olin, J.S.; LeRiche, W.H.; Kornaczewski, A.; Schmidt, W.; Rankin, J.G.: Social class and morbidity in clinically treated alcoholics. Drug Alcohol Depend. *1:* 263–276 (1975–76).
210 Neville, J.N.; Eagles, J.A.; Samson, G.; Olson, R.E.: Nutritional status of alcoholics. Am. J. clin. Nutr. *21:* 1329–1340 (1968).
211 Hurt, R.D.; Higgins, J.A.; Nelson, R.A.; Morse, R.M.; Dickson, E.R.: Nutritional status of a group of alcoholics before and after admission to an alcoholism treatment unit. Am. J. clin. Nutr. *34:* 386–392 (1978).
212 Thomson, A.D.: Alcohol and nutrition. Clin. Endocrinol. Metab. *7:* 405–428 (1978).
213 Paul, A.A.; Southgate, D.A.T.: in McCance, Widdowson, The composition of foods; 4th revised ed. of the MRC Special Report, No. 297 (HMSO, London 1978).
214 Barboriak, J.J.; Rooney, C.B.; Leitschuh, T.H.; Anderson, A.J.: Alcohol and nutrient intake of elderly men. J. Am. diet. Ass. *72:* 493–495 (1978).
215 Gruchow, H.W.; Sobocinski, K.A.; Barboriak, J.J.; Scheller, J.G.: Alcohol consumption, nutrient intake and relative body weight among US adults. Am. J. clin. Nutr. *42:* 289–295 (1985).
216 Tanaka, K.: New light on biotin deficiency. New Engl. J. Med. *304:* 839–840 (1981).

217 Whitehead, C.C.: The assessment of biotin status in man and animals. Proc. Nutr. Soc. *40:* 165–172 (1981).

218 Baines, M.: Detection and incidence of B and C vitamin deficiency in alcohol-related illness. Ann. clin. Biochem. *15:* 307–312 (1978).

219 Majumdar, S.K.; Shaw, G.K.; O'Gorman, P.; Aps, E.J.; Offerman, E.L.; Thomson, A.D.: Blood vitamin status (B_1, B_2, B_6, folic acid and B_{12}) in patients with alcoholic liver disease. Int. J. Vitam. Nutr. Res. *52:* 266–271 (1982).

220 Lowenstein, S.R.; Gabow, P.A.; Cramer, J.; Oliva, P.B.; Ratner, K.: The role of alcohol in new-onset atrial fibrillation. Archs intern. Med. *143:* 1882–1885 (1982).

221 Esterp, H.; Shaw, W.A.; Watlington, C.; Hobe, R.; Holland, W.; Tucker, St. G.: Hypocalcemia due to hypomagnesemia and reversible parathyroid hormone unresponsiveness. J. clin. Endocr. Metab. *29:* 842–848 (1969).

222 McIntyre, N.: The effects of alcohol on water, electrolytes, and minerals; in Rosalki, Clinical biochemistry of alcoholism, pp. 117–134 (Churchill-Livingstone, New York 1985).

223 Morgan, M.Y.: Alcohol and the endocrine system. Med. Bull. *38:* 35–42 (1982).

224 Martin, H.E.; McCuskey, C., Jr.; Tupikova, N.: Electrolyte disturbance in acute alcoholism with particular reference to magnesium. Am. J. clin. Nutr. *7:* 191–196 (1959).

225 McCollister, R.J.; Flink, E.B.; Doe, R.P.: Magnesium balance studies in chronic alcoholism. J. Lab. clin. Med. *55:* 98–104 (1960).

226 Majumdar, S.K.; Shaw, G.K.; Thomson, A.D.: Serum zinc, magnesium, and calcium status in the Wernicke-Korsakoff syndrome. Drug Alc. Depend. *12:* 403–405 (1983).

227 Yajnik, C.S.; et al.: Fasting plasma magnesium concentrations and glucose disposal in diabetes. Br. med. J. *288:* 1032–1034 (1984).

228 McClain, C.J.; Su, L.-C.: Zinc dependency in the alcoholic: a review. Alcoholism clin. exp. Res. *7:* 5–10 (1983).

229 Prasad, A.S.: Zinc in human nutrition, pp. 17–18 (CRC Press, Boca Raton 1979).

230 Wu, C.-T.; Lee, J.-N.; Shen, W.W.; Lee, S.-L.: Serum zinc, copper, and ceruloplasmin levels in male alcoholics. Biol. Psychiat. *19:* 1333–1338 (1984).

231 Review: Liver vitamin A mobilization during zinc deficiency and restricted food intake. Nutr. Rev. *35:* 213–215 (1977).

232 Smith, J.C., Jr.: The vitamin A-zinc connection: a review. Ann. N.Y. Acad. Sci. *355:* 62–75 (1980).

233 Review: Mobilization of hepatic vitamin A by zinc supplementation in zinc deficiency associated with protein-energy malnutrition. Nutr. Rev. *38:* 275–277 (1980).

234 Sturtevant, F.M.: Zinc deficiency, acrodermatitis enteropathica, optic atrophy, subacute myelo-optic neuropathy, and 5,7-dihalo-8-quinolinols. Pediatrics *65:* 610–613 (1980).

235 Herlong, H.F.; Russell, R.M.; Maddry, W.C.: Vitamin A and zinc therapy in primary biliary cirrhosis. Hematology *1:* 348–351 (1981).

236 West, K.M.; Erdreich, L.J.; Stober, J.A.: A detailed study of risk factors for retinopathy and nephropathy in diabetes. Diabetes *29:* 501–508 (1980).

237 Young, R.J.; McCulloch, D.K.; Prescott, R.J.; Clarke, B.F.: Alcohol consumption and diabetic retinopathy. Diabetologia *25:* 206a (1983).

238 Allen, J.I.; Kay, N.E.; McCain, E.J.: Severe zinc deficiency in humans: association with a reversible T-lymphocyte dysfunction. Ann. intern. Med. *95:* 154–157 (1981).
239 Hartoma, T.R.; Sotaniemi, E.A.; Maatlanen, J.: Effect of zinc on some biochemical indices of metabolism. Nutr. Metab. *23:* 294–300 (1979).
240 Chandra, R.R.; Au, B.: Single nutrient deficiency and cell-mediated immune responses. 1. Zinc. Am. J. clin. Nutr. *33:* 736–738 (1980).
241 Mezey, E.: Metabolic effects of alcohol. Fed. Proc. *44:* 134–138 (1985).
242 McIntyre, N.: The effects of alcohol on water, electrolytes, and minerals; in Rosalki, Clinical biochemistry of alcoholism, pp. 117–134 (Churchill-Livingstone, New York 1985).
243 Pirola, R.C.; Lieber, C.S.: The energy cost of the metabolism of drugs, including ethanol. Pharmacology *7:* 185–196 (1972).
244 McDonald, J.T.; Margen, S.: Wine versus ethanol in human nutrition. I. Nitrogen and caloric balance. Am. J. clin. Nutr. *29:* 1093–1103 (1976).
245 Bebb, H.T.; Houser, H.B.; Witschi, J.C.; Littell, A.S.; Fuller, R.K.: Calorie and nutrient contribution of alcoholic beverages to the usual diets of 155 adults. Am. J. clin. Nutr. *24:* 1042–1052 (1971).
246 Morgan, M.Y.: Alcohol and nutrition. Br. med. Bull. *38:* 21–29 (1982).
247 Mezey, E.; Faillace, L.A.: Metabolic impairment and recovery time in acute ethanol intoxication. J. nerv. ment. Dis. *153:* 445–452 (1971).
248 Morgan, J.Y.: Enteral nutrition in chronic liver disease. Acta chirurg. scand. *507:* suppl., pp. 81–90 (1981).
249 Simko, V.; Connell, A.M.; Banks, B.: Nutritional status in alcoholics with and without liver disease. Am. J. clin. Nutr. *35:* 197–203 (1982).
250 Editorial: Alcohol and body weight. Alc. Alcoholism *19:* 1–6 (1984).
251 World, M.J.; Ryle, P.R.; Jones, D.; Shaw, G.K.; Thomson, A.D.: Differential effect of chronic alcohol intake and poor nutrition on body weight and fat stores. Alc. Alcoholism *19:* 281–290 (1984).
252 Hillers, V.N.; Massey, L.K.: Interrelationships of moderate and high alcohol consumption with diet and health status. Am. J. clin. Nutr. *41:* 356–362 (1985).
253 Lanier, D.C.: Familial alcoholism. J. Fam. Prac. *18:* 417–422 (1984).
254 Shuckit, M.A.; Parker, D.C.; Rossman, L.R.: Ethanol-related prolactin responses and risk for alcoholism. Biol. Psychiat. *18:* 1153–1159 (1983).
255 Schuckit, M.A.: Biological markers: metabolism and acute reactions to alcohol in sons of alcoholics. Pharmacol. Biochem. Behav. *13:* suppl. 1, pp. 9–16 (1980).
256 Schuckit, M.A.; Derby, J.: Alcohol-related flushing and the risk for alcoholism in sons of alcoholics. J. clin. Psychiat. *32:* 415–418 (1982).
257 Begleiter, H.; Poyesz, B.; Bihari, B.; Kissin, B.: Event-related brain potentials in boys at risk for alcoholism. Science *225:* 1493–1495 (1984).
258 Schuckit, M.A.: Ethanol-induced changes in body sway in men at high alcoholism risk. Archs gen. Psychiat. *42:* 375–379 (1985).
259 Schuckit, M.A.: Differences in plasma cortisol after ingestion of ethanol in relatives of alcoholics and controls: preliminary results. J. clin. Psychiat. *45:* 374–379 (1984).
260 Shigeta, Y.; Ishii, H.; Takagi, S.; Yoshitake, Y.; Hirano, T.; Takata, H.; Kohno, H.;

Tsuchiya, M.: HLA antigens as immunogenetic markers of alcoholism and alcoholic liver disease. Pharmacol. Biochem. Behav. *13:* suppl. 1, pp. 89–94 (1980).
261 Schuckit, M.A.: Genetics and the risk for alcoholism. J. Am. med. Ass. *254:* 2614–2617 (1985).
262 Editorial: Inborn alcoholism? Lancet *June 22:* 1427–1428 (1985).
263 Boyd, J.H.: Heredity and alcoholism. Med. Asp. Hum. Sexual. *19:* 23–35 (1985).
264 Editorial: Alcoholism, genetics, and society. Br. J. Addict. *79:* 353 (1984).
265 Reinhard, K.R.; Greenwalt, N.I.; Todd, A.L.; Madden, M.A.; Rabin, D.A.: Diabetes mellitus and alcoholic liver cirrhosis in an American Indian population. Proc. 105th Annu. Meet. Am. Public Health Association, (Indian Health Service, Tucson 1977).
266 Reinhard, K.R.; Klappenbach, R.S.; Rog, E.W.; Justice, J.W.: Alcohol-related mortality and morbidity in a southwestern United States Indian population. Proc. 10th Joint Meet. Prof. Ass. (US Public Health Service, Las Vegas 1975).
267 Goodwin, D.W.: Genetic component of alcoholism. Am. Rev. Med. *32:* 93–99 (1981).
268 Goodwin, D.W.: Alcoholism and genetics. Archs gen. Psychiat. *42:* 171–174 (1985).
269 Knop, J.: Risk factors in alcoholism. Lancet *Aug. 17:* 387–388 (1985).
270 Cook, B.L.; Winokur, G.: Separate heritability of alcoholism and psychotic symptoms. Am. J. Psychiat. *142:* 360–361 (1985).
271 Goodwin, D.W.; Schulsinger, F.; Moller, N.: Drinking problems in adopted and non-adopted sons of alcoholics. Archs gen. Psychiat. *31:* 164–169 (1974).
272 Volicer, L.; Volicer, B.J.; D'Angelo, N.: Assessment of genetic predisposition to alcoholism in male alcoholics. Alc. Alcoholism *20:* 63–68 (1985).
273 Saunders, J.B.; Wodak, A.D.; Haines, A.; Powell-Jackson, P.R.; Portmann, B.; Davis, M.; Williams, R.: Accelerated development of alcoholic cirrhosis in patients with HLA-B8. Lancet *i:* 1381–1384 (1982).
274 Jenkins, W.J.; Thomas, H.C.: Genetic factors in determining susceptibility to alcohol dependence and development of alcohol-induced liver disease. Clin. Gastroenterol. *10:* 307–314 (1981).
275 Agarwal, D.P.; Harada, S.; Goedde, H.W.: Racial differences in biological sensitivity to ethanol: the role of alcohol dehydrogenase and aldehyde dehydrogenase isozymes. Alcoholism: Clin. exp. Res. *5:* 12–16 (1981).
276 Zeiner, A.R.; Paredes, A.: Differential biological sensitivity to ethanol as a predictor of alcohol abuse. 4th National Drug Abuse Conf., San Francisco. A multicultural view of drug abuse. Proc. National Drug Abuse Conf., 1977, pp. 591–599 (Schenkman, Cambridge 1978).
277 Reed, T.E.; Kalant, H.; Gibbins, R.J.; Kapur, B.M.; Rankin, J.G.: Alcohol and acetaldehyde metabolism in Caucasians, Chinese, and Amerinds. Can. med. Ass. J. *115:* 851–855 (1976).
278 Farris, J.J.; Jones, B.N.: Ethanol metabolism in male American Indians and Whites. Alcoholism *2:* 77–81 (1978).
279 Farris, J.J.; Jones, B.N.: Ethanol metabolism in male American Indians and Caucasians. Proc. 8th Annu. NCA-AMSA Medical Scientific Session of the National Alcoholism Forum, San Diego 1977.

280 Ijiri, I.: Studies on the relationship between the concentrations of blood acetaldehyde and urinary catecholamine and the symptoms after drinking alcohol. Jap. J. Stud. Alc. *9:* 35–39 (1974).
281 Lehninger, A.L.; McKusick, V.A.; Santora, P.B.: Proceedings of the Conference on Genetic and Biochemical Variability in Response to Alcohol. Alcoholism: Clin. exp. Res. *5:* 435–463 (1981).
282 Robinson, S. (ed.): Knipe, self-help programs for Indians and native Alaskans. Alcohol Hlth Res. Wld *1:* 11–16 (1974).
283 Schaefer, J.M.: Firewater myths revisited. J. Stud. Alcohol *9:* suppl., pp. 99–117 (1981).
284 Zeiner, A.R.; Paredes, A.; Cowden, L.: Physiological responses to ethanol among the Tarahumara Indians. Ann. N.Y. Acad. Sci. *273:* 103–106 (1976).
285 Stratton, R.; Zeiner, A.R.: Variations in alcohol problems within the Oklahoma Indian population. Proc. 8th Annu. NCA-AMSA Meet. National Alcoholism Forum, San Diego 1977.
286 Zeiner, A.R.; Paredes, A.; Musicant, R.; Cowden, L.: Racial differences in psychophysiological responses to ethanol and placebo; in Seixas, Currents in alcoholism, vol. 1, pp. 271–286 (Grune & Stratton, New York 1977).
287 Rummelt, G.: Analysis of selected data of evaluation of community alcoholism services-Papago Indian reservation, Summer 1981 (Indian Health Service, Tucson 1982).

Mary E. Mohs, MS, RD, Department of Family and Community Medicine,
University of Arizona, Health Science Center, Tucson, AZ 85724 (USA)

Wld Rev. Nutr. Diet., vol. 56, pp. 173–216 (Karger, Basel 1988)

Vitamin D: Experimental Research and Its Practical Application

V.B. Spirichev, I.N. Sergeev[1]

Institute of Nutrition, Academy of Medical Sciences, Moscow, USSR

Contents

[1] We thank Mrs. I.V. Mecshanova for assistance in preparing the manuscript.

Introduction

The recent two-decade investigation into vitamin D function, metabolism and mechanism of its action has marked a considerable success in this field. These achievements, in the first place, are preconditioned by the discovery of active vitamin D forms, such as 25-hydroxyvitamin D (25-OHD), 1,25-dihydroxyvitamin D (1,25[OH]$_2$D), 24,25-dihydroxyvitamin D (24,25[OH]$_2$D), and other metabolites. After the key role of 1,25(OH)$_2$D in endocrine regulation and maintenance of the calcium homeostasis system had been established, a number of important new hypotheses appeared. As for their application, all of them were of certain scientific value, though they varied greatly and some of them were quite unexpected. The main findings have been covered in numerous reviews and monographs [DeLuca, 1979, 1980, 1982; DeLuca and Schnoes, 1983; Norman, 1979, 1980; Norman et al., 1982a, b; Norman and Miller, 1984; Lawson, 1978; Rajalakshmi, 1980; Fraser, 1980; Henry and Norman, 1984; Kumar, 1984; Spirichev, 1978, 1980, 1986].

The present work deals with some results of the research in this field that has been carried out during the past 15 years in the Laboratory of Vitamin and Mineral Metabolism, Institute of Nutrition, Academy of Medical Sciences, Moscow, USSR.

Vitamin D and Intestinal Calcium Absorption

One of the main physiological functions of vitamin D is to stimulate calcium absorption in the intestine. Though much research work has been done in this field, a great number of structural and biochemical aspects of vitamin-D-dependent calcium transport in the intestine have not been established yet [Wasserman, 1981; Wasserman and Fullmer, 1983; Norman et al., 1982a, b; Nemere and Norman, 1982].

According to widely spread theories, Ca^{2+} ion absorption passes three stages: the transport from the intestine throughout the brush border into the absorbing cell, intracellular Ca^{2+} transport to the basal-lateral surface, and Ca^{2+} output across the basal-lateral membrane to the blood stream [Bronner, 1982].

The principle difficulties in the problem of positive vitamin D effects on calcium absorption result from lack of knowledge on the structural and functional basis of ion transport itself in the intestine. That is why our laboratory has given full attention to the problem of specific ways of calcium transport across enterocytes and to the various subcellular structures' possible involvement in this process. The investigation has proved that in radioactive ^{45}Ca absorption, it binds mostly with the microvilli and microsomes, whereas in mitochondria and cytosol ^{45}Ca is present in a small amount [Morozov et al., 1980a, b]. ^{45}Ca accumulation in microsomes is accompanied by the marking enzyme of microvilli, e.g. saccharase, which may indicate vesicle formation from the microvillus membrane transporting calcium through the enterocyte [Morozov et al., 1980a, b; Fernandes et al., 1981].

The investigation of ^{45}Ca binding by intestinal epithelial microvilli in rats has revealed two types of Ca^{2+} binding sites: with high $K_a = (0.4–7.2) \cdot 10^4 M^{-1}$ and low $K_a = (2.7–5.7) \cdot 10^3 M^{-1}$ affinity to this ion, as well as phospholipids' key role as the Ca^{2+} acceptors by those membrane structures [Fernandes et al., 1981].

These findings correspond to electron microscopic observations which showed that in the Ca^{2+}-absorbing process this ion does not mix with enterocyte cytosol, but transfers inside the membrane vesicles in a sequestered form [Morozov et al., 1980a, b]. These Ca^{2+} transporting vesicles are displaced from the apical membrane at the microvillus base, taking up microvilli-bound calcium and transferring it through the enterocyte; they then uncover themselves at the lateral membrane, thus releasing Ca^{2+} into interecellular space.

Although electron microscopic and biochemical investigations have not proved direct mitochondria participation in Ca^{2+} transport through the enterocyte, an important role of the energy provided by Ca^{2+} absorption and a close dependence of these organelles' functional state on vitamin D uptake became evident [Adrianov et al., 1977]. Vitamin D deficiency, causing calcium absorption disorders in the small intestine in rats against electrochemical gradient (active transport), did not markedly influence microvilli enzyme activity, e.g. saccharase, but led to a considerable fall in microvilli phospholipids [Sokolova et al., 1983].

The investigation of an active calcium transport mechanism and its coupling with metabolic energy expenditure enabled us to suggest a theory of a membrane carrier that, being phosphorylated in the apical membrane, acquires the ability of binding Ca^{2+} and, when dephosphorylated in the lateral membrane, releases it into the intercellular space. The mechanism ensures coupling of Ca^{2+} transport with adenosine triphosphate (ATP) hydrolysis and Ca^{2+} anisotropic transport against the concentration gradient from the intestinal lumen to the blood stream.

The experimental test of the idea has shown that intestinal calcium absorption in rats is accompanied by simultaneous nonorganic phosphate output on the basal surface of the intestinal epithelium, e.g. on the surface where absorbed calcium is released [Sokolova et al., 1982]. Simultaneously, calcium absorption enhances the phosphoric acid residue metabolism in intestinal epithelium phospholipids and phosphoproteins, not affecting ^{32}P incorporation into nucleic acids [Sokolova et al., 1983]. These data correspond to the idea of a specific carrier of either phospholipid or phosphoprotein in the active calcium transport, and the transport of Ca^{2+} against the concentration gradient is accompanied by its cyclic phosphorylation and dephosphorylation [Spirichev and Kon, 1978; Sokolova et al., 1982, 1983].

Vitamin D and Bone Collagen

Though the major pathomorphological indication of rickets is bone mineralization disorder, the question of the positive role of vitamin D in osteogenesis is not yet clear. Lacking convincing proof of direct vitamin D involvement in mineralization, dependent mostly on the calcium and phosphorus-replete state, some researchers came to the conclusion that osteogenic defects in the vitamin-D-deficient state are of a secondary nature and that they are caused by calcium and phosphorus deficiency because of the disorders of a vitamin-D-dependent process in mineral absorption in the intestine and their mobilization from bone [Baylink et al., 1970; Parfitt, 1984; Underwood, 1984].

To maintain a calcium- and phosphorus-saturated concentration in blood and bone, intercellular liquid is one of the factors that determines the ongoing process in bone tissue mineralization. Another, hardly less important, factor is the state of the collagen's organic matrix, above all, which plays the role of a heterogeneous catalyst responsible for regulating formation and localization of hydroxyapatite crystals [Bourne, 1972b].

Studies of bone collagen fractional content provided with a different vitamin D state showed that vitamin D deficiency caused a remarkable lowering (3–4 times) of salt-soluble nonmatured collagen; meanwhile, nonsoluble collagen increased 10–20% in rat epiphyses and diaphyses. An optimum level of calcium and phosphorus in the diet of vitamin-D-deficient animals prevented hypocalcemia, but does not modulate changes in bone collagen fractional content [Isaeva et al., 1974]. It is possible to classify these changes as the osteogenetic defects which were not mediated by hypocalcemia and caused mostly by vitamin D deficiency [Spirichev and Isaeva, 1984] (table I).

Changes in bone collagen fractional content with vitamin D deficiency have been determined by the intensification of its maturity. Data in favor of this idea show a sharp increase (3–4 times) of aldehyde groups in salt-soluble collagen involved in cross-link formation in collagen maturation and a drop of relative content of monomeric α-chains; meanwhile, the content of dimeric β-chain and trimeric γ-chain subunits of salt and acid-soluble collagen increases in vitamin D deficiency [Isaeva and Spirichev, 1978] (fig. 1).

A growing number of cross-links in bone collagen can serve as a steric obstacle to mineralization and, thus, become one of the reasons for its defect in vitamin D deficiency. Since a newly formed salt-soluble collagen plays the leading role at the initial calcification stages, remarkably lowering this fraction and enhancing its maturation to nonsoluble collagen with quite a number of cross-links can also be one of the reasons for bone organic matrix mineralization disorder in vitamin D deficiency. On the other hand, enhanced formation and a growing number of cross-links

Table I. Collagen fractions and aldehyde groups content in bone of rats with different vitamin D status on the diet containing 0.9% of Ca and 0.6% of P. From Isaeva et al. [1974]

Bone fragment	Groups of animals	Collagen, μg of hydroxyproline/100 mg dry bone				Aldehyde groups nmol/mg of hydroxyproline
		total	salt-soluble	acid-soluble	nonsoluble	
Epiphyses	control	2,130±41	153±6	36±5	1,780±78	190±12
	−D	2,220±44	42±5[a]	20±1.5[a]	2.090±36[a]	810±96[a,b]
	−D+D	1,920±50[a,b]	143±6[b]	41±2[b]	1,850±54[b]	260±19[a,b]
Diaphyses	control	2,250±40	58±3	5±0.7	2,380±81	440±14
	−D	2,540±60[a]	14±0.6[a]	18±2[a]	2,590±37[a]	930±66[a]
	−D+D	2,290±53[b]	154±3[a,b]	37±7[a,b]	2,050±60[a,b]	560±91[b]

Here and in tables II–VIII values are means ± SE. [a] Significant differences from control; [b] from vitamin-D-deficient rats.

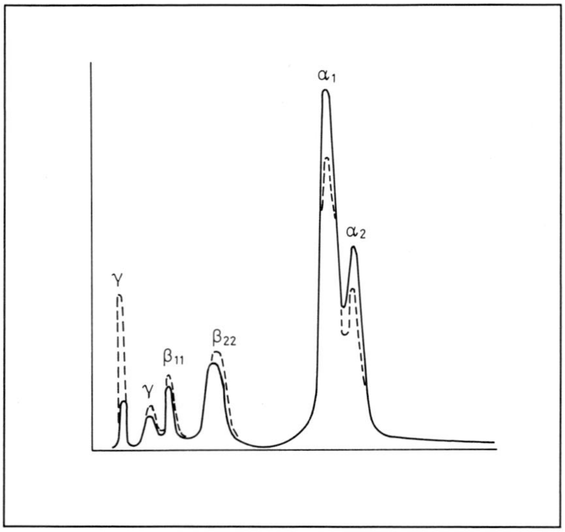

Fig. 1. PAGE densitogramms of rat bone salt-soluble collagen. From Isaeva and Spirichev [1978]. Solid line = control; dashed line = vitamin D deficiency.

Table II. Effects of vitamin D_3, $1,25(OH)_2D_3$ and $24,25(OH)_2D_3$ on serum Ca, intestinal Ca transport and bone parameters in vitamin-D-deficient rats. From Alexeeva et al. [1982]

Groups of animals	Dose, μg	Serum Ca mg/dl	Ca transport $^{45}Ca_{in}/^{45}Ca_{out}$	Diaphyses density g/cm³	Diaphyses Ca, mg/cm³	Epiphyses Ca, mg/g	Epiphyses hydroxyproline, mg/g
Control	vehicle	8.4±0.2	5.9±0.7	1.50±0.05	386±20	209±2	26.2±1.1
–D	vehicle	4.3±0.2^a	2.8±0.3^a	1.07±0.04^a	262±16^a	178±14^a	30.8±1.2^a
D_3	0.5	8.2±0.2^b	7.1±1.3^b	1.23±0.05^b	359±19^b	224±9^b	23.2±0.9^b
$1,25(OH)_2D_3$	0.03	5.6±0.6	4.4±0.7^b	1.40±0.10^b	373±22^b	197±6	25.0±1.9^b
$1,25(OH)_2D_3$	0.3	7.6±0.3^b	5.0±0.8^b	1.18±0.05^a	313±19^c	187±5^a	23.0±1.8^b
$24,25(OH)_2D_3$	0.25	5.1±0.3	6.0±0.6^b	1.27±0.09^b	332±33^b	223±8^b	33.6±1.3^a
$24,24(OH)_2D_3$	2.5	8.4±0.2^b	6.4±1.0^b	1.29±0.04^b	393±32^b	214±15^b	29.6±1.8^a

Significant differences: [a] from control; [b] from vitamin-D-deficient rats; [c] from group of animals, who got a lower dose of the metabolite.

in collagen can be a compensatory response to the disorder of mineralization that is to promote bone tissue integration by an increase in fibrillation.

Biological Activity of 1,25(OH)$_2$D$_3$ and 24,25(OH)$_2$D$_3$ in Rats

As stated above, the most important active vitamin D_3 metabolite which is directly responsible for increasing calcium and phosphorus absorption in the intestine and their mobilization from bone tissue is 1,25$(OH)_2D_3$.

Side by side with 1,25$(OH)_2D_3$ there is also an alternative metabolite – 24,25$(OH)_2D_3$ – synthesized in the kidneys. Biochemical functions of the latter are less clear.

The comparative investigation into biological activity of both 1,25$(OH)_2D_3$ and 24,25$(OH)_2D_3$ made it possible to expose a number of new and important problems. It was established [Alexeeva et al., 1982] that the administration of a physiological dose of 1,25$(OH)_2D_3$ (0.03 μg/day) during 5 days into vitamin-D-deficient rats increased calcium absorption in the intestine, enhanced the density of diaphyses and their calcium content, but did not ensure a normal calcium level in blood and epiphyses. An increased dose of 1,25$(OH)_2D_3$ to 0.3 μg/day by bringing up calcium level in blood led to a decreased diaphyses and epiphyses mineralization which is indicative of an excessive resorption intensification in bone tissue, when increased doses of this metabolite are used (table II).

Somewhat different results were obtained when administering 24,25$(OH)_2D_3$ at a physiological dose (0.25 μg/day). The metabolite completely restored the active calcium transport in the intestine, but did not correct hypocalcemia. In bone tissue the effect of 24,25$(OH)_2D_3$ in respect to the majority of indices was equal to that of vitamin D. Unlike 1,25$(OH)_2D_3$, which in no doses given led to a significant increase of calcium content in epiphyses, 24,25$(OH)_2D_3$ made this index entirely normal.

The increased dose of 24,25$(OH)_2D_3$ (2.5 μg/day) resulted in an entire normalization of not only calcium absorption in the intestine but also of its level in blood. In bone tissue the increased dose of 24,25$(OH)_2D_3$, unlike 1,25$(OH)_2D_3$, far from aggravating, even encouraged further improvement of patterns indicative of its state and, in particular, led to a marked increase of calcium content and a significant increase of the calcium/hydroxyproline ratio in diaphyses.

Thus, $24,25(OH)_2D_3$ ensured a better correction of the greater part of parameters indicative of the bone tissue state than $1,25(OH)_2D_3$ and, in particular, made the calcium content in epiphyses normal, which was not the case when $1,25(OH)_2D_3$ was administered. Along with this, unlike $1,25(OH)_2D_3$, $24,25(OH)_2D_3$ did not cause the collagen content to reduce in either epiphyses or diaphyses.

From our point of view, all these peculiarities can be indicative of the difference in the functions and mechanism of action of $1,25(OH)_2D_3$ and $24,25(OH)_2D_3$ in bone tissue and of the necessity of their combined application to ensure normal osteogenesis. This conclusion is to some extent supported by the results obtained when a combined administration of $1,25(OH)_2D_3$ and $24,25(OH)_2D_3$ was used, which led to full normalization of the active calcium transport in the intestine and of the majority of patterns indicative of the bone tissue state.

The general changes observed in bones when administering both of the metabolites was similar to those seen during vitamin D_3 administration, and the presence of $24,25(OH)_2D_3$ partially neutralized the resorptive effect of the increased $1,25(OH)_2D_3$ dose.

The data obtained by us correlate well with the results of histologic researches, which revealed an incomplete effectiveness of $1,25(OH)_2D_3$ and the need for $24,25(OH)_2D_3$ application to provide normal growth and mineralization of bone tissue [Ornoy et al., 1978, 1985; Edelstein and Ornoy, 1979; Binderman, 1984; Sömjen et al., 1985].

Apparently, the major differences in the effects of $1,25(OH)_2D_3$ and $24,25(OH)_2D_3$ on bone tissue lie in the fact that in the function of $1,25(OH)_2D_3$ the priority is given to its calcium-mobilizing effect on the bone. Moreover, according to our data, $1,25(OH)_2D_3$ is incapable of providing normal mineralization of epiphyses.

By contrast, $24,25(OH)_2D_3$ is devoid of a pronounced resorptive effect on the bone and efficiently encourages the mineralization of epiphyses. Along with this both of the metabolites are almost similar in their activity on calcium absorption in the intestine. Hence, we can probably consider $1,25(OH)_2D_3$ as an 'emergency' hormone, acting in calcium deficiency and severe hypocalcemia. The hormone possesses the capacity to quickly normalize the calcium level in blood, having the effect of increasing calcium absorption in the intestine and resorption of preformed bone tissue.

By contrast, $24,25(OH)_2D_3$ is a hormone showing its effect in physiological conditions of normocalcemia and providing not only calcium absorption in the intestine but also its utilization in the formation and mineralization of bone tissue.

Irrespective of the presence or absence of specific function in osteogenesis and the mechanism of function in $24,25(OH)_2D_3$, the peculiar combination of the metabolite's properties to stimulate intestinal absorption of calcium and to maintain its stable level in blood, with no indication of resorptive action evident in the bone, makes this compound a highly valuable potential therapeutic means in all cases when it is necessary to increase calcium absorption and bone tissue mineralization without stimulating bone resorption at the same time.

Vitamin D Metabolism and Receptor Binding in Deficiency of Vitamins C and B_2

Recent data concerning vitamin D have enabled us to elucidate the problem of rickets. But certain epidemiologic and clinical observations prove that an insufficient or unbalanced supply of a number of other nutrients, some vitamins in particular, may also play an essential role in rickets [Bourne, 1972a; Stewart, 1975; Tazibaev, 1984].

In connection with this, our laboratory has carried out research of vitamin-D-mediated mechanisms via certain nutrients that can be involved in the pathogenesis of the disease. This chapter deals with the data on the effect of ascorbic acid and riboflavin deficiency on vitamin D metabolism and receptor binding in experimental animals (rats and guinea pigs) [Sergeev et al., 1987c; Sergeev and Spirichev, 1986].

To study vitamin D metabolism, we have determined the serum concentration of 25-OHD, the main circulating metabolite of vitamin D, forming in the liver under the action of vitamin D 25-hydroxylase, and the activity of 1- and 24-hydroxylase of $25\text{-}OHD_3$ (1- and 24-OHase) in kidneys in vitro [Armbrecht et al., 1981; Gray and Napoli, 1983; Sergeev et al., 1984]. Since the biological responses of $1,25(OH)_2D_3$ are realized via its interaction with the specific receptor-like binding protein that may have a nuclear localization in vivo [Norman et al., 1982a, b], we carried out differential quantisation of endogenously (in vivo) occupied and unoccupied chromatin receptors for $1,25(OH)_2D_3$ in intestinal mucosa by methods worked out previously [Hunziker et al., 1980; Wilhelm and Norman, 1985].

The rats and guinea pigs raised on a vitamin-D-deficient diet gave a picture of common biological symptoms of deficiency in that vitamin, such as a decreased serum concentration of 25-OHD down to an undetectable level, hypocalcemia and hypophosphatemia development, and a marked decrease of active calcium transport in the small intestine. The changes typical of osteoid accumulation appeared in bone tissue; more precisely, a decreased density of femur diaphyses and epiphyses, a reduced calcium and phosphorus content in them and some increase of hydroxyproline (collagen) content. Those disorders were characterized by pronounced changes on the part of vitamin D_3 dihydroxymetabolite production in the kidneys in vitro, brought about by an increased 1-OHase activity and a decreased 24-OHase activity. The concentration of $1,25(OH)_2D_3$-filled receptors in the chromatin fraction of intestinal mucosa fell to minimum, and there was a tendency of a reduced concentration of $1,25(OH)_2D_3$-unfilled receptors (tables III, IV).

Table III. 25-OHD serum concentration, renal 1- and 24-hydroxylases activity and intestinal chromatin receptors for $1,25(OH)_2D_3$ in vitamin-B_2-deficient rats. From Sergeev et al. [1987c]

Groups of animals	Serum 25-OHD ng/ml	Renal metabolites 25-OHD_3 $pmol \cdot h^{-1} \cdot g^{-1}$		Receptors for $1,25(OH)_2D_3$ $fmol \cdot mg^{-1}$ nuclear protein	
		$1,25(OH)_2D_3$	$24,25(OH)_2D_3$	unoccupied	occupied
I +D+B_2	15.4 ± 1.7	136 ± 16	479 ± 99	83.2 ± 24.0	20.0 ± 2.5
II +D–B_2	6.9 ± 0.8[a]	120 ± 24	176 ± 36[a]	48.7 ± 8.4	16.3 ± 3.3
III –D+B_2	< 2.5	297 ± 23[b]	144 ± 15[b]	63.2 ± 21.5	3.7 ± 0.5[b]
IV –D–B_2	< 2.5	214 ± 13[a, b]	86 ± 11[a, b]	44.6 ± 10.6	4.2 ± 1.1[b]
V –D+B_2, +D, 1 day	5.2 ± 0.4[b]	284 ± 27[b]	237 ± 21[b]	65.0 ± 8.5	20.1 ± 3.3
VI –D–B_2, +D, 1 day	2.9 ± 0.2[a, b]	226 ± 29[b]	133 ± 17[a]	54.3 ± 7.7	15.2 ± 3.9
VII –D+B_2, +D, 6 days	19.8 ± 1.6	230 ± 25[b]	293 ± 44	73.2 ± 9.3	22.4 ± 1.4
VIII –D–B_2, +D, 6 days	22.0 ± 2.2[b]	151 ± 22	227 ± 47[a]	52.9 ± 18.3	17.4 ± 2.8[a]

[a] Significant differences from a vitamin B_2- (or C)-replete group of animals.
[b] From respective control group (I or II). 25-OHD_3 metabolism has been investigated in vitro using renal cortex slies in substrate saturating concentrations (2.5–5.0 μ*M*). 25-OHD_3 metabolites were purified and resolved by HPLC. The level of intestinal chromatin $1,25(OH)_2D_3$ receptors were determined in saturating concentration of $[^3H]$-$1,25(OH)_2D_3$ (2.0–2.5 n*M*) high specific radioactivity (100–160 Ci/mmol). When measuring occupied receptor level, unoccupied binding sites were blocked by preincubation with TPCK.

Similar but less pronounced disorders of calcium metabolism were observed in the deficiency of vitamins B_2 and C in experimental animals, such as moderate hypocalcemia, a tendency of decreased calcium absorption in the small intestine, mineral and collagen contents in bone tissue (the latter seen only in vitamin C deficiency). A considerable fall (2.2-fold) of serum 25-OHD concentration and a reduced amount of $1,25(OH)_2D_3$-unfilled receptors in mucosa, accompanied by a less pronounced fall of its filled binding sites, were typical of vitamin B_2 deficiency, whereas $1,25(OH)_2D_3$ production in kidneys did not change, but $24,25(OH)_2D_3$ fell 2.7-fold.

Quite different changes were observed in ascorbic acid deficiency: 1-OHase activity fell 2-fold, but 24-OHase activity increased 1.6-fold. The concentration of $1,25(OH)_2D_3$-unoccupied receptors in mucosa decreased and the level of the occupied receptors fell from 12–17 to 6–8%.

Combined deficiency of vitamins D and B_2 did not augment disorders typical of rickets. But ascorbic acid deficiency enhanced hypophosphatemia and led to a more pronounced delay of bone mineralization in vitamin-D-deficient guinea pigs. It was accompanied by a marked lowering of 25-OHD serum concentration, the lack of a typical increase of 1-OHase activity and a low level of unfilled and filled receptors for $1,25(OH)_2D_3$.

The administration of cholecalciferol into vitamin-D-deficient animals either 24 h or 4–6 days before decapitation led to partial or almost

Table IV. 25-OHD serum concentration, renal 1- and 24-hydroxylases activity and intestinal chromatin receptors for $1,25(OH)_2D_3$ in vitamin-C-deficient guinea pigs. From Sergeev et al. [1987b]

Groups of animals	Serum 25-OHD ng/ml	Renal metabolites $25\text{-}OHD_3$ pmol·30 min^{-1}·g^{-1}		Receptors for $1,25(OH)_2D_3$ fmol·mg^{-1} nuclear protein	
		$1,25(OH)_2D_3$	$24,25(OH)_2D_3$	unoccupied	occupied
I +D+C	18.6±1.9	75.2±11.7	169±30.8	177±28.3	23.7±4.79
II +D–C	12.5±2.6	37.0±5.94[a]	272±45.9[a]	138±7.04	13.1±1.23[a]
III –D+C	3.5±0.5[b]	191±24.3[b]	117±20.7	149±13.4	4.79±1.64[b]
IV –D–C	1.2±0.35[a,b]	45.4±2.60[a]	155±9.74[b]	96.9±7.90[a,b]	2.62±2.07[b]
V –D+C, +D, 1 day	9.2±1.3	88.2±11.4	125±13.6	109±3.38	20.2±1.68
VI –D–C, +D, 1 day	6.0±1.0[a,b]	47.4±6.42[a]	154±8.12	99.1±13.0[b]	9.23±1.26[a,b]
VII –D+C, +D, 4 days	14.2±4.8	102±3.94[b]	164±30.3[b]	123±33.6[b]	26.2±4.28
VIII –D–C, +D, 4 days	9.7±3.1	59.1±21.8[a]	240±59.6	85.2±18.5[b]	5.68±1.72[a,b]

total normalization of calcium metabolism and bone tissue state. It is essential that in animals with vitamin B_2 and C deficiency the above-mentioned restoration was less complete. It corresponds well to the vitamin D endocrine system of those animals: absence or lack of increase of 25-OHD serum concentration and 1-OHase activity in kidneys, as well as a decreased concentration of occupied receptors of $1,25(OH)_2D_3$.

To date, the role of vitamin B_2 and C deficiency in the pathogenesis of rickets has not been studied closely. The data obtained permit us to make a concept that the role of these vitamins in calcium metabolism is evidently to a great extent conditioned by changes in vitamin D metabolism and receptor binding.

Vitamin B_2 deficiency has turned out to manifest itself in a pronounced decrease of 24-OHase activity as well as a less considerable stimulation of 1-OHase when administering cholecalciferol to vitamin-D-deficient animals. Preincubation of kidney slices from vitamin-D- and B_2-deficient animals in the medium with riboflavin has led to a 5-fold increase of 24-OHase activity, whereas $1,25(OH)_2D_3$ production has not significantly increased. Possibly, the essential role in this case is played by the filling of flavin adenine dinucleotide (FAD), coferment renal flavoprotein constituting a part of 25-OHD mixed function monooxygenase.

Vitamin C deficiency has led to a pronounced decrease of 1-OHase activity and a reciprocal increase of 24-OHase activity. Evidently, a replete ascorbic acid status of an organism is essential for the maximum activity of 1-OHase as in deficiency of this vitamin there was no noticeable increase of $1,25(OH)_2D_3$ production in vitamin-D-deficient animals when they were administered cholecalciferol. The decrease of microsomal and mitochondrial mixed function monooxygenase activity, in particular cholesterol and its derivative hydroxylases as well as the level of cytochrome P-450 in vitamin C deficiency is well known, though the biochemical mechanism of the phenomenon is still unclear [Peterson et al., 1983]. It is likely that the protective role of ascorbic acid can be of a certain significance for monooxygenases of vitamin D and 25-OHD.

However, the high activity of 24-OHase in vitamin-C-deficient animals makes it possible to surmise a more specific influence of ascorbic acid on 1-hydroxylation of $25\text{-}OHD_3$, which may be related to its acting as a cofactor of 1-OHase.

The data obtained tell us also that vitamin B_2 and C deficiency affects the receptor binding of $1,25(OH)_2D_3$ in the intestinal mucosa of rats and guinea pigs.

The first thing worthy of note is the decreased concentration of receptors (occupied and unoccupied) for 1,25$(OH)_2D_3$, more pronounced in vitamin C deficiency, as well as a strong correlation for the level of occupied binding sites of this receptor to 1,25$(OH)_2D_3$ production in kidneys.

The receptor protein for 1,25$(OH)_2D_3$ is apparently autoregulated under the positive feedback mechanism; in this case the decrease of the circulating level of 1,25$(OH)_2D_3$ can lead to a decrease in the concentration of its receptor.

In vitamin C deficiency, binding performances of the receptors for 1,25$(OH)_2D_3$ decreased due to the lowering of positive cooperativity as well. In that case a decrease of the Hill coefficient (from 1.7 to 1.4) occurred without average dissociation constant (K_d) changes, calculated for two binding sites (0.22–0.26 n*M*), and without K_{d2} changes, determined for the second binding site (0.06–0.10 n*M*). This indicates a decreased effectiveness of ligand binding with receptor because of the limit of maximum receptor capacity, but not its affinity (fig. 2).

An important effector in the specific binding of 1,25$(OH)_2D_3$ in target tissues, diminishing affinity and cooperativity in hormone-receptor interaction, is 24,25$(OH)_2D_3$ [Wilhelm et al., 1985]. The increased production of this metabolite in vitamin C deficiency, accompanied by dropping the level of cooperativity but not affinity in the binding of 1,25$(OH)_2D_3$ to its receptor, resulted in a more pronounced decrease of the number of its occupied binding sites under these conditions.

Unlike vitamin C depletion, in vitamin B_2 deficiency there was observed a relative increase of 1,25$(OH)_2D_3$-occupied receptors that was correlated to a decreased 24,25$(OH)_2D_3$ production in the kidneys.

It is also not excluded that riboflavin and ascorbic acid can be directly involved in the functioning of 1,25$(OH)_2D_3$ receptors; for example, by producing a stabilizing or modifying effect on the receptor protein for this hormone.

Viewing the matter in the aspect of the receptor-mediator interaction, it is possible to explain the decrease of 24,25$(OH)_2D_3$ production in vitamin-B_2-deficient animals. The binding of 1,25$(OH)_2D_3$ with its renal receptor augments the production of 24-OHase. In the case of a decreased concentration of 1,25$(OH)_2D_3$ receptors, the amount of enzyme is left reduced, and stimulation of 24-OHase by riboflavin can be determined by its influence on the concentration and binding ability of 1,25$(OH)_2D_3$ receptors in the kidneys.

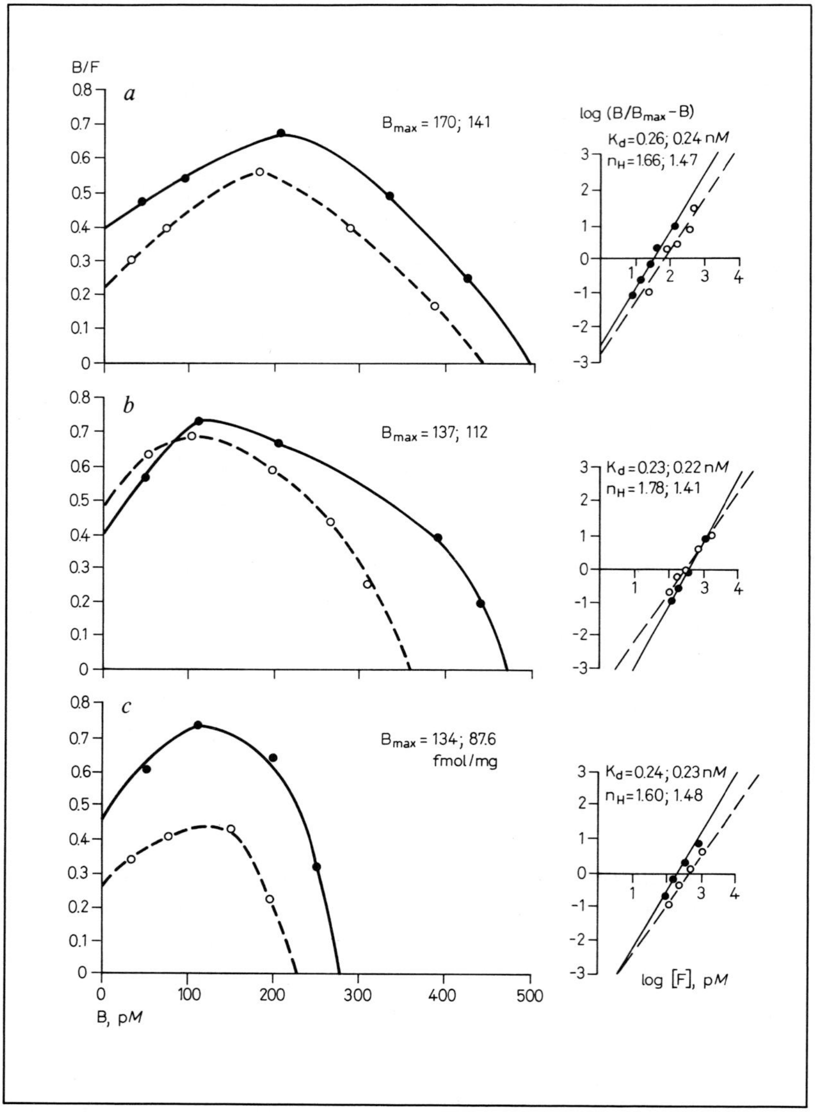

Fig. 2. Saturation analysis and Hill plot of chromatin guinea pig intestinal receptor for $1,25(OH)_2D_3$: effect of vitamin C. From Sergeev et al. [1987a]. Solid line and black circles = vitamin C supplied animals; dashed lines and open circles = vitamin-C-deficient animals. *a* I and II, *b* III and IV, *c* V and VI groups of animals (table IV). B_{max} = Maximum binding capacity; B = concentration of bound and F = free ligand; K_d = average dissociation constant; n_H = Hill coefficient. The first and second values in the line refer to the vitamin-C-supplied and vitamin-C-deficient animals, respectively.

The reciprocal change of 1- and 24-OHase activity in the kidneys which is analogous to the observed one in animals devoid of vitamin C is apparently the result of the change of the functional state of one isoform of cytochrome P-450 hydroxylating 25-OHD in the C-1 or C-24 position [Ghazarian, 1979].

To sum it up, it is necessary to emphasize that the deficiency of vitamin B_2, and especially vitamin C, causing disorders in calcium homeostasis, makes it impossible to achieve a complete restoration of this mineral metabolic pattern in ricketic animals, when administering vitamin D. These effects are apparently realized via the changed production of active vitamin D_3 metabolites in kidneys (the decrease of $1,25[OH]_2D_3$ formation in ascorbic acid deficiency, the compensated functioning of 1-OHase and the decrease of $24,25[OH]_2D_3$ synthesis in vitamin B_2 deficiency) as well as the decrease of the receptor binding of the hormonal form of vitamin D_3 – $1,25(OH)_2D_3$ – in the intestinal mucosa.

The Role of Vitamin-D-Active Metabolites in Calcium Metabolism and Bone Tissue State in Hypokinesia

Long-term limitation of motor activity results in disorders of calcium metabolism and bone tissue structure in experimental animals and human beings [Kovalenko and Gurovsky, 1980]. The investigation into those disorders' mechanisms and working out optimal ways of their correction as well as their prevention are very important for the people who lack motor activity due to illness or old age or under specific working conditions. Finally, in the broadest sense, the problem concerns the majority of people, because there is less manual labor now, and it is marked by a sharp fall of motor activity under social advances.

The role of the vitamin D endocrine system in calcium metabolism regulation and bone tissue state is essential now, but no research work has been done to find out the role of vitamin D regulation in hypokinesia.

In our experiments with young and adult rats with hypokinesia, we used special box panels, providing rigid immobilization of animals for a 4- to 5-week period. Under those hypokinetic conditions, we observed changes in calcium metabolism and bone tissue, e.g. hypocalcemia, a decrease of intestinal calcium absorption, a tendency to nephro- and arteriocalcinosis, a sharp delay of bone growth and mineralization with the

Table V. Serum Ca, 25-OHD, PTH, CT concentration and intestinal Ca transport in long-term hypokinetic rats. From Sergeev et al. [1984]

Parameter	Control	Hypokinesia
Serum Ca, mg/dl	10.1 ± 0.1	9.0 ± 0.3*
^{45}Ca transport, $nmol \cdot h^{-1} \cdot cm^{-1}$	52.8 ± 2.1	38.9 ± 4.8*
25-OHD, ng/ml	32.9 ± 3.7	44.9 ± 6.1
PTH, IU/l	21.3 ± 2.4	11.5 ± 4.1*
CT, pg/ml	13.0 ± 1.3	21.4 ± 4.2*

* Significant differences from control.

following osteoporosis of the spongy substance [Sergeev and Spirichev, 1986; Sergeev et al., 1985; Kabitskaya et al., 1984] (table V).

The study of the metabolism of the 1,25$(OH)_2D_3$ and 24,25$(OH)_2D_3$ precursor 25-OH[26(27)^3-H]D_3 in vivo in rats with hypokinesia showed [Sergeev et al., 1983, 1984] that ^{3}H-1,25$(OH)_2D_3$ production in kidneys fell 21.3 and 35.3% due to the immobilization for one and 4 weeks, respectively, and ^{3}H-24,25$(OH)_2D_3$ rose 32.0 and 57.1%, respectively. After 4 weeks of hypokinesia, the ^{3}H-25-OHD_3 level increased in intestinal mucosa and bones of rats; this might suggest the inhibition of 25-OHD_3 metabolism in those tissues. A slight increase of serum 25-OHD_3 concentration in rats with hypokinesia could be brought about by its slower metabolism in the kidneys (fig. 3).

After 4 weeks of hypokinesia, ^{3}H-1,25$(OH)_2D_3$ and ^{3}H-24,25$(OH)_2D_3$ levels fell by 29.0 and 27.5% in intestinal mucosa and 42.3 and 42.2% in bones, respectively, though the formation of the latter metabolite rose in the kidneys. Evidently, the reduction of the accumulation of ^{3}H-24,25$(OH)_2D_3$ in bones and mucosa was caused by a decrease of metabolite binding in those tissues; meanwhile, a proportional lowering of the ^{3}H-1,25$(OH)_2D_3$ level in tested tissues was, primarily, the result of its decrease in synthesis in the kidneys. The changes of ^{3}H-25-OHD_3 metabolism in rats with hypokinesia could be connected with a long-term parathyroid hormone (PTH) secretion suppression and cyclic 3′:5′-adenosine monophosphate (cyclic AMP) content lowering in the kidneys [Sergeev et al., 1984].

It should be noted here that the hypocalcemia-stimulating effect on 25-OHD_3 1-hydroxylation is, evidently, connected with PTH to a great extent, and hypocalcemia itself can be the result of a long-term decrease of

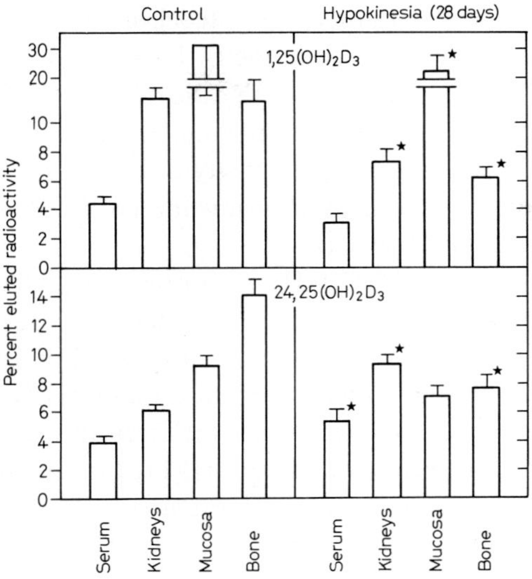

Fig. 3. [^{3}H]-Metabolite D_3 content in serum kidneys, intestinal mucosa, and bone of long-term (1 month) hypokinetic rats. From Sergeev et al. [1984]. * Significant differences from control.

serum PTH content. Serum calcitonin (CT) content in rats with hypokinesia was high, which might suppress 1,25(OH)$_2$D$_3$ formation under those conditions.

Besides similar changes of 25-OHD$_3$ metabolism could be observed in the case of hyperglucocorticoidism as well as in a decreased growth hormone level [Fraser, 1980; Henry and Norman, 1984]. The changes of hormone content in blood were detected in the case of hypokinesia [Kovalenko and Gurovsky, 1980].

The administration of 1,25(OH)$_2$D$_3$ and 24,25(OH)$_2$D$_3$ prophylactically to rats, under a long-term rigid hypokinetic condition, normalized calcium metabolism and produced positive effects on bone tissue, depending on the dose and their combination [Ushakov et al., 1982, 1983a, 1984; Kabitskaya et al., 1984; Sergeev, 1987b]. The administration of 1,25(OH)$_2$D$_3$ at a dose of 0.03 μg per animal stimulated effectively calcium absorption in the small intestine, corrected hypocalcemia, partially increased bone tissue density and bone calcium and phosphorus content, volume of spongiosa, the width of epiphyseal growth plate (EGP) and the number of osteoclasts. An increased dose of the metabolite (0.15 μg) caused hypercalcemia, hyperphosphatemia, bone tissue resorption intensification, a marked increase of the number of osteoclasts and ectopic calcification. The administration of combined $1,25(OH)_2D_3$ and $24,25(OH)_2D_3$ (0.03 and 0.25 or 1.25 μg), or a high dose of $24,25(OH)_2D_3$ alone (1.25 μg), restored calcium absorption in intestine as well as its concentration in blood, mineral composition and density of bone tissue, the volume or primary and secondary spongiosa; meanwhile the EGP width and number of osteoclasts remained low (fig. 4).

It should be emphasized that the $24,25(OH)_2D_3$ normalizing effect on bone tissue is, apparently, connected mostly with this metabolite's specific activity in bone tissue mineralization [Sergeev et al., 1982a, b]. Normalization of spongiosa volume in rats which received $24,25(OH)_2D_3$ occurred in the first place, due to the bone trabecule thickness and size but not their number. That ossiferous effect of $24,25(OH)_2D_3$ prevented the development of spongiosa osteoporosis, but its structure became more rough. We should not neglect the possible modulating effect of $24,25(OH)_2D_3$ on the influence of $1,25(OH)_2D_3$ in bone tissue, caused by the $1,25(OH)_2D_3$ resorbing activity inhibition by that metabolite and, consequently, an enhanced ossific effect of the latter in young animals. The number of osteoclasts did not rise in the case of a combined administration of $1,25(OH)_2D_3$ and $24,25(OH)_2D_3$, proving the above-mentioned idea.

A combined administration of $1,25(OH)_2D_3$ and $24,25(OH)_2D_3$ to rats with hypokinesia favored a more perfect normalization of calcium metabolism and bone tissue structure than the administration of one of the two metabolites alone. Apparently, under those conditions, $1,25(OH)_2D_3$ stimulates calcium absorption in the intestine and regulates its concentration in blood, while $24,25(OH)_2D_3$ ensures calcium utilization in ossification. $1,25(OH)_2D_3$, probably, ensures enough resorption of a formed bone, thus accelerating bone remodelling and growth. However, physiological overdose of $1,25(OH)_2D_3$ apparently enhances simultaneously both bone formation and resorption, but the latter prevails. That is why osteoporosis is more pronounced in this case than under hypokinetic conditions.

Fig. 4. Tibial epiphyseal growth plate and metaphyseal spongy bone. Upper left = control; upper right = hypokinesia: plate thickness decreases, primary and secondary spongiosa loosen, and their volume diminishes; lower left = hypokinesia + $24,25(OH)_2D_3$ (at a dose of 1.25 μg): plate thickness decreases, volume of primary and secondary spongiosa is close to the control; lower right = hypokinesia + $1,25(OH)_2D_3$ (at a dose of 0.15 μg): plate thickness diminishes, volume of primary and secondary spongiosa decreases. HE. × 3.5 lens, × 7 eye-piece. From Ushakov et al. [1984].

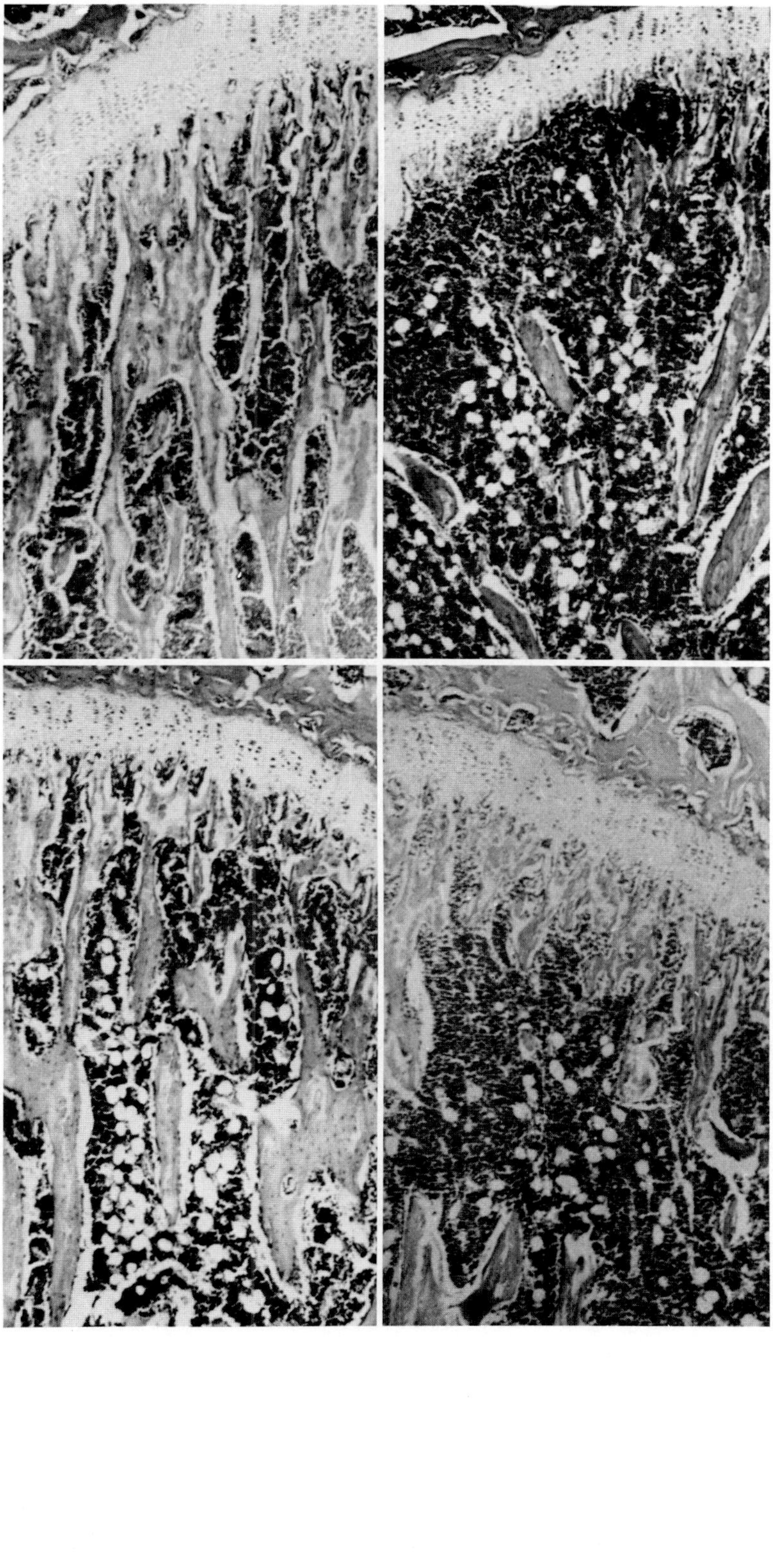

4

Thus, the data obtained enable us to come to the conclusion that changes in synthesis and secretion of calcium-regulating hormones (PTH, $1,25(OH)_2D_3$, $24,25(OH)_2D_3$, CT) in rats with a long-term hypokinesia are to maintain calcium homeostasis and bone tissue structure according to skeletal functions under these conditions. Preventive use of $1,25(OH)_2D_3$ and $24,25(OH)_2D_3$ in hypokinesia stimulates calcium absorption in the intestine and ensures sufficient modelling and remodelling of a bone tissue in growing animals. Interaction of $1,25(OH)_2D_3$ and $24,25(OH)_2D_3$ is, probably, brought about by their different functional roles in calcium metabolism regulation, bone tissue growth and remodelling, which favors their combined use in hypokinesia.

Vitamin D and Bone Repair

The vitamin D endocrine system may play an important part in calcium metabolism rearrangement and osteogenesis of reparative bone tissue regeneration. In this connection, we have carried out an investigation on vitamin D metabolism and the effect of $1,25(OH)_2D_3$ and $24,25(OH)_2D_3$ on reparative osteogenesis in rats with femoral fractures.

The investigation has shown that callus formation at the site of femoral fracture in vitamin-D-replete rats is accompanied by the mineral content and density increase of the noninjured twin bone, which in its turn indicates a rise of systemic ossification at this period, whereas there is a slight osteopenia in epiphyses of the injured bone [Blazheevich et al., 1982a].

Vitamin D deficiency leads to retardation of callus mineralization and significant demineralization of intact femur; this proves a pathological enhancement of bone resorption under these conditions [Blazheevich et al., 1982]. Thus, in the case of adequate vitamin D intake, calcium requirements are satisfied by an outside supply with food to increase mineralization, but in vitamin D deficiency, brought about by calcium absorption disorders in the small intestine, the skeleton becomes the main source of calcium to meet the organism's need, resulting in an increase of bone resorption.

The determination of the serum concentration of vitamin D_3 metabolites in vitamin-D-replete rats in fracture consolidation has revealed an increased $25\text{-}OHD_3$ concentration, a decreased content of $1,25(OH)_2D_3$ and an unchanged level of $24,25(OH)_2D_3$ at the stage of callus formation

Table VI. Vitamin D_3 metabolites serum concentration and intestinal Ca transport in rats with femur fracture. From Arkhapchev et al. [1986]

Day after fracture	Groups of animals	25-OHD_3 ng/ml	24,25$(OH)_2D_3$ ng/ml	1,25$(OH)_2D_3$ pg/ml	Active ^{45}Ca transport $nmol \cdot 15\ min^{-1} \cdot cm^{-2}$
3rd	control	5.6 ± 1.3	0.6 ± 0.3	78 ± 16	143 ± 17
	fracture	7.8 ± 1.1	0.9 ± 0.4	83 ± 17	130 ± 17
10th	control	4.3 ± 0.9	0.8 ± 0.2	64 ± 16	118 ± 7
	fracture	6.5 ± 1.4	1.0 ± 0.3	44 ± 14	161 ± 16^{a}
28th	control	3.5 ± 1.0	0.8 ± 0.3	26 ± 2.2^{b}	100 ± 8^{b}
	fracture	5.5 ± 1.4	0.8 ± 0.2	$12 \pm 3.2^{a,b}$	138 ± 26

[a] Significant differences from control; [b] from respective '3rd day' group.

and mineralization [Arkhapchev and Sergeev, 1984; Arkhapchev et al., 1984]. It is paradoxical but these changes are accompanied by a slight serum calcium concentration and stimulation of the active (O_2-dependent) calcium absorption by duodenal slices. It should be noted here that 1,25$(OH)_2D_3$ concentration markedly decreases, depending on the age of rats both of intact animals and of rats with femoral fractures. However, active calcium transport in the intestine decreased only in intact rats but not in rats with femoral fractures (table VI).

The investigation of 25-OH[26,27-^{3}H]D_3 metabolism in vivo in rats at various stages of fracture consolidation (3, 10 and 28 days) has shown an increased label incorporation to vitamin D_3 dihydroxymetabolites, especially 1,25$(OH)_2D_3$, in serum and mucosa of the small intestine only 3 days after the fracture [Arkhapchev and Sergeev, 1984; Arkhapchev et al., 1984]. This may indicate a stimulation of 1,25$(OH)_2D_3$ synthesis in kidneys with a rapid yield into the blood flow and binding in the target tissue. ^{3}H-1,25$(OH)_2D_3$ content in mucosa has fallen by the 10th and 28th days after the fracture. The decrease of the content along with a simultaneous fall in the blood concentration of 1,25$(OH)_2D_3$ could be brought about by a distinctive rise of 1,25$(OH)_2D_3$-occupied receptors in target tissues with a consequent decrease of the endogenously formed ^{3}H-1,25$(OH)_2D_3$ change on 1,25$(OH)_2D_3$. At that period, an increased calcium absorption in the intestine can be possibly preconditioned by the high binding performance of 1,25$(OH)_2D_3$. There has been a 3-fold increase of ^{3}H-25-OHD_3 incorporation into diaphyses of the injured bone 3 days after the fracture and its

Table VII. [^{3}H]metabolites D_3 content in femur diaphyses of rats with fracture (in percent to control). From Arkhapchev et al. [1984]

Day after fracture	Groups of animals	Femur	25-OHD_3	24,25$(OH)_2D_3$	1,25$(OH)_2D_3$
3rd	control	sound	100±9	100±7	100±5
	fracture	sound	216±2*	294±3*	252±3
		fractured	322±2*	136±6	83±6
				(742±18)	(450±19)
10th	control	sound	100±17	100±16	100±7
	fracture	sound	127±10	206±15*	210±8*
		fractured	454±23*	106±20	90±21
				(591±26)	(471±19)
28th	control	sound	100±17	100±11	100±17
	fracture	sound	117±15	199±17*	152±9
		fractured	145±13	63±14	59±12
				(255±16)	(232±13)

* Significant differences from control. Figures in parentheses represent [^{3}H]metabolites D_3 content calculated for bone tissue diaphyses weight substracted nonossifying callus weight.

incorporation into the noninjured twin bone diaphyses doubled simultaneously. ^{3}H-25-OHD_3 incorporation into the diaphyses of the injured bone 3 times exceeded the norm and its level in the noninjured twin bone diaphyses has dropped to that of the intact control. By the 28th day, ^{3}H-25-OHD_3 incorporation into diaphyses of both injured and intact bones of rats with femoral fractures did not differ from the control. Incorporation of ^{3}H-25-OHD_3 into the epiphyses of the injured and intact bones changed the same way (table VII).

Thus, fracture of the femur in rats is characterized by a marked activation of 25-OHD_3 binding in bone tissue at the first stages (3–10 days) after the fracture, and it is quite systemic and occurs not only in diaphyses of the injured but epiphyses of the uninjured bone and intact parts of the skeleton too. The activation of 25-OHD_3 binding in bones of rats at the first stages of fracture consolidation may reflect proliferation of cartilage and bone cells binding this metabolite and taking an active part in modelling and remodelling of the bone tissue.

25-OHD_3 accumulation in bone tissue may stimulate synthesis of 1,25$(OH)_2D_3$ and 24,25$(OH)_2D_3$ in it. Indeed, label incorporated into

$1,25(OH)_2D_3$ and $24,25(OH)_2D_3$ in diaphyses of intact twin bone and in epiphyses of both intact and injured bone at all the stages after the fracture doubled. ^3H-$1,25(OH)_2D_3$ and ^3H-$24,25(OH)_2D_3$ content in diaphyses of an injured bone did not change significantly; however, the amount of label entering $1,25(OH)_2D_3$ and $24,25(OH)_2D_3$ from ^3H-$25(OH)D_3$ increased 2- to 3-fold in the whole bone injured, e.g. the total amount of those metabolites in the injured bone increased. We suppose that if $1,25(OH)_2D_3$ and $24,25(OH)_2D_3$ are not localized in fibrous cellular structures, performing a temporary compensatory supporting function, then their concentration in bone tissue of the damaged bone diaphyses should be an increased one.

However, specific ^3H-$1,25(OH)_2D_3$ and ^3H-$24,25(OH)_2D_3$ incorporation into callus can be difficult due to a high level of these steroid-occupied receptors in cartilage tissue. The fact that ^3H-$1,25(OH)_2D_3$ and ^3H-$24,25(OH)_2D_3$ concentration in diaphyses of the noninjured twin bone reaches 40–50% of its ^3H-25-OHD_3 content whereas in diaphyses of the injured bone the amount is reduced to 5–7% may indirectly prove the idea. Thus, the findings prove that $1,25(OH)_2D_3$ and $24,25(OH)_2D_3$ have a possible role in calcium metabolism regulation and bone tissue state in rats with fractures.

The increasing calcium concentration in blood and its high absorption in the intestine, when callus forms and mineralizes, is apparently determined by the enhanced binding of $1,25(OH)_2D_3$ in mucosa of the small intestine; meanwhile, renal production of this hormone does not increase. A similar accumulation of $1,25(OH)_2D_3$ and $24,25(OH)_2D_3$ in cartilage and bone tissues can be brought about by the same factors, and/or by their enhanced biosynthesis in these tissues. Apparently, $1,25(OH)_2D_3$ affects increased resorption of a preformed bone tissue because it is necessary to provide a newly formed bone with calcium, whereas $24,25(OH)_2D_3$ can serve as a modulator. This prevents a considerable increase of calcium mobilization from the skeleton or directly stimulates bone tissue formation and mineralization.

Control of $1,25(OH)_2D_3$ functions in fractures can take place due to the changes of their binding but does not cause biosynthetic changes in kidneys.

The data on vitamin D metabolism made it possible to stimulate bone tissue reparative regeneration in vitamin-D-replete rats by means of an additional supply of $1,25(OH)_2D_3$ or $24,25(OH)_2D_3$. It turned out that a month's administration of the metabolites in an approximately physiological dose (0.03 μg of $1,25[OH]_2D_3$ or 0.25 μg of $24,25[OH]_2D_3$), as well as their combined usage, did not affect callus mineralization, serum calcium and P_i concentration or alkaline phosphatase activity. An increased dose of $1,25(OH)_2D_3$ to 0.15 μg markedly retarded mineralization and led to high alkaline phosphatase activity. A pronounced toxicity was revealed high by simultaneous hypercalcemia, hyperphosphatemia, and kidney calcinosis.

Contrarily, an increased dose of $24,25(OH)_2D_3$ to 1.25 μg produced a pronounced stimulating effect on callus mineralization and normalized alkaline phosphatase activity. Unlike $1,25(OH)_2D_3$, a high dose of $24,25(OH)_2D_3$ did not cause kidney calcinosis or any other after-effects [Blazheevich et al., 1982b].

The data enables us to consider $24,25(OH)_2D_3$ as a potentially effective and harmless compound which stimulates bone repair. The use of the drug can be recommended when callus is forming and mineralizes, and $1,25(OH)_2D_3$ can be used when bone fragments resorb and newly formed callus remodel.

Vitamin D and Hyperglucocorticoidism

Serious disorders of calcium homeostasis and bone tissue state (characterized by lowering of calcium absorption in the intestine, hypercalcemia, and osteopenia) occur in Cushing's disease and exogenous hypercorticoidism, which in their turn are complications of glucocorticoid therapy. Calcium metabolism disorders and bone tissue changes after corticosteroid therapy can be imitated in experiments with young rats when they receive hydrocortisone (cortisol) for 2–4 weeks at a daily dose of 1.5–5.0 mg/100 g body weight. The injections of cortisol lead to a rapid lowering of calcium absorption in the small intestine, severe hypercalcemia, hypophosphatemia and osteoporotic changes of bones [Karatabanova et al., 1983].

The investigations carried out by our laboratory proved the disorders to be dependent on a disturbance of vitamin D metabolism [Karatabanova et al., 1987]. When rats (after they received cortisol for a week) were injected with $25\text{-}OH[26(27)\text{-}^3H]D_3$, the content of $^3H\text{-}1,25(OH)_2D_3$ significantly increased in the kidneys. Similar changes of that metabolite's concentration were observed in serum, liver, intestinal mucosa and, especially, in bones. The content of $^3H\text{-}24,25(OH)_2D_3$ did not change greatly at that time. In animals receiving cortisol, there was a marked lowering of $^3H\text{-}25\text{-}(OH)D_3$ content in the liver, which may indicate a high metabolic rate of vitamin D. There was a tendency to an accumulation of $^3H\text{-}25\text{-}OHD_3$ in

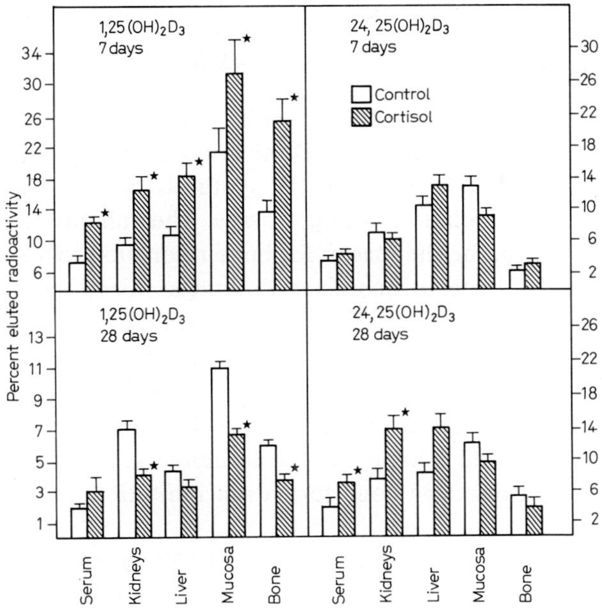

Fig. 5. [^{3}H]-Metabolite D_3 content in serum, kidneys, liver, intestinal mucosa, and bone of rats injected cortisol for 7 or 28 days. From Karatabanova et al. [1987]. * Significant differences from control.

mucosa and bones of rats on cortisol. A considerable increase of the ^{3}H-1,25(OH)$_2$D$_3$ level in serum, kidneys, mucosa and bones at the initial stage of hypercorticoidism indicates a stimulation of the metabolite's synthesis at that time (fig. 5).

Prolonged injections of cortisol produced other changes of ^{3}H-25-OHD$_3$ metabolism. At that time, the level of 1,25(OH)$_2$D$_3$ incorporation into serum did not differ from that of the control, whereas the ^{3}H-24,25(OH)$_2$D$_3$ level increased twice as much, which pointed to a considerable rise of that metabolite's synthesis. Tendencies to a decreased content of ^{3}H-1,25(OH)$_2$D$_3$ and a simultaneous increased content of ^{3}H-24,25(OH)$_2$D$_3$ were seen in the kidneys. It should be noted that a suppressed 1,25(OH)$_2$D$_3$ formation in the kidneys also appeared against a background of hypercalcemia and hyperparathyroidism.

A significant fall of both ^{3}H-1,25(OH)$_2$D$_3$ and ^{3}H-24,25(OH)$_2$D$_3$ levels was observed in mucosa and bones, and ^{3}H-25OHD$_3$ tended to accuate. This suggests a decrease of D_3 dihydroxymetabolite binding in these target tissues, conditioned by a fall in the performance of $1,25(OH)_2D_3$ receptors in hypercorticoidism.

The data obtained demonstrated a biphasic pattern of the effect of glucocorticoids on vitamin D metabolism. At the initial stage of exogenous hypercorticoidism there is stimulation of the synthesis of $1,25(OH)_2D_3$ and an increase of its accumulation in target tissue. The enhancement of $1,25(OH)_2D_3$ formation can be the reason for bone resorption increasing, even at the initial stage of hypercorticoidism. Prolonged injections of cortisol causes inhibition of the synthesis of $1,25(OH)_2D_3$ in the kidneys and a lowering of its binding in the intestinal mucosa and bones. Suppression of $1,25(OH)_2D_3$ formation in kidneys at the following stages of hypercorticoidism results in a fall of calcium absorption in the small intestine. A decrease of $1,25(OH)_2D_3$ and $24,25(OH)_2D_3$ accumulation in bone tissue at this time can be caused by bone formation inhibition and osteodystrophy.

Research of the activity of $1,25(OH)_2D_3$ and $24,25(OH)_2D_3$ in exogenous hyperglucocorticoidism revealed a high effectiveness of those D_3 metabolites in the prevention of calcium-phosphorus metabolism disorders and osteopenia [Karatabanova et al., 1985a, b]. Additional administration of $1,25(OH)_2D_3$ and $24,25(OH)_2D_3$ alone as well as their combined use in cortisol-injected rats normalized calcium concentration in the blood. Administration of a physiological dose of $1,25(OH)_2D_3$ (0.03 μg) alone and a combination of $1,25(OH)_2D_3$ and $24,25(OH)_2D_3$ normalized P_i in serum. The administration of $1,25(OH)_2D_3$ at a dose of 0.15 μg caused considerable hyperphosphatemia. Physiological and high doses of $1,25(OH)_2D_3$ completely restored calcium absorption in the small intestine, whereas $24,25(OH)_2D_3$ was less effective. A combined administration of $1,25(OH)_2D_3$ and $24,25(OH)_2D_3$ normalized calcium absorption in rats injected cortisol, and its level was a bit higher than that of the control.

A physiological dose of $1,25(OH)_2D_3$ favors the rise in density of diaphyses and epiphyses and increases calcium, phosphorus and hydroxyproline content in them. Increased doses of the metabolite lead to a rapid osteoporotic change in bones. A physiological dose of $24,25(OH)_2D_3$ was less effective, but the administration of that metabolite in an increased dose considerably improved bone tissue density and mineralization. The administration of a combination of $1,25(OH)_2D_3$ and $24,25(OH)_2D_3$ was most effective in the normalization of bone tissue density and calcium, phosphorus and hydroxyproline content.

The results of the above-mentioned investigations show that 1,25$(OH)_2D_3$ and 24,25$(OH)_2D_3$ produce positive effects on calcium homeostasis in rats on cortisol. Besides, 24,25$(OH)_2D_3$ is evidently more safe, since a 5-fold increase of its dose does not enhance bone resorption. A combination of 1,25$(OH)_2D_3$ and 24,25$(OH)_2D_3$ turned out to be most effective in normalizing calcium-phosphorus metabolism and bone tissue state in exogenous hypercorticoidism; this is why the combination of the two metabolites is advisable. A high effectiveness of this composition is brought about by the very reasons we have mentioned on page 190; more precisely stated, 1,25$(OH)_2D_3$ increases calcium absorption in the intestine and bone tissue remodelling, while 24,25$(OH)_2D_3$ stimulates bone mineralization and, perhaps, its formation.

Mechanism of Vitamin D Toxicity

The use of heavy doses of vitamin D, e.g. exceeding physiological levels, results in hypervitaminosis and its serious side effects. A systematic investigation on biochemical changes and metastatic calcification development in the dynamics of vitamin D intoxication has taken place in our laboratory. Based on these findings, we have come to the conclusion that there are three consecutive stages of vitamin D hypervitaminosis. We characterized them from a biochemical point of view and provided confirmation to the suggestions aimed at differential diagnosis, prevention, and treatment [Spirichev et al., 1978; Spirichev and Barkova, 1974].

The first stage of vitamin D hypervitaminosis is characterized by rapidly developing and rapidly passing hyperphosphatemia without marked calcium changes in the blood. At the second stage, there are hypercalcemia, metastatic calcification of the internal organs, and hyperphosphatemia. During the third stage, after vitamin D has been discontinued, there is a rapid normalization of calcium concentration in blood with a steady hypophosphatemia and metastatic calcification.

An increased phosphorus content in blood is seen earlier than other changes, thus serving as a more reliable parameter for intoxication than hypercalcemia. But hypophosphatemia indicating the second and third stages of hypervitaminosis is a more stable disorder compared to hypercalcemia [Spirichev et al., 1969].

The investigation of the vitamin D toxic effect mechanism enables us to suggest a conception of vitamin D free radical conversions and vitamin-

D-induced lipid peroxidation in the course of the vitamin D damaging effect on biological membranes and vitamin D hypervitaminosis pathogenesis [Spirichev and Blazheevich, 1969]. An increased concentration of free radicals in animal tissues during the first hours after administration of high doses of vitamin D (results from electron-spin resonance, ESR), a tendency of the tissue lipids to peroxidation in vitamin D hypervitaminotic animals, an increasing vitamin-D-induced metastatic calcification in vitamin E deficiency, a protective effect after the animals have been given antioxidants – all these factors speak in favor of the concept [Spirichev et al., 1974].

Finding out the free radicals' role in the toxic effect mechanism of vitamin D and its dependence on the vitamin E supply of an organism makes it possible to recommend the use of tocopherol alone, as well as its combination with other antioxidants – selenium, for instance – in the complex treatment of vitamin D hypervitaminosis.

High vitamin D toxicity, a pronounced membrane-damaging effect, an irreversible calcinosis of internal organs and tissues induced by vitamin D are convincing proofs of the inadmissibility of using vitamin D doses higher than physiological ones to prevent rickets.

Free radicals changed concentration in tissues in vitamin D hypervitaminosis; high reactive properties of free radical forms in that case enabled Spirichev et al. [1974] to suggest that free radicals could play a certain role in vitamin D metabolism.

The concentration of free radicals and other paramagnetic centers in liver, kidneys, and mucosa of the small intestine as well as the concentration changes after vitamin D administration into rachitic animals in certain periods of time have been detected in vitamin-D-deficient rats [Spirichev et al., 1976].

Vitamin D deficiency was characterized by a 20% fall in free radicals' concentration in liver and a 30% drop in kidneys compared to the control. Simultaneously, there was a significant decrease of ESR signal intensity (30–50%) preconditioned by a nonheme iron complex with mitochondrial protein, and a considerable decrease of the anisotropic signal determined by a low-spin heme iron state in the microsome cytochrome P-450. A single 25-μg administration of vitamin D normalized completely the concentration of free radicals and paramagnetic centers in kidneys 6 h and in liver 16 h after the preparation had been given. The free radicals content in mucosa of the small intestine in vitamin-D-deficient rats did not differ from the control.

These data confirm the concept of the possible role of free radicals in vitamin D metabolism, and hydroperoxides formed on their base can be intermediators of the formation of 25-OHD_3, 1,25$(OH)_2D_3$, and other hydroxylate vitamin D metabolites. This point of view has been confirmed by the work of Warner [1983], who proved the formation of 1,25$(OH)_2D_3$ as the result of dioxygenase reaction.

Toxicologic and Pharmacologic Effects of the Acute and Chronic Administration of 1-OHD_3 and 24,25$(OH)_2D_3$

The use of active vitamin D metabolites in clinical practice enables us to correct differentially various calcium-phosphorus impairments in a number of pathologies which are characterized by the partial biosynthesis disability of vitamin D hydroxymetabolites and their resistance to traditional therapy. The experience of using 1-OHD_3, a synthetic analogue of 1,25$(OH)_2D_3$, shows that its application is limited by a pronounced hypercalcemic effect, leading to calcification of soft tissues.

Unlike 1-OHD_3, 24,25$(OH)_2D_3$ does not cause hypercalcemia and it is apparently capable of increasing bone tissue mineralization and formation, not effecting its resorption [Edelstein and Ornoy, 1979; Sergeev et al., 1982a]. These factors prove 24,25$(OH)_2D_3$ to be more effective and safe in application, and it is advisable to analyze its toxic and pharmacologic properties compared to 1-OHD_3.

Since 1-OHD_3 toxicity was revealed by hypercalcemia, soft tissue metastatic calcification and bone resorption, we investigated the effect of both metabolites according to the same indices [Spirichev et al., 1978].

Daily per os administration of 1-OHD_3 at doses 0.25, 2.5, and 25 μg per animal to young and adult rats for 5 days caused hypercalcemia and hyperphosphatemia regardless of the dose. Loss of body weight and the worsening of bone density appeared at a dose of 2.5 μg. A high dose of the compound leads to numerous lethal cases and severe calcium accumulation in soft tissues. Unlike 1-OHD_3, 24,25$(OH)_2D_3$ (we used the same doses) did not produce hypercalcemic or hyperphosphatic effects but, on the contrary, a high dose of it (25 μg) favored a decrease of calcium and P_i levels in blood. None of the doses of 24,25$(OH)_2D_3$ caused ectopic calcium accumulation or lowering of bone density. But 25 μg of the compound led to retardation of growth.

Long-term daily (6 months) administration of physiological (0.025 μg) and 5-fold (0.125 μg) doses of 1-OHD_3 to the rats did not cause changes of growth rate in the animals and low doses of the compound did not influence the calcium-phosphorus metabolism. A high dose of 1-OHD_3 did not affect the calcium concentration in serum, but increased P_i level, and also led to calcium accumulation in heart and kidneys. An increased dose of the compound brought about osteoporotic-like disorders of bones; however, the degree of mineralization of the remaining parts of bones increased.

Chronic (6 months) daily administration of 24,25$(OH)_2D_3$ to adult rats at physiological (0.25 μg) and 5-fold (1.25 μg) doses did not influence body weight gain during the first half of the experiment. But later, the rats on 1.25 μg showed more rapid weight stabilization. After 3 months metabolite administration to rats, no significant change of calcium-phosphorus metabolism happened. Six months later, there was a considerable decrease of distal epiphyses density of femur bones in control animals. Chronic administration of a physiological dose of the metabolite favored epiphyses density maintenance for a 3-month period and a marked increase of calcium and phosphorus content in them. 24,25$(OH)_2D_3$ administration at a dose of 1.25 μg did not greatly influence those indices which were, probably, determined by certain toxic effects of surplus amounts of the metabolite, bringing to naught its positive effect on bone tissue. Thus, the data prove the following: a short use of 24,25$(OH)_2D_3$ at a dose 10-fold higher than the physiological one is quite possible and a long-term administration of a physiological dose is absolutely safe.

1,25$(OH)_2D_3$ and 24,25$(OH)_2D_3$ Application in Chronic Renal Insufficiency

The lowering of active vitamin D metabolite formation in kidneys plays an important role in the impairment of calcium-phosphorus metabolism at later stages of chronic renal insufficiency (CRI) [Seino et al., 1985]. Hemodialysis may also influence vitamin D metabolite concentration in blood [Furlong et al., 1985].

1,25$(OH)_2D_3$ and its synthetic analogue, 1-OHD_3, are widely used now to prevent and treat renal osteodystrophia in cases of CRI. The use of these drugs stimulates calcium absorption in the intestine and they possess the capacity to normalize calcemia in renal patients, producing an inhibiting effect on renal osteodystrophia progression in a number of cases [Coburn and Massry, 1980; Nielsen et al., 1980].

However, the required effect does not occur in all the cases and does not normalize completely bone tissue state. Besides, the use of $1,25(OH)_2D_3$ and $1\text{-}OHD_3$ may lead to hypercalcemia, hyperphosphatemia and an enhanced soft tissue calcification; this makes it necessary to sharply reduce the available dose of the drug and sometimes to stop further treatment with it. The main reason of the adverse effect of the drug is mostly brought about by the pronounced resorbing effect on bones of $1,25(OH)_2D_3$. Taking into account the above-mentioned, we should develop a suitable compound, capable of preventing these disorders in CRI and having no these side effects.

We have carried out a comparative investigation on the effects of $1,25(OH)_2D_3$, $1\text{-}OHD_3$, and $24,25(OH)_2D_3$ on calcium-phosphorus metabolism and bone tissue state in rats under conditions of experimental CRI for 2 and 6 months [Blazheevich et al., 1980; Alexeeva et al., 1983; Alexeeva, 1984]. We imitated experimental CRI by partial excision, e.g. five sixths, of renal tissue and it was characterized by a severe increase of blood urea nitrogen, hyperphosphatemia, a decrease of diaphyses density, calcium, phosphorus, and hydroxyproline content in them and calcium content in the epiphyses. $1,25(OH)_2D_3$ or $1\text{-}OHD_3$ administration to these animals produced no normalizing effect in respect of the mentioned indices. Simultaneously, $1,25(OH)_2D_3$ and $1\text{-}OHD_3$ enhance hyperphosphatemia and epiphyses demineralization and cause moderate hypercalcemia, and sharply increase calcinosis of the aorta and kidney remnants.

Unlike $1,25(OH)_2D_3$, the administration of $24,25(OH)_2D_3$ at a dose of 0.25 μg/day produced a normalizing effect on the majority of parameters: increasing diaphyses density and their calcium and phosphorus content. $24,25(OH)_2D_3$ simultaneously increased collagen content in diaphyses and epiphyses. The increased dose of $24,25(OH)_2D_3$ (1.25 μg/day) was not more effective. None of the $24,25(OH)_2D_3$ doses caused hypercalcemia and ectopic calcification. The combination of $1,25(OH)_2D_3$ and $24,25(OH)_2D_3$ (0.025 plus 1.25 μg) partially reduced $1,25(OH)_2D_3$ effect on hypercalcemia, hyperphosphatemia and calcinosis (table VIII).

What really is quite important is that $24,25(OH)_2D_3$ not only prevented hypocalcemia and osteopenia, but simultaneously normalized phosphorus concentration in blood, thus preventing hyperphosphatemia and favoring a decrease of azotemia. The latter proves the correcting effect of $24,25(OH)_2D_3$ on the secondary impairment of calcium and phosphorus metabolism, osteogenesis in CRI, as well as, on the primary defect of the pathology, accompanied by the disorders of secretory renal function.

The data obtained prove $24,25(OH)_2D_3$ to be a more effective and safer compound for the control of metabolic bone disorders in CRI than $1,25(OH)_2D_3$.

Clinical Use of 1-OHD$_3$ and 24,25(OH)$_2$D$_3$

The discovery of active vitamin D forms allows us to use them for calcium-phosphorus impairment correction. In this connection, $1\text{-}OHD_3$ is of a special interest, since it represents a synthetic analogue of $1,25(OH)_2D_3$ – the hormonal form of vitamin D.

A comprehensive pharmacological test of the $1\text{-}OHD_3$, made by our laboratory, has shown its high biological activity; more precisely, its capability of normalizing calcium absorption in nephrectomy [Spirichev et al., 1978; Blazheevich et al., 1980].

The administration of a physiological dose of $1\text{-}OHD_3$ with phosphorus restriction prevented hypocalcemia, osteoporosis, and metastatic calcification in experimental CRI [Blazheevich et al., 1980]. These findings enabled us to use successfully the home-produced compound $1\text{-}OHD_3$ to correct calcium metabolism disorders caused by a biosynthesis defect of $1,25(OH)_2D_3$ in the case of CRI, hypoparathyroidism, vitamin-D-dependent rickets (type I), hypokinesia, bone fractures, hypercorticoidism, and other pathologies. Today this preparation, called 'Oxidevit', is widely used in this country.

Table VIII. Effects of $1,25(OH)_2D_3$ and $24,25(OH)_2D_3$ administration on serum and bone parameters in rats with a 6-month CRI. From Alexeeva et al. [1983]

Groups of animals	Dose of metabolite, µg	Serum Ca mg/dl	Serum P_i mg/dl
Control	vehicle	10.7 ± 0.03	7.3 ± 0.1
CRI	vehicle	10.4 ± 0.2	9.1 ± 0.4^{a}
$1,25(OH)_2D_3$	0.025	11.6 ± 0.2^{a}	10.3 ± 0.7^{a}
$24,25(OH)_2D_3$	0.25	10.6 ± 0.08	7.7 ± 0.2^{b}
$1,25(OH)_2D_3 + 24,25(OH)_2D_3$	0.025 + 1.25	$11.2 \pm 0.1^{a,b}$	8.9 ± 0.2^{a}

[a] Significant differences from control; [b] from CRI group; [c] from $1,25(OH)_2D_3$ group.

Comprehensive data, obtained in our laboratory [Alexeeva et al., 1982, 1983; Blazheevich et al., 1982b; Sergeev et al., 1982a; Ushakov et al., 1984; Karatabanova et al., 1985a, b], and some other laboratories [Ornoy et al., 1978; Edelstein and Ornoy, 1979; Sömjen et al., 1985] proved the high biological activity and peculiar functions of the vitamin D_3 metabolite, capable of regulating osteogenesis. These functions can be realized by means of genomic or nongenomic mechanism analogues to $1,25(OH)_2D_3$ as well as by action modification of other calcium-regulating hormones ($1,25[OH]_2D_3$, PTH, CT probably). Regardless of the positive effects of $24,25(OH)_2D_3$, e.g. capability of stimulating calcium absorption in the intestine, formation and mineralization of bone without a pronounced effect on bone resorption, the compound can be used effectively in treatment against a great number of metabolic and other bone disorders.

In particular, our laboratory has proved the high effectiveness of $24,25(OH)_2D_3$ when used alone, or in combination with $1,25(OH)_2D_3$, to correct calcium metabolism disorder and bone tissue state in chronic renal failure, hypokinesia, hypercorticoidism, and bone fractures. It should be noted here that sufficient doses of the drug (physiological or multiples of up to 5–10 times) are essential.

Vitamin D and Optimum Phosphorus Intake

Experimental, clinical and epidemiological research of the 1970s showed that excessive phosphorus intake, typical of the modern diet, produced unfavorable effects, such as hyperphosphatemia, hypocalcemia,

Blood urea nitrogen, mg/dl	Diaphyses density, g/cm³	Diaphyses Ca mg/cm³	Diaphyses P mg/cm³	Diaphyses hydroxyproline, mg/cm³
32 ± 1	1.92 ± 0.01	479 ± 8	241 ± 4	40.1 ± 0.6
105 ± 8[a]	1.69 ± 0.02[a]	412 ± 11[a]	215 ± 7[a]	36.4 ± 1.2[a]
121 ± 5[a]	1.74 ± 0.03[a]	420 ± 16[a]	210 ± 9[a]	38.4 ± 1.5
82 ± 7[a,c]	1.89 ± 0.02[b]	440 ± 15[a]	231 ± 9	44.0 ± 1.8[a,b]
106 ± 15[a]	1.90 ± 0.01	437 ± 11[a]	221 ± 8[a,b]	43.5 ± 2.2[b]

osteoporosis and soft tissue calcinosis. These findings have been covered in the corresponding reviews [Draper and Bell, 1979; Draper and Scythes, 1981; Chinn, 1981].

Experimental research work has been done by our laboratory since the early 1970s and has revealed a similar effect of a high phosphorus consumption in intact animals (1.8% of the diet with 0.6% Ca content) as well as those effects occurring under certain physiological and pathological conditions, such as pregnancy, lactation, chronic renal insufficiency, hypokinesia, and hypercorticoidism [Blazheevich et al., 1974a, b, 1975, 1978; Belakovsky et al., 1982; Spirichev et al., 1984]. A restricted phosphorus intake (0.3% of the diet) produced a positive effect on calcium-phosphorus metabolism and bone tissue under the above-mentioned conditions, enhanced effectiveness or, in a number of cases, was an indispensible condition of the harmless use of active vitamin-D_3 metabolites 1-OHD_3, 1,25$(OH)_2D_3$, and 24,25$(OH)_2D_3$ to a lesser extent [Blazheevich et al., 1982c; Isaeva et al., 1979; Ushakov et al., 1980, 1983b].

The most pronounced negative effect in a high phosphorus content in the diet has been registered in rats with experimental chronic renal insufficiency administered 1-OHD_3. The use of the compound at a dose close to the physiological one (0.05 μg/day) along with a diet with 1.2% of phosphorus content (calcium-phosphorus ratio = 1:2) worsened sharply mineral metabolism disorders [Blazheevich et al., 1980]. It revealed itself in a marked hyperphosphatemia, hypocalcemia, osteoporotic changes of bones and soft tissue calcinosis, especially in kidney remnants. A rapid development of renal insufficiency and the death of animals (100% of lethal cases 2 months later) were the results of those disorders.

The experimental data on 1-OHD_3 pronouncing a negative effect in CRI when a large amount of phosphorus is used correspond to the clinical observations showing an increase of calcinosis in internal organs in CRI when patients were recommended 1-OHD_3 without a restriction of phosphorus intake [Coburn and Massry, 1980]. This effect can be preconditioned by increased hyperphosphatemia which, in its turn, may play a key role in the pathogenesis of mineral metabolism disorders in CRI.

The data obtained prove that it is inadmissible to recommend 1-OHD_3 in CRI without appropriate measures aimed at regulating the phosphorus intake, and the drug should not be recommended in the initial stages of CRI before the breakdown of endogenous 1,25$(OH)_2D_3$ production in the kidneys.

The possible consequences of an unbalanced phosphorus intake were seen, for example, in the Nenetsky national region. People there eat traditionally much raw fish and meat and little dairy products; thus, their diet is poor in calcium (300–400 mg) and rich in phosphorus (2,100–2,600 mg), e.g. a calcium-phosphorus ratio of 1.0 : 7.0–7.5. The investigation showed a low calcium and a high phosphorus content in the serum of children and adults (pregnant women among them) compared to the same groups of people in central Russia [Blazheevich et al., 1983]. It should be noted that even women in childbirth and newborns of the region give a picture of decreased 25-OHD concentration. From our point of view, these changes, similar to those in the experiment, can be one of the reasons for nephrolithiasis occurring much more frequently among northern people than among people of the temperate areas. The findings confirm the idea of a pronounced negative effect in high phosphorus intake in the pathogenesis of arteriocalcinosis and urolithiasis. It is necessary to keep up an optimum calcium-phosphorus ratio in our diet.

Based on investigation, the recommended daily allowances (RDA) for phosphorus were reconsidered in this country. Information and RDA for other minerals and vitamins may be of interest to the foreign readers and is given in the Appendix.

Conclusion

The questions discussed cannot exhaust all the problems on the physiological functions of vitamin D, the effects of its active forms, mechanisms of action and their possible application for the improvement of various forms of calcium metabolism and osteogenetic disorders. In particular, the investigation of vitamin D metabolism and the use of its metabolites against endocrinopathies, senile and postmenopausal osteoporosis, malignant tumors, malabsorption syndrome, and parenteral nutrition has not been discussed here. The research of other nutrients' (vitamins, especially) effects on metabolism, binding, and biochemical functions of vitamin D is of special interest. These directions of research are being carried out or planned in our laboratory now.

A comprehensive research of vitamin D and application of the findings in this field, along with an investigation into the fundamental effects of vitamin D are the most interesting and promising spheres of this research work and attract more and more attention of not only theorists but also keen practitioners.

Appendix: Recommended daily allowances for vitamins in the USSR (1982)

Age groups years	Vitamins									
	thiamine mg	riboflavin mg	B_6, mg	B_{12} µg	folacin µg	niacin (niacin equiv.), mg	ascorbic acid, mg	A (retinol equiv.), µg	E IU	D IU
Male adults										
18–29	1.7–2.2 (1.8)	2.0–2.6 (2.1)	2.0–2.6 (2.1)	3	200	18–24 (20)	70–92 (75)	1,000	15	100
30–39	1.6–2.2 (1.7)	1.9–2.5 (2.0)	1.9–2.5 (2.0)	3	200	18–23 (19)	68–90 (72)	1,000	15	100
40–59	1.5–2.1 (1.7)	1.8–2.4 (1.9)	1.8–2.4 (1.9)	3	200	17–22 (18)	64–89 (69)	1,000	15	100
60–75	1.4	1.6	1.6	3	200	15	58	1,000	15	100
75+	1.2	1.4	1.4	3	200	13	50	1,000	15	100
Female adults										
18–29	1.4–1.9 (1.5)	1.7–2.2 (1.8)	1.7–2.2 (1.8)	3	200	16–20 (17)	60–79 (64)	1,000	12	100
30–39	1.4–1.8 (1.5)	1.6–2.1 (1.7)	1.6–2.1 (1.7)	3	200	15–20 (16)	58–76 (61)	1,000	12	100
40–59	1.3–1.7 (1.4)	1.5–2.0 (1.6)	1.5–2.0 (1.6)	3	200	14–19 (15)	55–73 (59)	1,000	12	100
60–75	1.3	1.5	1.5	3	200	14	52	1,000	12	100
75+	1.1	1.3	1.3	3	200	12	48	1,000	12	100
Pregnant	1.7	2.0	2.0	4	600	19	72	1,250	15	500
Lactating	1.9	2.2	2.2	4	600	21	80	1,500	15	500

Appendix (cont.)

	Vitamins									
	B_1	B_2	B_6	B_{12}	folacin	niacin	C	A	E	D
Children										
0–29 days, neonates	0.3	0.4	0.4	0.3	40	4	30	400	5	400
1–3 months	0.3	0.4	0.4	0.3	40	5	30	400	5	400
4–6 months	0.4	0.5	0.5	0.4	40	6	35	400	5	400
7–12 months	0.5	0.6	0.6	0.5	60	7	40	400	6	400
1–3 years	0.8	0.9	0.9	1	100	10	45	450	7	400
4–6 years	1.0	1.3	1.3	1.5	200	12	50	500	10	100
7–10 years	1.4	1.6	1.6	2	200	15	60	700	10	100
11–13 years, males	1.6	1.9	1.9	3	200	18	70	1,000	12	100
11–13 years, females	1.5	1.7	1.7	3	200	16	60	1,000	10	100
14–17 years, males	1.7	2.0	2.0	3	200	19	75	1,000	15	100
14–17 years, females	1.6	1.8	1.8	3	200	17	65	1,000	12	100

Minimum and maximum figures represent the requirement of adults involved mainly in brain work or manual labor, respectively. Figures in parentheses represent values for moderately active people.

Appendix (cont.): Recommended daily allowances for minerals in the USSR (1982)

Age groups	Minerals			
	calcium, mg	phosphorus, mg	magnesium, mg	iron[1], mg
0–29 days, neonates	240	120	50	1.5
1–3 months	500	400	60	5
4–6 months	500	400	60	7
7–12 months	600	500	70	10
1–3 years	800	800	150	10
4–6 years	1,200	1,450	300	15
7–10 years	1,100	1,650	250	18
11–13 years, males	1,200	1,800	350	18
11–13 years, females	1,100	1,650	300	18
14–17 years, males	1,200	1,800	300	18
14–17 years, females	1,100	1,650	300	18
Adult males	800	1,200	400	10
Adult females	800	1,200	400	18
Pregnant females	1,000	1,500	450	20
Lactating females	1,000	1,500	450	25

[1] Taking into account 10% utilization of intaken iron.

References

Adrianov, N.V.; Shyppe, N.G.; Blazheevich, N.B.; Spirichev, V.B.: The functional activity of mitochondria and the intensity of nucleic acids and protein synthesis in rat intestinal mucosa and liver under conditions of various supplies of vitamin D. Vopr. med. khimii *23:* 537–545 (1977).

Alexeeva, I.A.: Effect of 24,25-dihydroxycholecalciferol on calcium-phosphorus metabolism and bone tissue in rats with experimental renal failure. Vopr. pitan. *3:* 55–58 (1984).

Alexeeva, I.A.; Spirichev, V.B.; Blazheevich, N.V.; Bogoslovsky, N.A.: Biological activity of 1,25-dihydroxycholecalciferol and 24,25-dihydroxycholecalciferol in rats. Vopr. med. khimmi *28:* 71–78 (1982).

Alexeeva, I.A.; Spirichev, V.B.; Bogoslovsky, N.A.: Effects of 1,25-dihydroxycholecalciferol and 24,25-dihydroxycholecalciferol on calcium-phosphorus metabolism and bone tissue in rats with experimental renal insufficiency. Vopr. med. khimii *29:* 103–112 (1983).

Arkhapchev, Yu.P.; Sergeev, I.N.: 25-Hydroxyvitamin D_3 metabolism in rats with experimental femoral fracture. Vopr. pitan. *4:* 54–57 (1984).

Arkhapchev, Yu.P.; Sergeev, I.N.; Blazheevich, N.V.; Spirichev, V.B.: Metabolism of ^{3}H-25-hydroxycholecalciferol in rats with experimental femur fracture. Vopr. med. khimii *30:* 96–103 (1984).

Arkhapchev, Yu.P.; Sergeev, I.N.; Spirichev, V.B.; Blazheevich, N.V.: Calcium metabolism and vitamin D_3 active metabolites serum concentration in rats with bone tissue reparative regeneration. Vopr. med. khimii *32:* 122–129 (1986).

Armbrecht, H.J.; Zenser, T.V.; Davis, B.B.: Conversion of 25-hydroxyvitamin D_3 to 1,25-dihydroxyvitamin D_3 and 24,25-dihydroxyvitamin D_3 in renal slices from the rat. Endocrinology *109:* 218–222 (1981).

Baylink, D.J.; Stauffer, M.; Wergedal, J.E.; Rich, C.: Formation, mineralization and resorption of bone in vitamin D deficient rats. J. clin. Invest. *49:* 1122–1134 (1970).

Belakovsky, M.S.; Blazheevich, N.V.; Spirichev, V.B.; Sergeev, I.N.; Spitsyna, N.E.: Effect of excessive phosphorus consumption on phosphorus-calcium metabolism and bone state in hypokinetic rats. Kosm. biol. *5:* 70–73 (1982).

Binderman, I.: 24,25-Dihydroxycholecalciferol induces the growth of chick cartilage in vitro. Endocrinology *115:* 430–432 (1984).

Blazheevich, N.V.; Fernandes, R.; Isaeva, V.A.; Spirichev, V.B.: Effect of 1-hydroxycholecalciferol on the mineral metabolism in chronic kidney insufficiency. Vopr. med. khimii *26:* 13–23 (1980).

Blazheevich, N.V.; Matveichuk, N.B.; Spirichev, V.B.: Effect of vitamin D_2 and 1-hydroxycholecalciferol on the bone tissue in rats with femoral fracture. Vopr. pitan. *5:* 66–71 (1982a).

Blazheevich, N.V.; Sergeev, I.N.; Arkhapchev, Yu.P.; Isaeva, V.A.; Spirichev, V.B.; Bogoslovsky, N.A.: Effect of vitamin D_3 and its metabolites: 1,25-dihydroxycholecalciferol and 24,25-dihydroxycholecalciferol on callus mineralization in rats with femur fracture. Vopr. med. khimii *28:* 98–105 (1982b).

Blazheevich, N.V.; Spirichev, V.B.; Gazdarov, A.K.; Isaeva, V.A.: A possible role of excessive phosphorus consumption in the pathogenesis of nephrocalcinosis. Urol. nephrol. *4:* 11–14 (1974a).

Blazheevich, N.V.; Spirichev, V.B.; Pereverzeva, O.G.: Calcium-phosphorus metabolism and vitamin D status under the conditions of the extreme North. Vopr. pitan. *1:* 17–22 (1983).

Blazheevich, N.V.; Spirichev, V.B.; Pozdnyakov, A.L.: Role of excessive phosphorus consumption in development of aortic calcinosis. Cardiologia *6:* 67–71 (1975).

Blazheevich, N.V.; Spirichev, V.B.; Pozdnyakov, A.L.: Development and mechanism of mineral metabolism disorders in excessive phosphorus content in the diet. Vopr. pitan. *3:* 19–26 (1978).

Blazheevich, N.V.; Spirichev, V.B.; Pozdnyakov, A.L.; Isaeva, V.A.; Gazdarov, A.K.: Development of the kidneys and aortic calcinosis in rats with varying Ca:P ratio in their diet. Vopr. pitan. *5:* 28–34 (1974b).

Blazheevich, N.V.; Spirichev, V.B.; Ushakov, A.S.; Belakovsky, M.S.; Pozdnyakov, A.L.; Sergeev, I.N.: Effect of 1-hydroxycholecalciferol and varying phosphorus content in the diet on phosphorus-calcium metabolism in hypokinetic rats. Kosm. biol. *2:* 34–40 (1982c).

Bourne, G.H.: Vitamin C and bone; in Bourne, The biochemistry and physiology of bone; 2nd ed., vol. 2, chap. 6 (Academic Press, New York 1972a).

Bourne, G.H. (ed.): The biochemistry and physiology of bone; 2nd ed., vol. 3 (Academic Press, New York 1972b).

Bronner, F.: Intestinal calcium absorption and transport; in Caratoli, Membrane transport of calcium, pp. 237–262 (Academic Press, London 1982).

Chinn, H.I.: Effect of dietary factors on skeletal integrity in adults: calcium, phosphorus, vitamin D, and protein. FASEB Life Science Office, technical report 223-79-2275, pp. 1–75 (1981).

Coburn, J.W.; Massry, S.G. (eds): Used an action of 1,25-dihydroxyvitamin D_3 in uremia (Karger, Basel 1980).

DeLuca, H.F.: Vitamin D metabolism and function. Monogr. Endocr. *13:* 1–80 (1979).

DeLuca, H.F.: Some new concepts emanating from a study of the metabolism and function of vitamin D. Nutr. Rev. *38:* 169–182 (1980).

DeLuca, H.F.: Metabolism and molecular mechanism of action of vitamin D. Biochem. Soc. Trans. *10:* 147–158 (1982).

DeLuca, H.F.; Schnoes, H.K.: Vitamin D: recent advances. A. Rev. Biochem. *52:* 411–439 (1983).

Draper, H.H.; Bell, R.R.: Nutrition and osteoporosis. Adv. Nutr. Res. *2:* 79–106 (1979).

Draper, H.H.; Scythes, C.A.: Calcium, phosphorus and osteoporosis. Fed. Proc. *40:* 2434–2438 (1981).

Edelstein, S.; Ornoy, A.: 24,25-Dihydroxyvitamin D: the preferred metabolite for bone; in Norman, Vitamin D: basic research and its clinical application, pp. 381–389 (de Gruyter, Berlin 1979).

Fernandes, R.R.; Spirichev, V.B.; Blazheevich, N.V.; Pereverseva, O.G.; Knyzeva, T.A.: Calcium binding by rat small intestine epithelium microvilli at different contents of vitamin D. Biochimia *46:* 172–180 (1981).

Fraser, D.R.: Regulation of the metabolism of vitamin D. Physiol. Rev. *60:* 551–613 (1980).

Furlong, T.J.; Ibels, L.S.; Mason, R.S.: Serum 25-hydroxyvitamin D concentrations in chronic renal failure; in Norman, Vitamin D: chemical, biochemical, and clinical update, pp. 1141–1142 (de Gruyter, Berlin 1985).

Ghazarian, J.G.: The 1- and 24-hydroxylases of 25-hydroxycholecalciferol: one or two enzymes? in Norman, Vitamin D: basic research and its clinical application, pp. 587–596 (de Gruyter, Berlin 1979).

Gray, R.W.; Napoli, J.L.: Dietary phosphate deprivation increases 1,25-dihydroxyvitamin D_3 synthesis in rat kidney in vitro. J. biol. Chem. *258:* 1152–1155 (1983).

Henry, H.L.; Norman, A.W.: Vitamin D: metabolism and biological actions. Annu. Rev. Nutr. *4:* 493–520 (1984).

Hunziker, W.; Walters, M.R.; Norman, A.W.: 1,25-Dihydroxyvitamin D_3 receptors. Differential quantitation of endogenously occupied and unoccupied sites. J. biol. Chem. *255:* 9534–9537 (1980).

Isaeva, V.A.; Alexeeva, I.A.; Blazheevich, N.V.; Spirichev, V.B.: Experimental deficiency of vitamin D at various ratios Ca:P in a diet. Vopr. med. khimii *25:* 86–92 (1979).

Isaeva, V.A.; Bazanov, E.A.; Spirichev, V.B.: Investigation of the role played by the vitamin D in the metabolism of the bone tissue collagen of albino rats. Vopr. pitan. *1:* 45–49 (1974).

Isaeva, V.A.; Spirichev, V.B.: Relative content of α,β and γ-chains of solluble collagen fractions from bone tissue under various supplay of vitamin D. Vopr. med. khimii *24:* 270–274 (1978).

Kabitskaya, O.E.; Savik, Z.F.; Kaplansky, A.S.; Shvets, V.N.; Sergeev, I.N.; Spirichev, V.B.: Effect of 1,25-dihydroxyvitamin D_3 and 24,25-dihydroxyvitamin D_3 on the growth and remodelling of rat bones during hypokinesia (histomorphometric investigation). Kosm. biol. *4:* 49–55 (1984).

Karatabanova, N.A.; Arkhapchev, Yu.P.; Sergeev, I.N.; Spirichev, V.B.; Linberg, L.F.: Vitamin D metabolism in rats with exogenous hypercorticoidism. Vopr. med. khimii *34:* 83–86 (1988).

Karatabanova, N.A.; Sokolova, S.V.; Bogoslovsky, N.A.; Spirichev, V.B.: Effect of 1,25-dihydroxycholecalciferol and 24,25-dihydroxycholecalciferol on calcium homeostasis in rats treated with hydrocortisone. Vopr. med. khimii *31:* 112–116 (1985a).

Karatabanova, N.A.; Spirichev, V.B.; Sokolova, S.V.; Bogoslovsky, N.A.: Effect of 1,25-dihydroxycholecalciferol and 24,25-dihydroxycholecalciferol on calcium homeostasis in rats given hydrocortisone and the diet with varying phosphorus content. Vopr. pitan. *2:* 52–56 (1985b).

Karatabanova, N.A.; Spirichev, V.B.; Sokolova, S.V.; Isaeva, V.A.: Effect of varying phosphorus consumption on calcium homeostasis and bone tissue state in rats given hydrocortisone. Vopr. pitan. *5:* 32–38 (1983).

Kovalenko, E.A.; Gurovsky, N.N.: Hypokinesia (Medicina, Moscow 1980).

Kumar, R. (ed.): Vitamin D – basic and clinical aspects (Nijhoff, Boston 1984).

Lawson, D. (ed.): Vitamin D (Academic Press, London 1978).

Morozov, I.A.; Spirichev, V.B.; Fernandes, R.R.; Blazheevich, N.V.: Effect of vitamin D on ultrastructure of rat duodenal enterocytes. Vopr. med. khimii *26:* 823–826 (1980a).

Morozov, I.A.; Spirichev, V.B.; Lysikov, Yu.A.: Study of subcellular localization of $^{45}Ca^{2+}$ during its absorption by the epithelium of the rat small intestine. Bull. exp. biol. med. *90:* 736–738 (1980b).

Nemere, I.; Norman, A.W.: Vitamin D and intestinal cell membranes. Biochim. biophys. Acta *694:* 307–327 (1982).

Nielsen, H.E.; Romer, F.K.; Melsen, F.: 1-Hydroxyvitamin D_3 treatment of nondialyzed patients with chronic renal failure: effects on bone, mineral metabolism and kidney function. Clin. nephrol. *13:* 103–108 (1980).

Norman, A.W.: Vitamin D: the calcium homeostatic steroid hormone (Academic Press, New York 1979).

Norman, A.W. (ed.): Vitamin D: molecular biology and clinical nutrition (Dekker, New York 1980).

Norman, A.W.; Miller, B.E.: Vitamin D: in Machlin, Handbook of vitamins. Nutritional, biochemical, and clinical aspects, pp. 45–97 (Dekker, New York 1984).

Norman, A.W.; Putkey, J.A.; Nemere, I.: Intestinal calcium transport: pleiotropic effects mediated by vitamin D. Fed. Proc. *41:* 78–83 (1982a).

Norman, A.W.; Roth, J.; Orci, L.: The vitamin D endocrine system: steroid metabolism, hormone receptors, and biological response (calcium binding proteins). Endocr. Rev. *3:* 331–366 (1982b).

Ornoy, A.; Goodwin, D.; Noff, D.; Edelstein, S.: 24,25-Dihydroxyvitamin D is a metabolite of vitamin D essential for bone formation. Nature *276:* 517–519 (1978).

Ornoy, A.; Lidor, C.; Atkin, I.; Edelstein, S.: Effects of intraepiphyseal injection of vitamin D metabolites on healing of rickets in chicks; in Norman, Vitamin D: chemical, biochemical, and clinical update, pp. 314–315 (de Gruyter, Berlin 1985).

Parfitt, A.M.: Calcitriol but not other metabolites of vitamin D is essential for normal bone growth and development in the rat. J. clin. Invest. *73:* 576–586 (1984).

Peterson, F.; Holloway, D.E.; Duquette, P.H.; Rivers, J.M.: Dietary ascorbic acid and hepatic mixed function oxidase activity in the guinea pigs. Biochem. Pharmacol. *32:* 91–96 (1983).

Rajalakshmi, R.: Some naive questions and thoughts on vitamin D and its relatives. Wld Rev. Nutr. Diet., vol. 34, pp. 102–132 (Karger, Basel 1980).

Seino, Y.; Satomura, K.; Tanaka, Y.; De Luca, H.F.: Renal 25-OHD_3-1-hydroxylase and 24-hydroxylase in a patient with renal disease; in Norman, Vitamin D: chemical, biochemical and clinical update, pp. 515–520 (de Gruyter, Berlin 1985).

Sergeev, I.N.; Afonin, B.V.; Blazheevich, N.V.; Morukov, B.V.; Belakasky, M.S.: Role of vitamin D_3 active metabolites in the regulation of calcium metabolism in hypokinetic rats. Kosm. biol. *6:* 46–50 (1985).

Sergeev, I.N.; Arkhapchev, Yu.P.; Kim Ren Kha; Kodensova, V.M.; Spirichev, V.B.: Effect of ascorbic acid on 25-hydroxyvitamin D_3 metabolism in kidneys and 1,25-dihydroxyvitamin D_3 receptor-like binding in intestinal mucosa of guinea pigs. Biokhimia *52:* 1867–1874 (1987a).

Sergeev, I.N.; Arkhapchev, Yu.P.; Linberg, L.F.; Blazheevich, N.V.; Ushakov, A.S.; Spirichev, V.B.: 25-Hydroxyvitamin D_3 metabolism and its regulation in hypokinetic rats. Biockimia *49:* 590–598 (1984).

Sergeev, I.N.; Arkhapchev, Yu.P.; Spirichev, V.B.: Effect of hypokinesia on vitamin D metabolism in rats. Kosm. biol. *2:* 68–73 (1983).

Sergeev, I.N.; Blazheevich, N.V.; Belakovsky, M.S.; Spirichev, V.B.; Ushakov, A.S.: The role of 24,25-dihydroxycholecalciferol in bone mineralization of hypokinetic rats. Kosm. biol. *5:* 74–77 (1982a).

Sergeev, I.N.; Blazheevich, N.V.; Kaplansky, A.S.; Shvets, V.N.; Belakovsky, M.S.; Spirichev, V.B.: Comparative study of 1,25-dihydroxyvitamin D_3 and 24,25-dihydroxyvitamin D_3 effects upon calcium homeostasis and bone tissue state in hypokinetic rats. Vopr. med. khimii *33:* 100–107 (1987b).

Sergeev, I.N.; Blazheevich, N.V.; Spirichev, V.B.: Effect of 24,25-dihydroxycholecalciferol on the chemical composition of rat bone tissue in hypokinesia. Vopr. med. khimii *28:* 102–108 (1982b).

Sergeev, I.N.; Kim Ren Kha; Arkhapchev, Yu.P.; Spirichev, V.B.: 25-Hydroxyvitamin D_3 metabolism in kidneys and chromatin receptors for 1,25-dihydroxyvitamin D_3 in intestinal mucosa in vitamin B_2-deficient rats. Vopr. med. khimii *33:* 96–103 (1987c).

Sergeev, I.N.; Spirichev, V.B.: Calcium absorption in the intestine of hypokinetic rats. Vopr. pitan. *4:* 50–54 (1986).

Sokolova, S.V.; Spirichev, V.B.; Adrianov, N.V.: Mechanism of vitamin-D-dependent Ca^{2+} intestinal absorption. Interrelationship between active transport of Ca^{2+} and liberation of inorganic phosphate on the basal membrane of intestinal epithelium. Vopr. med. khimii *28:* 99–108 (1982).

Sokolova, S.V.; Spirichev, V.B.; Adrianov, N.V.: Active transport of Ca^{2+} and phosphorus compounds metabolism in rat enterocytes. Biokhimia *48:* 559–564 (1983).

Sömjen, D.; Weisman, Y.; Berger, E.: A comparison of the responses to 24,25$(OH)_2D_3$ and 1,25$(OH)_2D_3$ by developing skeletal tissue; in Norman, Vitamin D: chemical, biochemical, and clinical update, pp. 284–293 (de Gruyter, Berlin 1985).

Spirichev, V.B.: Rickets pathogenesis and prophilaxis in view of modern concepts on vitamin D metabolism and mechanism of action. Pediatria *12:* 69–72 (1977); *1:* 70–71 (1978).

Spirichev, V.B.: Investigations on vitamins biochemistry and its practical aspects. Vopr. pitan. *5:* 67–74 (1980).

Spirichev, V.B.: Investigations in vitaminology: theoretical and practical aspects. Vest. Akad. med. Nauk SSSR *11:* 84–90 (1986).

Spirichev, V.B.; Alexeeva, I.A.; Blazheevir, N.V.; Pereverzeva, O.G.: Effects of excessive phosphorus consumption on calcium-phosphorus metabolism and vitamin D status in perinatal period. Vopr. ochr. materinstva detstva *9:* 72–73 (1984).

Spirichev, V.B.; Barkova, L.V.: The alterations in serum phosphorus and calcium concentrations and metastatic calcification of some tissues in rats under administration of various doses of vitamin D_2. Vopr. med. khimii *20:* 207–215 (1974).

Spirichev, V.B.; Blazheevich, N.V.: On the study of toxic action mechanism of vitamin D. Int. Z. VitamForsch. *39:* 30–36 (1969).

Spirichev, V.B.; Blazheevich, N.B.; Bogoslovsky, N.A.: Comparison of biological activity and toxic effect of 1-hydroxycholecalciferol and ergocalciferol in rats. Vopr. med. khimii *24:* 679–690 (1978).

Spirichev, V.B.; Blazheevich, N.V.; Raskin, I.M.: Biochemical diagnostics of D-hypervitaminosis and its treatment. Vopr. med. khimii *15:* 123–127 (1969).

Spirichev, V.B.; Gazdarov, A.K.; Saprin, A.N.; Belyakov, V.A.: On the participation of free radicals in oxidative transformations and on the action mechanism of vitamin D. Biophysica *19:* 692–696 (1974).

Spirichev, V.B.; Gazdarov, A.K.; Saprin, A.N.; Blazheevich, N.V.: On the possible role of free radicals in transformations and mechanism of action of vitamin D. Biophysica *21:* 676–678 (1976).

Spirichev, V.B.; Isaeva, V.A.: Vitamin D and bone collagen. Vopr. med. khimii *30:* 5–17 (1984).

Spirichev, V.B.; Kon, I.Ya.: Fat-soluble vitamins and biological membranes. Zurnal Vsesousn. khim. obcsh. *23:* 425–434 (1978).

Stewart, R.J.C.: Bone pathology in experimental malnutrition. Wld Rev. Nutr. Diet., vol. 21, pp. 1–74 (Karger, Basel 1975).

Tazibaev, Ch.S.: The role of nutrition in etiology, pathogenesis and prophylaxis of rickets; Dr. Med. Sci. thesis, Moscow (1984).

Underwood, J.L.: Vitamin D is not directly necessary for bone growth and mineralization. Am. J. Physiol. *246:* E493–E498 (1984).

Ushakov, A.S.; Sergeev, I.N.; Belakovsky, M.S.; Spirichev, V.B.; Kaplansky, A.S.; Shvets, V.N.: Specific regulation of calcium-phosphorus metabolism during hypokinesia and weightlessness by vitamin-D_3-active metabolites. Physiologist *26:* S112–S113 (1983a).

Ushakov, A.S.; Spirichev, V.B.; Belakovsky, M.S.; Blazheevich, N.V.; Pozdnyakov, A.L.: Effect of 1-alpha-hydroxycholecalciferol and varying phosphorous content in the diet on calcium-phosphorous metabolism in hypokinetic rats. Aviat. Space Envir. Med. *51:* 24–28 (1980).

Ushakov, A.S.; Spirichev, V.B.; Belakovsky, M.S.; Sergeev, I.N.; Kaplansky, A.S.; Shvets, V.N.: Vitamin-D_3-active metabolites as a countermeasure against disorders of calcium-phosphorus metabolism in hypokinetic rats. Aviat. Space Envir. Med. *55:* 534–537 (1984).

Ushakov, A.S.; Spirichev, V.B.; Belakovsky, M.S.; Sergeev, I.N.; Kondratyev, Yu.I.: Calcium-phosphorus metabolism and prevention of its disorders in hypokinetic rats. Physiologist *25:* S45–S48 (1982).
Ushakov, A.S.; Spirichev, V.B.; Sergeev, I.N.; Belakovsky, M.S.; Blazheevich, N.V.; Bogoslovsky, N.A.: Bone tissue of hypokinetic rats: effects of 24,25-dihydroxycholecalciferol and varying phosphorous content in the diet. Aviat. Space Envir. Med. *54:* 447–451 (1983b).
Warner, M.: 25-Hydroxyvitamin D hydroxylation. Evidence for a dioxygenase activity of solubilized renal mitochondrial cytochrome P-450. J. biol. Chem. *258:* 11590–11593 (1983).
Wasserman, R.H.: Intestinal absorption of Ca^{2+} and phosphorus. Fed. Proc. *40:* 68–72 (1981).
Wasserman, R.H.; Fullmer, C.S.: Calcium transport proteins, calcium absorption and vitamin D. A. Rev. Physiol. *45:* 375–385 (1983).
Wilhelm, F.; Norman, A.W.: Biochemical characterization of positive cooperativity in the binding of 1,25-dihydroxyvitamin D_3 to its chick intestinal chromatin receptor. J. biol. Chem. *280:* 10087–10092 (1985).
Wilhelm, F.; Ross, F.P.; Norman, A.W.: $24R,25(OH)_2D_3$: an allosteric effector of $1,25(OH)_2D_3$ binding to its chick intestinal receptor; in Norman, Vitamin D: chemical, biochemical, and clinical update, pp. 129–130 (de Gruyter, Berlin 1985).

Dr. V.B. Spirichev, Department of Vitaminology, Laboratory of Vitamin and Mineral Metabolism, Institute of Nutrition, Academy of Medical Sciences, Ustinsky proesd, 2/14, Moscow 109240 (USSR)

Wld Rev. Nutr. Diet., vol. 56, pp. 217–258 (Karger, Basel 1988)

Nutritional and Health Properties of Yogurt

P. Bourlioux, P. Pochart

Laboratoire de Microbiologie industrielle, Centre d'études Pharmaceutiques, Châtenay-Malabry, France

Contents

Introduction

According to the *Codex alimentarius* definition (Standard No. A-11/a/1975), yogurt is: 'A coagulated milk product produced by lactic acid fermentation by *Lactobacillus bulgaricus* and *Streptococcus thermophilus* from milk... In the finished product, microorganisms must be in a viable state and in substantial amounts.' The Codex alimentarius also provides for the possiblity to combine other lactic bacteria species with *L. bulgaricus* and *S. thermophilus* for fermentation.

A great number of national regulations agree with the 'yogurt' definition of the *Codex alimentarius* as regards its principle. However, as far as concerns the ferments that must or can be used, the Spanish, Italian, French, Dutch and USA regulations only apply the 'yogurt' denomination to milk fermented by *L. bulgaricus* and *S. thermophilus* whereas the Canadian regulation is closer to the Codex standard since it authorizes the combination of other lactic bacteria species with *L. bulgaricus* and *S. thermophilus* for fermentation.

In recent years, researchers have been taking a growing interest in the 'health' value of yogurt, a fermented milk containing live ferments and for which regulatory definitions nearly agree all over the world. Therefore, the present document only takes account of works dealing with yogurt (nutritional aspect and 'health' value) or its constituent microflora.

The 'Nutritional' Aspect of Milk Conversion into Yogurt

From the nutritional point of view, milk and yogurt are rather similar products [Odet, 1973].

During its conversion into yogurt, the milk composition undergoes two types of changes, namely:

- changes resulting from a possible fortification of the initial milk achieved before fermentation by addition of milk powder, of caseinates for instance (increase in the proteins and/or lactose content)
- changes resulting from the fermentation of milk or of milk fortified with milk powder (decrease in the lactose, vitamin B_{12} content – lactic acid and galactose development – increase in the content of peptides, free amino acids, free fatty acids and folic acid) [Deeth et al., 1981].

Vitamins and Minerals

The yogurt vitamin composition depends on several factors: (a) The initial milk vitamin content more or less modified by the heat treatment undergone by this milk as well as the heat treatment undergone by the milk powder that can be added. (b) The used ferments strains. (c) Fermentation conditions.

During fermentation, a consumption of vitamins B_{12} and C as well as a folic acid production can be observed. The fermentation effect on the contents of vitamins B_1, B_2, B_6, PP, biotin and pantothenic acid is not so marked (different data according to the authors). This probably results from the use of different strains for fermentation [Rasic and Kurmann, 1978; Deeth and Tamine, 1981; Gurr, 1983]. Yet, these modifications are only of a slight interest when taking account of the low percentage of contribution of a 125-gram yogurt to the vitamins' recommended intakes.

The milk minerals' composition is not changed by fermentation. The amounts of calcium provided by a yogurt manufactured from a milk fortified with milk powder are of prime interest since they can reach 180 mg for 100 g of yogurt [Deeth and Tamine, 1981].

According to Blanc [1981], the minerals' distribution between ionic and colloidal forms could probably vary during milk transformation into yogurt, these changes being likely to influence these minerals' bioavailability. It has been shown by a study carried out in the INRA, in Rennes [Terre, 1985], that acidification results in a complete solubilizing of calcium, magnesium, phosphorus and a partial solubilizing of trace elements. Besides, on the one hand, the distribution of calcium, magnesium, zinc and phosphorus between the soluble phase and the proteic one only depends on the pH (similar distribution for yogurt and for milk acidified by hydrochloric acid at pH 4). On the other hand, the iron and copper contents of the yogurt-soluble phase are greater than those of the acidified milk-soluble phase.

Blanc's above-mentioned assumption, according to which fermentation might exert some effect on the minerals bioavailability, was backed up by the works of Balasubramanya et al. [1984]. Indeed, these works demonstrated that, in rats, calcium and phosphorus show higher levels of bioavailability when fed in the form of yogurt than when fed in the form of milk.

Besides, in rats previously fed with a calcium-deficient diet, Dupuis [1974] demonstrated that, as compared with calcium carbonate, yogurt enhances the calcium intestinal absorption as well as its retention. In addition, the calcium intakes recovery achieved through calcium carbonate do not allow the low calcemia to return to normal, whereas in rats given a 'yogurt' diet for 3 weeks, the calcemia recovers its normal value.

Pointillart et al. [1986] reported that, in pigs, a diet with a high yogurt content administered for 6 weeks results in an increased resistance to bone fracture, as compared to a diet of a similar calcium level with a lower – or no – yogurt content.

Lactose – Lactic Acid

During milk fermentation, a portion of lactose (20–30%, sometimes more) is hydrolyzed by ferments to glucose and galactose, glucose being subsequently converted into lactic acid [Rasic and Kurmann, 1978].

Therefore, the yogurt lactose content is:

– lower than that of the initial milk if no milk powder is added to this last before fermentation

– close to that of the initial milk if milk powder is added to this last (around 3%) before fermentation.

When considering the traditional case of a yogurt manufactured from a whole milk 'fortified' with skim milk powder, it can be observed that the lactose content is reduced from 6.5% in the fortified milk to 5.2% in yogurt just after the fermentation. Concurrently, the galactose and lactic acid

Table I. Changes in the composition of the carbohydrate portion when milk is fermented by one kind of yogurt culture strain

	Lactose	Galactose	Lactic acid
Milk 13 g/l fat	4.75%	0	0
	5.9 g/pot[a]	0	0
Milk + 3% skim milk powder	6%	0	0
	7.5 g/pot[a]	0	0
Yogurt + 24 h (4 °C)	4%	1%	1%
	5 g/pot[a]	1.25 g/pot	1.25 g/pot
Yogurt + 24 days (4 °C)	3.4%	1.3%	1.3%
	4.3 g/pot[a]	1.6 g/pot	1.6 g/pot

[a] 1 pot = 125 g of yogurt.

Analysis made by Syndifrais, 37, rue du Général-Foy, 75008 Paris.

contents change from 0 to 0.7% [Toba et al. 1983]. Table I shows the variations undergone by the carbohydrate portion during milk fortification with skim milk powder as well as during fortified milk fermentation.

According to Cochet et al. [1983], lactose enhances calcium absorption in non-lactase-deficient subjects whereas it decreases this absorption in lactase-deficient subjects (lactose oral load associated to calcium in this study: 50 g).

The yogurt lactic acid amounts to 1% approximately. Just after yogurt manufacture, the *L*(+)-lactic acid content ranges from 50 to 70%, the remaining being *D*(–)-lactic acid. The *L*(+) form is generated by *S. thermophilus,* the *D*(–) form by *L. bulgaricus.* During storage, the *L*(+)-relative proportion decreases for the benefit of the *D*(–) form [Rasic and Kurmann, 1978; Alm, 1982b; Klupsch, 1983].

In man, the *L*(+) form is metabolized into pyruvic acid, and subsequently into oxaloacetic acid before following one of the two following courses: Krebs' cycle or the glyconeogenesis course. It can also be excreted in urine. The *D*(–) form is either slowly metabolized into pyruvic acid through the *D*-α-hydroxy acid dehydrogenase or eliminated by urine [Blanc, 1981; De Waard et al., 1983; Oh et al., 1985].

In man, after racemic perfusion, Connor et al. [1983] reported a higher urinary excretion of the *D*(–) form than of the *L*(+) form (the amount of excreted *D*(–) being 14 times as high as that of the *L*(+) per time unit). In addition, the *L*(+) perfusion resulted in an increased *D*(–) urinary elimination, whereas the *D*(–)-isomer was found neither in the perfusate nor in blood.

The *D*(–) and *L*(+)-lactic acids are naturally found in the human subjects' urines, the amount of *D*(–)-lactic acid representing 24% of the total amount of excreted lactic acid. Besides, physical exercise results in a higher *L*(+)-lactic acid urinary excretion, whereas the *D*(–)-form urinary excretion is only increased to a very small extent [Judge et al., 1962]. Furthermore, after studying the two lactic acid isomers urinary excretion following the racemic perfusion, Oh et al. [1985] concluded that there is no evidence that the metabolic use of *D*(–)-lactic acid has any harmful effect on adults.

In rats, Cori et al. [1929] demonstrated that *L*(+)-lactic acid consumption or subcutaneous injection causes a significant hepatic glycogen synthesis whereas the urinary excretion is low. *D*(–)-lactic acid entails no glycogen synthesis and a significant part of the administered dose is excreted in urines. The *L*-isomer is utilized 4 times as fast as the *D*-isomer. On the basis of their experiments carried out in rabbits, Drury and Wick [1965] concluded that the two isomers are oxidized, the *L*-isomer being oxidized in a larger proportion than the *D*-isomer.

In short, if it has been admitted that the *D*(–)-isomer can be consumed by adults with no harmful effect, the case is different for infants. Indeed, since the infants enzymatic systems are not yet provided with all the required enzymes, the Joint FAO/WHO Committee of Food Additives Experts [JECFA, 1974] recommended that food preparations for infants under 3 months of age should be completely free from *D*(–)-lactic acid.

Proteins and Free Amino Acids

Casein can be found in milk in the form of micelles (a casein/calcium and phosphates complex) whose stability is altered by the acidification produced during lactic fermentation. During this fermentation, calcium and phosphorus are salted out of the casein micelles and appear in a soluble form [Rasic and Kurmann, 1978] while micelles are destabilized and the casein precipitation begins. This precipitation is completed at pH 4.6–4.7.

Milk heating, achieved before fermentation, provokes a 'denaturation' of part of the lactoserum proteins. This results in a reduction of their solubility in an acid medium and, in fact, the yogurt-coagulated proteins are a 'coprecipitate' of casein and lactoserum denatured proteins. This precipitate forms a 'gel' type three-dimensional lattice characterized by hydrophilic proteins. This lattice includes the lipidic globules as well as the lactoserum containing the dissolved constituents. Therefore, casein can be found in yogurt in the 'decalcified' form, precipitated in a fine flocculence which, according to Blanc [1981], offers a double advantage:

– on the one hand, casein is better penetrated by gastric medium, thus enhancing the proteolytic enzyme action,

– on the other hand, there is an easier access to the sites of action for these enzymes; therefore, lactic acid exerts an effect on the proteins' gastric digestibility.

Regarding the ferments' proteolytic activity, *L. bulgaricus* demonstrates a much stronger activity than *S. thermophilus.* The amount of amino acids released by *L. bulgaricus* during fermentation is higher than the amount of amino acids consumed by the two species during this fermentation. This is the reason why there is a significant increase in the free amino acid concentration during the manufacture of yogurt. Thus, the total amount of free amino acids raises from 5.9 mg for 100 g of cow's milk to 23.6 mg for 100 g of yogurt prepared from cow's milk [Rasic et al., 1971; Rasic and Kurmann, 1978] (fig. 1). Yet, one must bear in mind that these

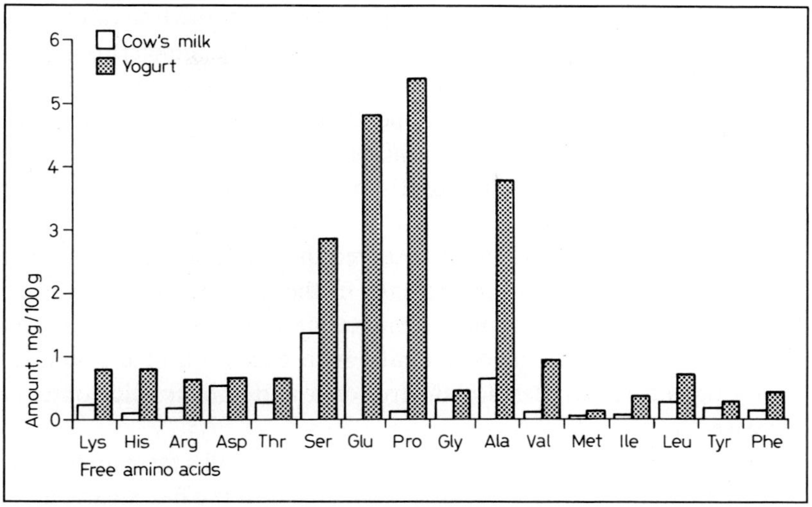

Fig. 1. Amount of free amino acids in cow's milk and in yogurt. From Rasic and Kurmann [1978].

values can differ according to the used *L. bulgaricus* strain. In an in vitro study (gastric digestion simulation) carried out in 1973, Breslaw et al. reported that yogurt has a better digestibility than the milk from which it is made. Indeed, at each digestion stage, and as compared with milk, yogurt demonstrates a smaller proteinic particle size, a greater amount of 'non-proteinic nitrogen' as well as a higher free amino acids content. These results were confirmed in a study by Vass et al. [1984].

Lipids and Free Fatty Acids

The total fatty acids content of milk includes around 60–70% of saturated fatty acids, 25–35% of monounsaturated fatty acids and 4% of polyunsaturated fatty acids [Anon, 1976; mentioned in Rao and Reddy, 1984]. Souci's [1981] tables give a similar composition. The triglyceride fatty acids composition is not altered by milk fermentation whatever milk is used (cow's or goat's milk) [Boccignone et al., 1984].

With cow's milks fermented either by *L. bulgaricus* or by *S. thermophilus* (fermentation time: 48 h), Rao and Reddy [1984] reported a slight increase in the contents of saturated fatty acids and oleic acid of the 'glyceride' portion as well as a slight decrease in the linoleic and linolenic acid contents of this same portion.

Alm et al. [1982c] reported a slight increase in the free fatty acid content during cow's milk conversion into yogurt. Yet, concerning milk free fatty acid composition, it should be noted that the changes undergone by milk during fermentation highly depend on the origin of the used milk and ferment strains. Moreover, after milk fermentation, some new compounds are detected in the 'free fatty acid' portion [Rasic and Kurmann, 1978; Boccignone et al., 1984].

Rasic and Kurmann [1978] observed that milk fermentation by a 'yogurt' symbiosis results in an increase in the amount of free fatty acids. They reported that cow's milk fermentation demonstrates an increase in the free saturated fatty acid contents, with exception of the stearic acid level which decreases. Besides, the free oleic and linoleic acid contents also decrease.

Rao and Reddy [1984] reported, with cow's milks fermented either by *L. bulgaricus* or by *S. thermophilus,* an increase in the free stearic and oleic acid concentrations (+10 to 20 mg for 100 g of fermented milk). However, one must bear in mind that free fatty acids only account for a small portion of the total amount of the fatty acids in milk (ranging from 1/30 to 1/100 according to the fatty acids). Concerning oleic acid, it can be observed that despite hydrolysis (free oleic acid increase), there is an increase in the oleic acid content of the 'glyceride' portion. The main reason for this increase could be a partial saturation of the linoleic and linolenic acids of the 'glyceride' portion due to the bacterial enzyme action.

Rao's results concerning the free fatty acids differ from those of Rasic, which gives evidence of different behaviors specific to the very strains. According to Rao and Reddy [1984], cholesterol levels (around 100 mg/l) undergo no modifications through milk fermentation.

The 'Physiology' Aspect of Milk Conversion into Yogurt

Gastric Emptying Kinetics

Mourot et al. [1985] compared milk gastric emptying kinetics with that of yogurt. The assumption was that yogurt will be cleared from the stomach more slowly than milk, taking account of its semi-fluid consistency, its higher energetic value and its greater osmolarity (the yogurt used in this study was manufactured from a milk fortified with milk powder). The study was carried out in man by means of an isotopic method. Healthy adults were given either 250 g of yogurt or 250 g of milk labelled with

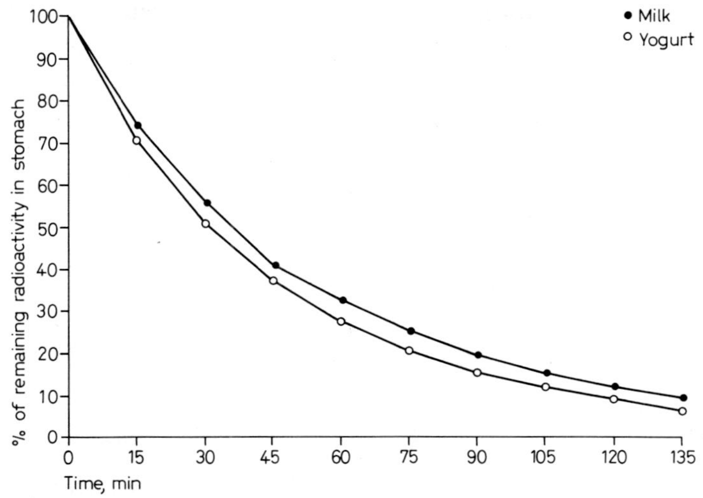

Fig. 2. Kinetics of yogurt and milk gastric emptying. From Mourot et al. [1985].

^{99m}Tc. The scintigraphy recordings achieved during 3 h did not reveal any difference between milk gastric emptying kinetics and that of yogurt (fig. 2).

Glycemic Index

Yogurt glycemic index is similar to that of milk [34 according to Jenkins et al., 1981]. It must be remembered that the glycemic index is obtained by dividing the area under the blood glucose response curve after yogurt ingestion (an amount corresponding to a 50-gram carbohydrate portion) by the area under the glucose response curve after a 50-gram glucose intake.

The Influence of Yogurt Intake on Urine Acidity

De Vries et al. [1986] studied the effect exerted by a morning intake (between 8 and 10 a.m.) of at least 1.5–2 liters of various drinks, such as yogurt, coca-cola, and orange juice, on urine acidity. During the remainder of the day, subjects were only given water and tea as drinks and bread,

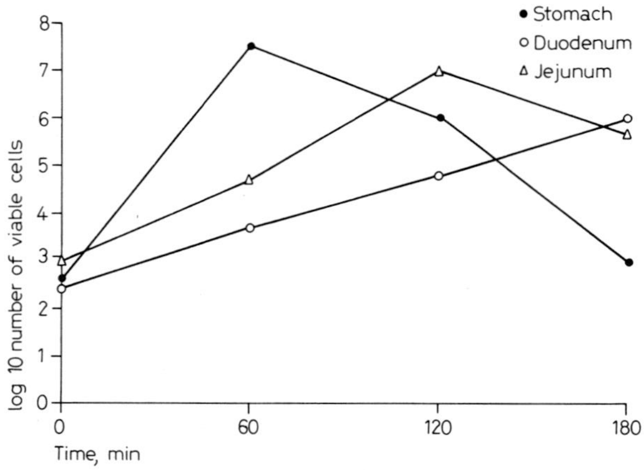

Fig. 3. Viable cell counts of gastrointestinal segments after yogurt intake. From Goodenough and Kleyn [1976].

biscuits, rice and sugar as food – a diet selected with the aim of reducing the intake of proteins and acid substances other than the tested ones. Urines were collected throughout a 24-hour period in several portions. The control group drink was tea and water. The acid urinary excretion induced by yogurt and coca-cola ingestion was more significant than the acid urinary excretion produced by the control drink consumption, this last excretion being also more important than the acid urinary excretion induced by orange juice ingestion.

The 'Health' Aspect of Milk Conversion into Yogurt

Yogurt Ferments Survival in the Alimentary Tract

In adults and infants, Bianchi Salvadori et al. [1967] as well as Salvadori et al. [1973] demonstrated the presence of live *L. bulgaricus* and *S. thermophilus* in the feces, after yogurt ingestion. Bianchi Salvadori et al. [1978] also reported that the administration to infants of 3–20 months of age, of a suspension of 100 billions per day of *L. bulgaricus* and *S. thermophilus* (the equivalent of 100 g of yogurt) during 15 days and before the last

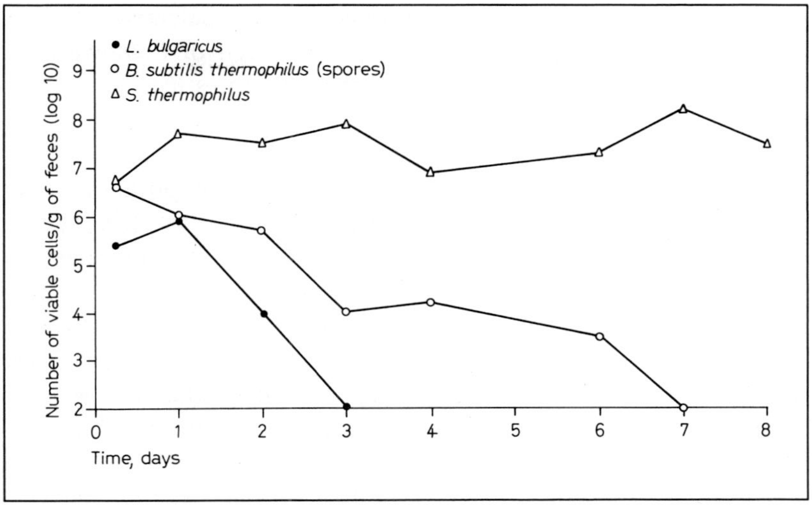

Fig. 4. Viable cell counts in the feces of gnotoxenic mice after ingestion of yogurt and spores of *Bacillus subtilis thermophilus.* From Besnier et al. [1983].

evening meal results in the survival of the two species that can be found in the feces. Therefore, the survival ability of ferments during their passage through the alimentary tract is not due – or not only due – to the possible protective part that could have been played by the yogurt proteins and fats.

In rats, a study carried out by Goodenough and Kleyn [1976] revealed, after yogurt consumption, a transient increase (2–3 h) in the number of live bacteria in stomach, jejunum and duodenum (fig. 3). Besides, Pacini et al. [1979] demonstrated, in mice, that 1 ml of yogurt administered by gavage twice a day during 30 days results in the presence, in the cecum, of live *L. bulgaricus* at the rate of 10 millions per liquid gram during treatment.

According to Besnier et al. [1983], in germ-free mice, a single gavage including yogurt and *B. subtilis thermophilus* spores (a transit tracer) results in a rapid fecal excretion of *L. bulgaricus* whereas *S. thermophilus* is not eliminated (high and constant concentration in the feces) (fig. 4). When mice are fed ad libitum with yogurt during one week, at the end of that week, the presence of the two species is demonstrated in the feces at rates close to those existing in yogurt.

After inoculation in germ-free mice, Bianchi Salvadori et al. [1984] demonstrated the implantation and proliferation of *L. bulgaricus* cells, especially at the level of stomach and the large intestine.

Providing a Lactase Activity

From weaning, the intestinal lactase activity disappears more or less rapidly and even sometimes completely according to race. The lactase activity of 70–100% of black or yellow race subjects disappears at the adult age, whereas in Europe this disappearance only affects the Mediterranean countries in which it reaches 40% in the Nice area [Costet et al., 1985]. A large part of the world adult population is lactase-deficient. The major determinant of this deficiency is 'ethnic' and not 'geographic'. Thus, Chinese populations in Asia, Australia and the USA have a very high prevalence of this deficiency (90%). In the same way, Jews, Arabs and other Mediterraneans have also high prevalences (60–100%), again irrespective of their geographic location. In the black population, the 'Fulani' and the 'Tutsi' are the only ones who have a low prevalence of this deficiency (7–20%) whereas the deficiency percentage of the other black populations is close to 90% [Gilat, 1979]. Newborn infants have a significant lactase activity and lactase deficiency is a 'normal' phenomenon at the adult age. Gilat, as well as Costet, suggested that in the adult a normal enterocytic lactase rate results from a genetic mutation which is thought to affect the regulation gene inhibiting lactase activity after weaning. Therefore, the lactase activity expression gene would be a controlled gene.

Wagh et al. [1984] showed lactase concentrations in the brush border, in infants under 3 years of age, children above 3 years of age and adults. Indeed, a significant decrease can be observed as the subject gets older.

A great number of articles aimed at determining the lactase deficiency prevalence and we have gathered these results in figure 5. Besides the previously mentioned researches, we have referred to the works of Jia Ju Zheng and Rosenberg [1984], Brand et al. [1985], Flatz et al. [1982], Burgio et al. [1984], Ferguson et al. [1984], Cuddenec et al. [1982], Bujanover et al. [1985], Dillon et al. [1982], Simoons [1978], Guix Garcia et al. [1974], and Alm [1982a].

In lactase-deficient adults, Kolars et al. [1984] as well as Savaiano et al. [1984] and Dewit [1985] demonstrated – for a similar amount of ingested lactose – a better absorption of the yogurt lactose than that of milk (fig. 6). This observation cannot be explained by a difference in gastric

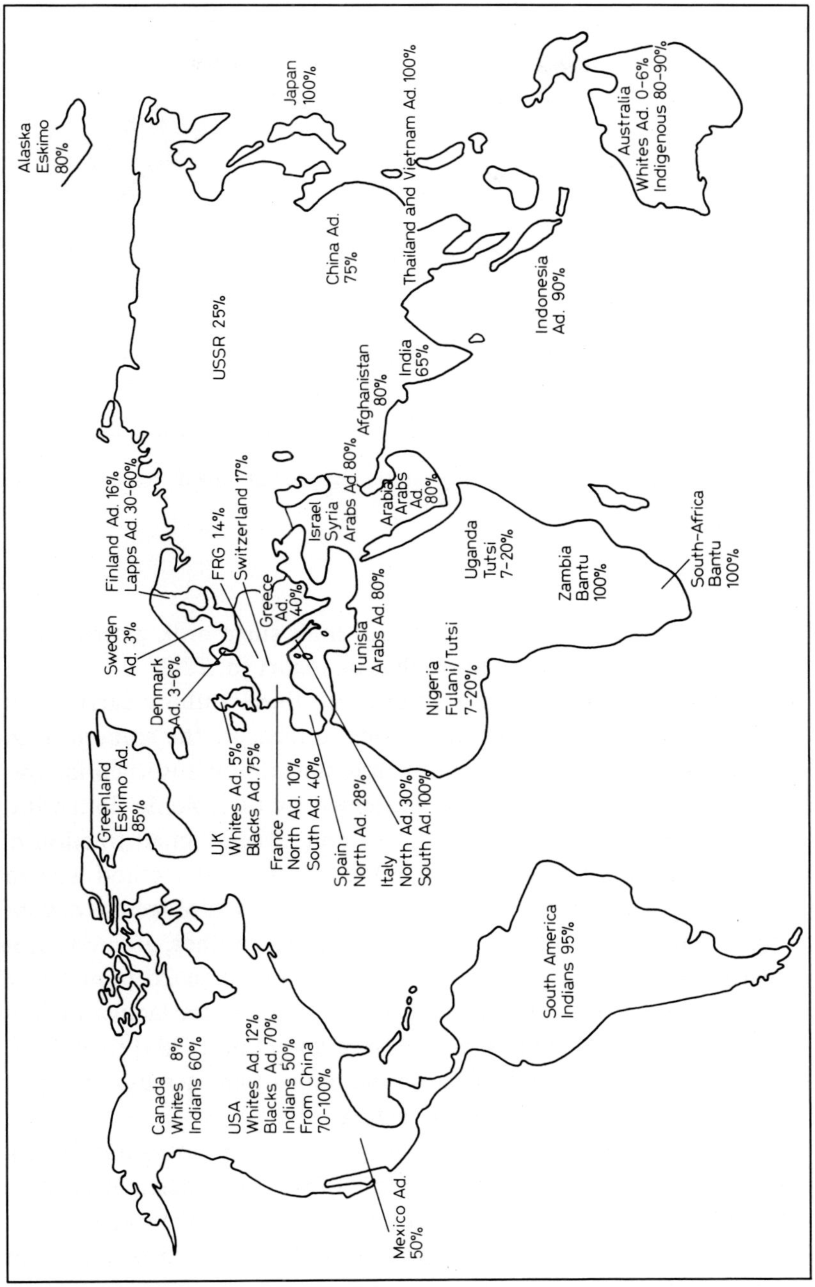

Fig. 5. Prevalence of lactose malabsorption. Ad. = Adults.

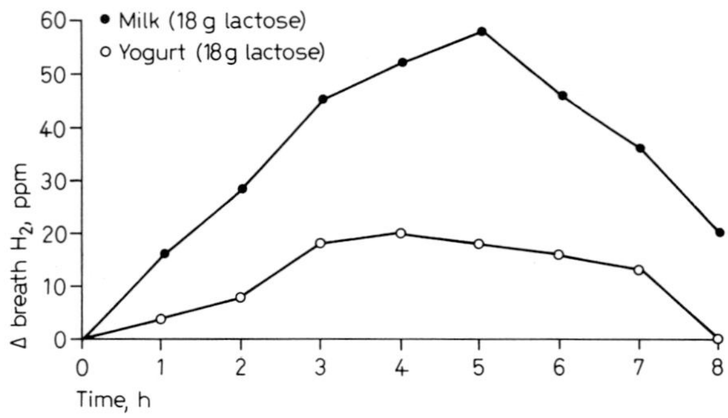

Fig. 6. Changes in breath hydrogen after ingestion of milk or yogurt in lactase-deficient subjects. From Kolars et al. [1984].

emptying kinetics between yogurt and milk since milk gastric emptying kinetics can be superimposed on that of yogurt (p. 224).

In order to study lactose absorption, these authors carried out the 'breath hydrogen test' which allows one to measure the amount of breath hydrogen expelled as indicating the amount of non-absorbed lactose and therefore the amount of lactose fermented by the colonic flora with production of gas, especially of CO_2, H_2, and CH_4. A small fraction of gas diffuses in blood and is excreted in the breath. This method is acknowledged as being sensitive and specific to the detection of lactose malabsorption [Parente et al., 1983]. According to this last author, an increase in the expelled breath hydrogen concentration greater than 20 ppm above the basic level after ingestion of 50 g of lactose indicates the lactose malabsorption. Kolars et al. [1984] as well as Savaiano et al. [1984] identified subjects with lactose malabsorption on the basis of an increase of more than 20 ppm after ingestion of 20 g of lactose.

Flatz et al. [1984] insisted on the precautionary measures to be taken when using the 'breath hydrogen test'. Indeed, in intestinal lactase-deficient subjects, this test validity can be altered by two variables:

– a late surge of the curve representing the expelled breath hydrogen concentration after an oral lactose load,

– and a high expelled breath hydrogen when fasting.

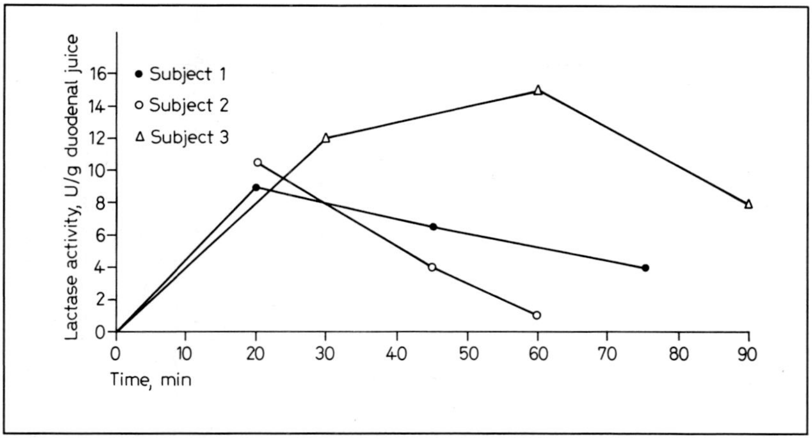

Fig. 7. Lactase activity in duodenal contents at various intervals after yogurt ingestion in 3 lactase-deficient subjects. ○ = First value not registered. From Kolars et al. [1984].

According to Kolars et al. [1984], the amount of breath hydrogen excreted by lactase-deficient subjects after ingestion of 10 g of lactulose (non-absorbable dissacharide) is comparable to that expelled after 20 g of lactose ingested as such or 18 g of lactose ingested in the form of milk. Thus, only 50% of the lactose is absorbed by these subjects.

Besides, Kolars demonstrated that incubation of yogurt at 4 °C and pH 4 reveals a negligible lactase activity whereas when sonicated yogurt is incubated at 37 °C and pH 7, a highly significant lactase activity is observed. This amount of activity is sufficient to hydrolyze 95% of the lactose content in a 4-hour period.

In 3 subjects, Kolars measured the lactase activity in the duodenal contents. A negligible activity was observed before yogurt ingestion. However, for 1 h afterwards, an appreciable lactase activity was present in the duodenal content (measurement at pH 7; fig. 7). Samples obtained during the first hour after yogurt ingestion had sufficient activity to hydrolyze from 50 to 100% of the measured lactose content in a 4-hour period. According to these authors, this demonstrates that the bacterial lactase in yogurt survives the passage through the stomach. This is close to the study of Kilara and Shahani [1976] and, in addition, it backs up Kolars' assumption according to which the lactic ferments' lactase would act in vivo and would substitute for the lack of endogenous lactase.

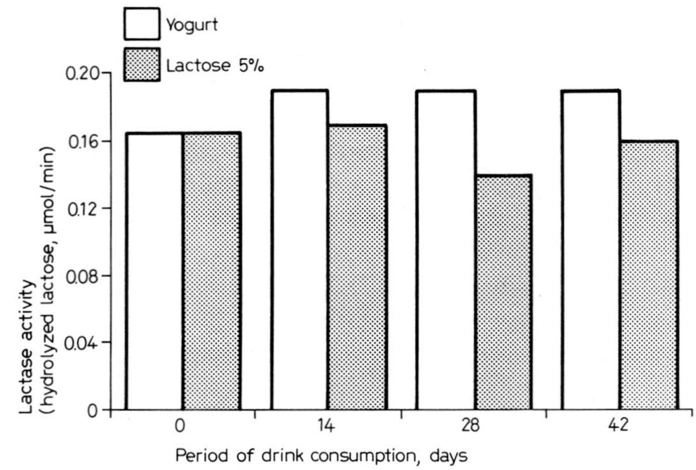

Fig. 8. Total lactase activity of the small intestine wall in axenic or gnotoxenic mice according to the drink consumed. From Besnier et al. [1983].

Since, in lactase-deficient subjects, lactose is better absorbed in the form of yogurt than in that of milk, it can be assumed that in these subjects, a calcium dose will be better absorbed when ingested in yogurt than in milk, considering that, in normal subjects, lactose enhances calcium absorption [Cochet et al., 1983].

When Besnier et al. [1983] administered to germ-free or conventional, just-weaned mice either a 5% lactose solution or yogurt diluted 3:5 in this lactose solution, given as drinks, they observed the following results: in the two sets of mice, regular yogurt ingestion resulted in an increase in the total lactase activity of the small intestine wall. This increase remained constant to the end of the experiment (42 days after weaning), whereas the initial lactase activity was not changed by the lactose solution ingestion (fig. 8).

The analysis achieved at the intestinal contents level demonstrated total lactase activities negligible there, but following the variations measured at the wall level. What is assumed is that yogurt ingestion enhances mice intestinal lactase activity both in germ-free and conventional sets of mice.

Furthermore, the lactase contained in ferments seems to be salted out during (in vitro) gastric digestion since the lactase activity measured by Kilara and Shahani [1976] is multiplied by five when yogurt is placed in a restored gastric medium and increases slightly for the 3 h afterward of in vitro digestion (lactase activity evaluated at pH 7). Thus, the salted-out lactase does not seem to be destroyed by the gastric environment. On the contrary, concerning milks fermented by only one species of yogurt ferments, after the lactase activity increase following the introduction into the gastric medium, they demonstrate a gradual reduction of this very activity during digestion. This difference gives evidence of the significance of the 'yogurt' symbiosis as compared to the two species considered separately. According to Kilara, as compared to *L. bulgaricus, S. thermophilus* contains three times as much lactase.

The Effect of Yogurt Microflora against the Alimentary Tract Infections

Such an effect was demonstrated by Niv et al. [1963] in 45 children, 75% of whom being infants below one year of age, who were admitted to hospital for cases of diarrhea. The '100 ml of yogurt three times per day' treatment appeared to be of a higher efficiency than the 'one teaspoon of neomycin-kaolin-pectin three times per day' treatment (each teaspoon containing 50 mg neomycin sulfate, 15 g kaolin, 0.3 g pectin). The means for days to recovery were 2.7 for the 'yogurt' group and 4.8 for the 'neomycin-kaolin-pectin' group (fig. 9).

The 4-week administration of 250 ml yogurt per day to adult subjects resulted in a few changes at the level of the intestinal flora of the subjects: a slight reduction of enterobacteria with a significant reduction of *E. coli* along with an increase in the number of mesophile lactic bacteria [Salvadori et al., 1973].

The 15-day administration of 100 billions of *L. bulgaricus* and 100 billions of *S. thermophilus* (ferments in saline suspension) to infants from 3 to 20 months of age, before the last evening meal, resulted in an increase in the lactic (mesophile and thermophile) and bifid flora. The number of enterobacteria did not undergo any change [Bianchi Salvadori et al., 1978].

Shapiro [1960] demonstrated the interest of yogurt in the treatment of antibiotic-induced diarrhea, an effect of lactic ferments will known and widely used in our country.

Mitchell and Kenworthy [1976] infested part of some weaned young pigs with a strain of enteropathogenic *E. coli* while the other part was kept

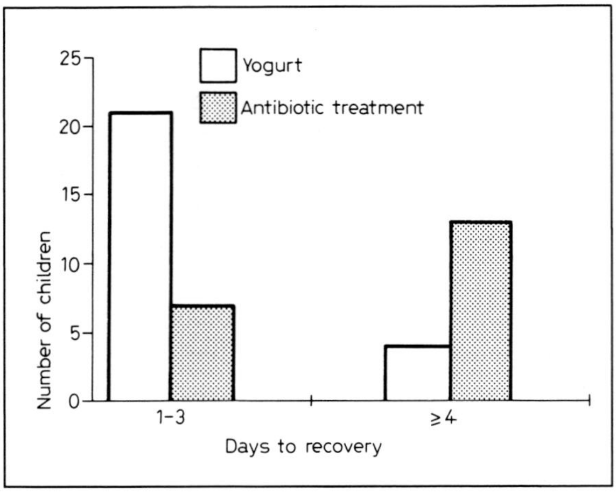

Fig. 9. Effect of yogurt compared with an antibiotic treatment on infantile diarrhea (45 children: 75% = infants less than one year). From Niv et al. [1963].

in a usual medium. In addition to their basic diet, these pigs received either a *L. bulgaricus* broth (live ferments) or an autoclaved *L. bulgaricus* broth during 2 weeks. As regards the diarrhea severity and mortality, no difference was observed between the 'infested' and 'non-infested' groups. As compared to the autoclaved broth, the *L. bulgaricus* broth (live ferments) seemed to enhance growth and survival in the young pigs. According to Mitchell, the *L. bulgaricus* broth's beneficial action cannot be ascribed to acidity, since all diets are provided with the same pH, nor to the anti-*E. coli* action which is minimal during fermentations of more than 24 h, as in the case of the used broths, but would rather result from an anti-enterotoxin activity.

In rats fed with milk (a milk fortified with skimmed milk powder and partially supplemented with iron, copper and vitamins just before freeze-drying), Hitchins et al. [1985a] observed a lower resistance to an intragastric inoculation of *Salmonella enteritidis* (carried out after a 1-day, 1-, 2- or 3-week diet) than in yogurt-fed rats (a yogurt manufactured from the above-mentioned milk, and freeze-dried). Rats were kept on 'milk' and 'yogurt' diets for 3 weeks after inoculation. As compared to milk, yogurt demonstrated a lower mortality (fig. 10) (the disease having not been avoided) and a less significant growth-retarding effect, mainly during the first week after inoculation.

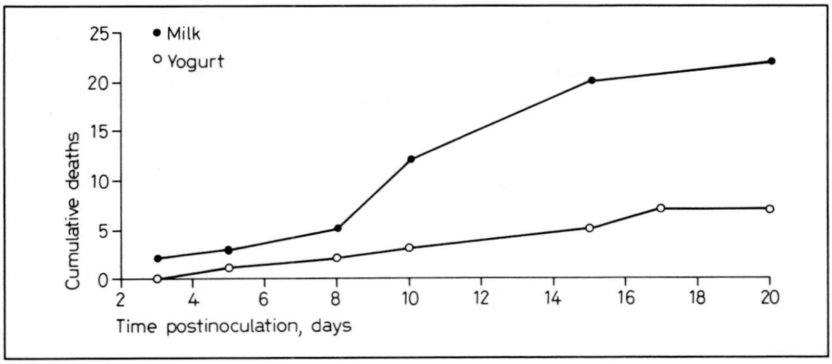

Fig. 10. Cumulative mortality according to the diet after intragastric inoculation with *Salmonella enteritidis.* From Hitchins et al. [1985a].

In another study, Hitchins et al. [1985b] supplemented the initial milk with the recommended amounts of vitamins and minerals, which did not alter the preceding results. Moreover, an intraperitoneal inoculation of this same Salmonella demonstrated no difference between the 'milk' and 'yogurt' groups, which suggests that the protective effect of yogurt against infectious challenge originates at the gastrointestinal level.

In addition, when two groups of rats were challenged intragastrically with *S. enteritidis* (after 7 days on a 'milk' or 'yogurt' diet) and then fed either with the same diet (milk/milk), (yogurt/yogurt) or with the other diet (yogurt/milk), (milk/yogurt), it was shown that the group kept continuously on a yogurt diet survives best, while the other dietary groups show greater mortality incidences. Therefore, the authors concluded that the continuous consumption of yogurt, both pre- and postinoculation, was necessary for it to play a protective role.

In a third study, Hitchins et al. [1986] demonstrated that the previously observed resistance to infectious challenge is not due to yogurt acidity but seems to be related to the lactose content. Thus, a milk with hydrolyzed lactose prevents weight gain deceleration and the death of inoculated animals, contrarily to the milk consumption. In other words, the consumption of milk with hydrolyzed lactose exerts a protective effect in animals inoculated with *S. enteritidis.* It can be concluded that the presence of lactose in their diet renders rats more susceptible to gastrointestinal salmonellosis, an effect which, according to the authors, is probably related to the low digestibility of lactose in rats after weaning.

The yogurt antimicrobial effect against numerous pathogenic species was shown in some in vitro studies [Yazicioglu and Yilmaz, 1966]. What should be mainly mentioned is the sensitivity to yogurt, demonstrated by an *E. coli* pathogenic strain and a *P. aeruginosa* strain, which are both resistant to a great number of antibiotics. The filtrate obtained through a gauze is also active.

The in vitro *S. typhimurium* growth is inhibited by yogurt, as well as that of other Salmonella and *S. sonnei*. This inhibition is enhanced by the adjunction of human gastric juice to the medium [Alm, 1983] whereas it is decreased by the addition of saline.

Wong et al. [1983] reported that yogurt, in vitro, is provided with antimicrobial proprieties as well as milk supplemented with *L. bulgaricus* or *S. thermophilus*.

The study of the yogurt-isolated ferments' effects gives evidence of inhibitory activities of high interest: the *L. bulgaricus* culture supernatant demonstrates an anti-*E. coli* activity. In addition, *L. bulgaricus* also exerts an anti-*E. coli* enterotoxin activity and half of this activity is found in the supernatant after centrifugation [Mitchell and Kenworthy, 1976]. Furthermore, *S. thermophilus* exerts an in vitro inhibitory effect against a great number of pathogenic organisms [Dubois et al., 1982; Rao et al., 1981; Pulusani et al., 1979] as well as *L. bulgaricus* [Pulusani et al., 1979; Shanani et al., 1976] and the mixed cultures of *S. thermophilus* and *L. bulgaricus* [Abou-Donia et al., 1980].

Effect on Cholesterolemia

Mann [1977] demonstrated that, in adults, the daily supplementation of 2 and 4 liters of whole yogurt, during 12 days, results in a drop of cholesterolemia which reaches its minimal level at day 16 and at day 20, respectively, and returns to its initial value at day 28. A daily consumption of 2 liters of skimmed yogurt during 12 days results in a more significant decrease in cholesterolemia whereas the daily intake of 2 liters of whole milk does not modify cholesterolemia.

According to Mann, yogurt would contain an agent inhibiting the cholesterol synthesis from acetate. He suggests that the hydroxymethylglutarate (HMG) present in yogurt would inhibit the HMG-CoA reductase. In a thorough analysis of the yogurt and initial milk constituents, Haggerty et al. [1984] demonstrated that, in fact, HMG cannot be found in milk nor in yogurt. On the contrary, a coeluant HMG can be found in yogurt in a higher or lower amount than in milk according to the strains used for fermentation.

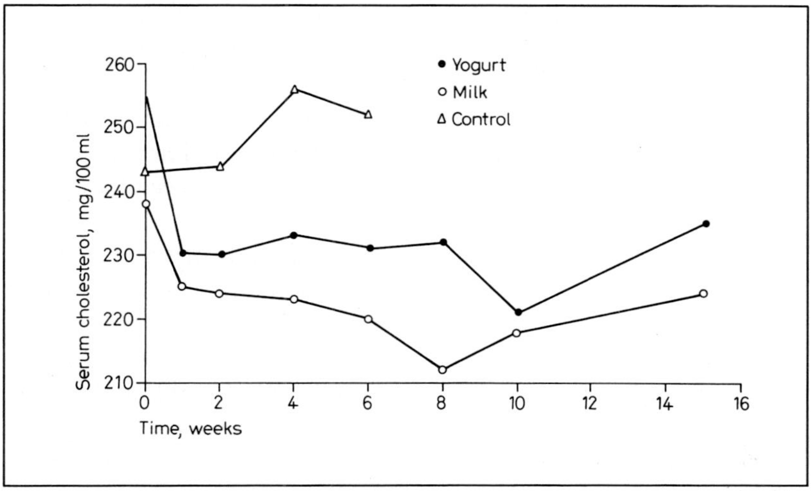

Fig. 11. Effect of milk or yogurt supplementation (12 weeks) on cholesterolemia in man (lipid and cholesterol intakes are the same for the three groups). From Hepner et al. [1979].

In man, Hepner et al. [1979] demonstrated that the supplementation of the regular diet with three 240-ml cups of yogurt (2% fat) or milk (2% fat) per day for 12 weeks results, as compared to the control group (no supplementation) in a significant reduction of the serum cholesterol level at the end of one week, a reduction being higher with yogurt than with milk (fig. 11). There are no significant changes in the triglycerides nor in the subjects' weight. The three groups received a similar diet (calories, cholesterol, lipids and fibers, proteins and carbohydrates) except for calcium intakes. This suggests that the effects obtained are independent of alterations in the major dietary constituents.

Rossouw et al. [1981] compared the effects in young boys of a daily diet supplemented with 2 liters of skimmed milk, whole milk or yogurt (1.8% fat) for 3 weeks. The 'skimmed' milk supplementation resulted in a drop of the serum cholesterol level correlated with a decrease in the amount of ingested lipids. Yogurt and whole milk caused an increase in the serum cholesterol level followed by a return to normal, while the amounts of cholesterol and lipids ingested during this time rose significantly. The serum triglyceride level tended to decrease in the three groups. One week after the end of supplementation, all values returned to normal, except total cholesterol in the 'skimmed milk' group and triglycerides in the three groups (values lower than those recorded before supplementation).

According to Rossouw, the serum cholesterol level's return to normal, occurring after the second week of supplementation with whole milk and yogurt, results from a physiological process of adaptation to an uncommon cholesterol and lipid load rather than from the presence of a hypocholesterolemic factor.

Thompson et al. [1982] supplemented the daily diet of their subjects (a diet including 250 ml of 2% fat milk) with either 1 liter of skimmed milk, or 1 liter of 2% fat milk, or 1 liter of whole milk, or 1 liter of 2% fat yogurt, for 3 weeks. The various types of supplementation resulted in an increase in the energy intake (which is the case of whole milk and yogurt), an increase in the lipid intake (as for whole milk) or a decrease in this last intake (which is the case of skimmed milk). The cholesterol intakes were not quantified. Total cholesterol, high-density lipoprotein cholesterol (HDL-cholesterol) and low-density lipoprotein cholesterol (LDL-cholesterol) remained unchanged, whereas a slight increase in the triglyceride level was observed with yogurt.

In a study achieved by Bazzarre et al. [1983] in 16 young women assigned for one week to a diet supplemented with around 750 g of (1% fat) yogurt per day (in three doses), then for one week to the regular diet, and then for one week to a diet including three doses of 250 mg of calcium carbonate per day, and at last to a regular diet again for one week, the following results were obtained: the 'yogurt' supplementation resulted in a reduction of total cholesterol; the 'yogurt' and 'calcium' supplementations resulted in an increase in the HDL-cholesterol level and in the HDL/total cholesterol ratio. The lipid and cholesterol ingesta were unknown.

Jaspers et al. [1984] carried out a 21-day study on the effect of the consumption of three types of non-fat yogurts corresponding to different symbioses in man. Subjects were asked to consume 680 g of yogurt per day in addition to their 'regular' diet. Diets were balanced in such a way that there was no difference between the usual diet and the 'yogurt' diets as far as concerns the energy intakes, proteins, carbohydrates, lipids, saturated, polyunsaturated fatty acids, and cholesterol levels. The difference mainly lay in the calcium (and phosphorus) level, since the intakes provided by the regular diet represented half of those provided by the 'yogurt' diets.

The three types of yogurts demonstrated a reduction of total cholesterol within 7 or 14 days according to the strains, followed or not by a return to the initial value during the study. For one of the yogurts, within 7 days, HDL-cholesterol decreased significantly before increasing, whereas it remained unchanged with the two other types of yogurts. Within 14 days, LDL-cholesterol demonstrated a significant reduction for two types of yogurt, whereas it underwent no change with the third type of yogurt. Triglycerides underwent no change. Therefore, these results suggest that the effect on total cholesterolemia and the cholesterol of various lipoproteins depends upon the ferment strains used for yogurt manufacture (fig. 12a–c).

Thakur and Jha [1981] gave rabbits for 16 weeks a diet with a high cholesterol content, on the one hand, and the same diet supplemented either with milk, or with yogurt (fat content not specified), or with calcium, on the other hand. The calcium contents of the diets with a high cholesterol content and supplemented with milk or yogurt were similar to and twice as high as that of the diet with a high cholesterol content and supplemented with calcium. The calcium content of the diets with a high cholesterol content and supplemented with milk or yogurt was three times as high as that of the diet with a high cholesterol content and with no supplementation. In the 'cholesterol + milk' group, the cholesterolemia underwent a less significant increase than in the 'cholesterol only' group, but a more significant increase than in the 'cholesterol + yogurt' and 'cholesterol + calcium' groups which demonstrated a significant decrease in cholesterolemia after the 12th week (fig. 13). There were significant aortic lesions in the 'cholesterol only' group, no lesions in the 'cholesterol + yogurt' group and intermediate lesions in the 'cholesterol + milk' and 'cholesterol + calcium' groups. Therefore, this study suggests that calcium may be one of the agents responsible for the yogurt hypocholesterolemic effect.

Boguslawski and Wrobel [1974] demonstrated that cow's milk exerts an inhibitory effect against cholesterol hepatic synthesis, both in vivo (in rats) and in vitro.

Effect on Immunity

Conge et al. [1980] supplemented the regular diet of mice with yogurt (amounting to 35% of their diet). After 10–13 weeks of supplementation, some of the animals were vaccinated (antitetanic vaccination) and kept on the 'yogurt'-supplemented diet until they were sacrificed on the 15th week. An effect specific to vaccination (increase in the IgG1, IgA) as well as an effect specific to yogurt ingestion (increase in the IgG2a) were observed. Besides, in the vaccinated animals, the spleens of the yogurt-fed mice were hyperactive as compared to those of the control animals. In the same way,

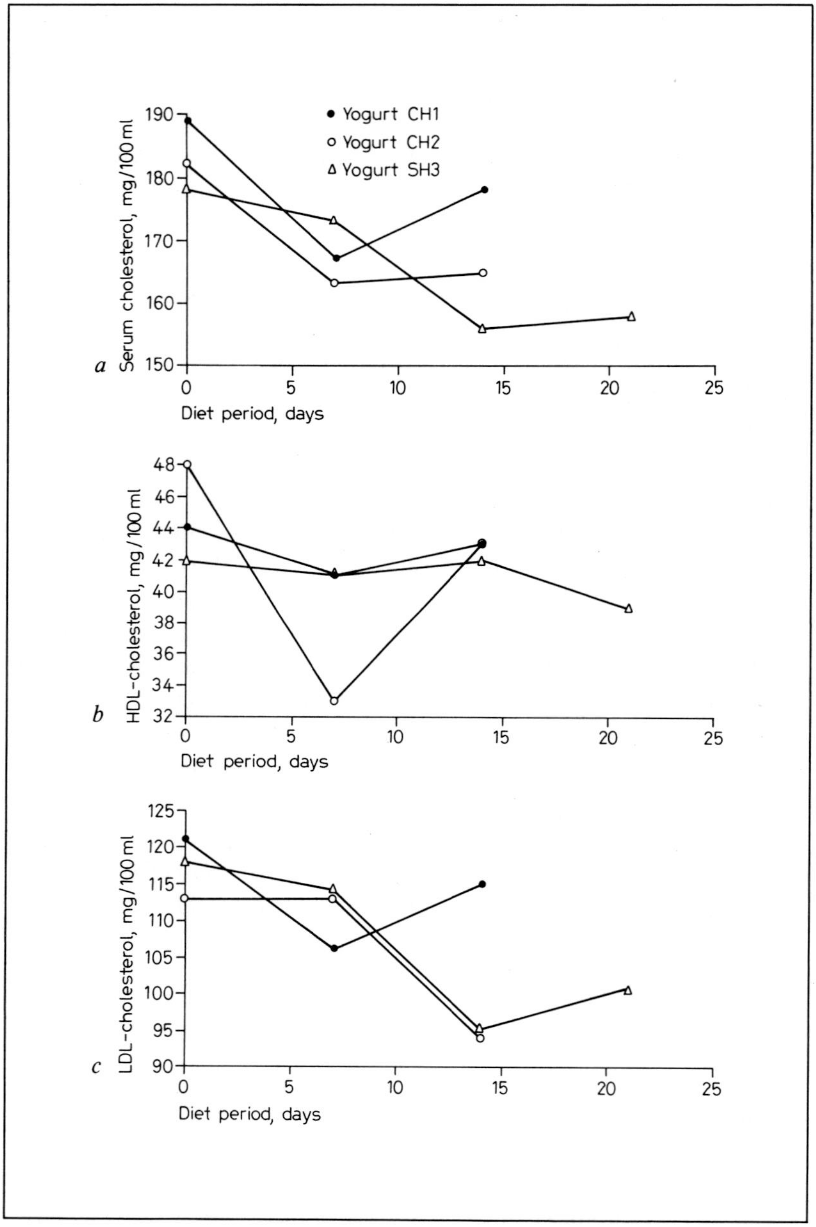

Fig. 12. Effect of consuming yogurts prepared with three culture strains: *a* on human serum cholesterol; *b* on human serum HDL-cholesterol; *c* on human serum LDL-cholesterol. From Jaspers et al. [1984].

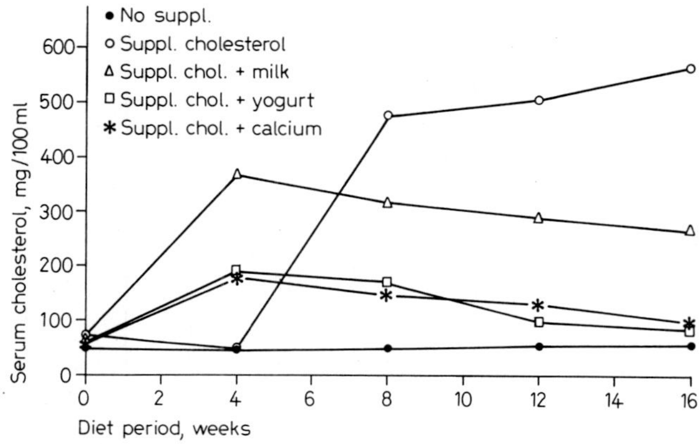

Fig. 13. Influence of various supplementations of rabbit diet on induced hypercholesterolemia. From Thakur et al. [1981].

in the non-vaccinated animals, the spleens of the yogurt-fed mice were less active than those of the corresponding vaccinated group, but remained nevertheless more active than the spleens of control mice (these differences involving both B and T cells). Thus, Conge et al. [1980] demonstrated that the two types of immunity responses are modified by the ingestion of yogurt. These effects were also shown by Vesely et al. [1985].

The addition of yogurt to a culture of human lymphocytes does not result, under the study conditions, in any increase in the production of γ-interferon (γIFN) by cells. On the contrary, the adjunction of concanavalin A to a culture of human lymphocytes enhances the production and salting-out of γIFN by cells. De Simone et al. [1986] demonstrated that the addition of yogurt to this medium increases significantly the amount of γIFN produced (fig. 14). Therefore, yogurt has the property of potentiating the production of γIFN by the human lymphocytes stimulated by the concanavalin A (a mitogen stimulus).

Moreover, the incubation of lymphocytes with the medium supernatant in which the γIFN production was achieved results in an increase in the NK activity ('natural killer'), an effect demonstrated against some tumorous cells. The authors give evidence of a relation between these effects of yogurt and ferments, since the yogurt filtrate exerts no stimulat-

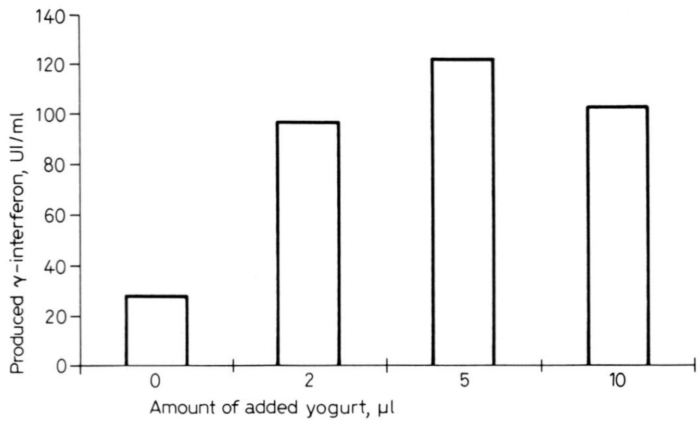

Fig. 14. The adjuvant effect of yogurt on the production of γ-interferon by concanavalin A-stimulated human peripheral blood lymphocytes (an in vitro study). From De Simone et al. [1986].

ing effect on the γIFN production. Though *L. bulgaricus* and *S. thermophilus* are both active, the former appears to be more active than the latter.

Effect on Growth

A 4-week study, carried out in rats by Hargrove and Alford [1978], showed that the 'yogurt' diet inducs a better growth than the 'milk' one (the initial milk being supplemented with iron and copper and fortified with skimmed milk powder), this effect being independent of the fat content of the initial milk (1.5 or 3.6% fat).

The initial milk supplementation with vitamins (in this case, a 1.5% fat milk) always resulted in a superior growth in the 'yogurt' group than in the 'milk' one. Besides, yogurt and milk supplemented with vitamins showed a higher growth-stimulating effect than that of the corresponding non-supplemented food products. As compared to milk, yogurt only demonstrated a superior 'feed efficiency' when considering food products containing 1.5% fat, with or without any vitamin supplementation.

In a 4-week study, in rats, McDonough et al. [1982] compared the effect on growth of milk fortified with iron, copper, vitamins and skimmed milk powder to that of the yogurt manufactured from this milk. They showed that the growth-stimulating effect (weight gain) and the feed efficiency were higher with yogurt than with milk. Similar results were obtained when using freeze-dried diets. The 'yogurt' and 'milk' diets gave respectively results similar to those of the freeze-dried 'yogurt' and freeze-dried milk diets. This is the reason why there is a growing tendency among the authors to use freeze-dried diets, for obvious practical reasons.

In a 4-week feeding experiment in rats, Wong et al. [1983] demonstrated higher values in 'yogurt'-fed rats than in 'milk'-fed rats (a milk supplemented with skimmed milk powder as well as iron and copper from which yogurt is manufactured) as fas as concerns weight gain and feed efficiency.

Milk added with the yogurt ferments (10^8/ml), either sonicated or not, also gave better weight gain and feed efficiency than milk. Milk added with *S. thermophilus* (either sonicated or not) gave similar results. The above-mentioned diets presented as being 'superior to milk' were approximately all equivalent. According to the authors, the superiority of milk with added *S. thermophilus,* as compared to milk, can only be demonstrated when the amount of live cells is at least 10^7/g. Therefore, *S. thermophilus* seems to lie at the roots of the yogurt superiority as compared to milk.

When considering freeze-dried products, it can be seen that yogurt, as well as milk with added *S. thermophilus,* increased significantly the 'feed efficiency' and the weight gain as compared to milk, whereas milk with added *L. bulgaricus* as well as the supernatants, either of *L. bulgaricus* or *S. thermophilus* cultures, demonstrated no growth-stimulating effect. From these results, the authors concluded that, in rats, the growth-stimulating effect of yogurt (as compared to milk) must be related to the *S. thermophilus* cells rather than to the changes undergone during milk fermentation.

During a 3-week experiment, Broussalian and Westhoff [1983] fed rats either with freeze-dried milk, or with freeze-dried 'yogurt', or with freeze-dried hydrolyzed lactose milk or yogurt. In this case, the freeze-dried milk contained 43.6% of lactose against 32.7% for freeze-dried 'yogurt'. The initial milk was supplemented with skimmed milk powder, iron, copper and vitamins. This study offered the advantage of specifying the lactose content of the freeze-dried products. With hydrolyzed products, no significant difference was observed, over the 3 weeks, between milk and yogurt as far as concerns weight gain and feed efficiency. During the first week, the 'yogurt'-fed group weight gain was similar to that of the 'milk'-fed group, but lower than that of the 'hydrolyzed diets'-fed rats. During the second week, the 'yogurt'-fed rats' weight gain became similar to that of the 'hydrolyzed diets'-fed groups, i.e. higher than that of the 'milk'-fed group, and during the third week, the weight gain was similar in all rats. At last, within the end of the third week, the 'yogurt'-fed group total weight gain became as important as the total weight gain of the 'hydrolyzed diets'-fed groups, contrarily to the 'milk' rats. During the first 2 weeks, the 'yogurt'-fed rats' 'feed efficiency' was higher than in the 'milk'-fed rats, and similar to that of the 'hydrolyzed diets'-fed groups, whereas during the third week, the 'yogurt'-fed rats' 'feed efficiency' was similar to that of the 'milk'-fed group but higher than those of the rats on 'hydrolyzed diets'.

In rats fed with 'non-hydrolyzed' diets, lactose-intolerance symptoms were observed during the first 2 weeks (diarrhea) which ended on the third week. When taking account of the weight gain and 'feed efficiency' results, it seems that the 'yogurt'-fed rats adapted themselves to the lactose load more rapidly than the 'milk'-fed rats. However, it must be kept in mind that the amount of lactose ingested in the yogurt form was less important.

Since a high concentration of lactose exerts an adverse effect against rats' growth, it seems that, as compared to milk, yogurt does not stimulate growth but rather retards it less significantly than milk. It can be suggested that the lower lactose content of yogurt, as compared to milk (see the above-mentionned lactose contents) as well as the lactase activity provided by yogurt (an assumption of a great number of authors) could account for the fact that rats' growth is higher with the 'yogurt' diet than with the 'milk' one, the growth of 'yogurt'-fed rats being close to that of 'hydrolyzed diets'-fed rats.

During a 6-week feeding experiment, as part of a diversified diet, supplemented with vitamins and minerals, Vass et al. [1984] gave rats either some freeze-dried 'yogurt' or milk, or casein as a protein source, in proportions forming a similar macronutriment composition. In the 'yogurt'-fed rats, weight gain was higher than in the rats of a 'milk' diet, these last demonstrating also a higher weight gain than in the 'casein'-fed animals (fig. 15). The calculation of the proteic utilization index (weight gain/total proteic intake) gave results that can be superimposed. Therefore, the yogurt biological value is higher than that of milk which is itself higher than that of casein (see also p. 222).

In a 4-week study in rats, McDonough et al. [1985] compared the effect of freeze-dried diets on growth (milk fortified with skimmed milk powder and supplemented or not with vitamins and minerals, as well as the yogurt manufactured from this milk).

When products were not supplemented with vitamins and minerals, the diets were vitamins D-, E-, B_1-, PP-, B_6-, and B_{12}-deficient as well as

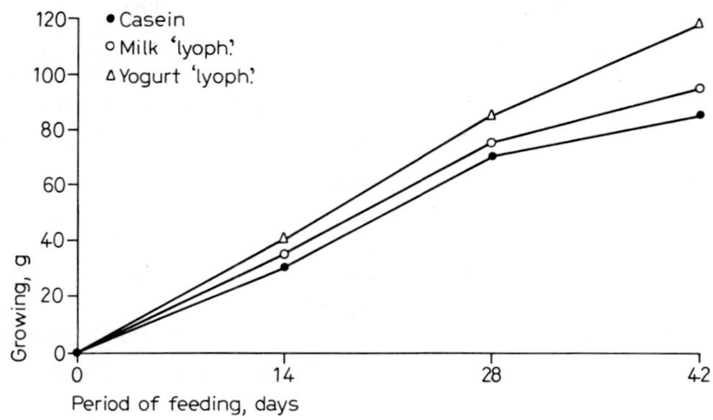

Fig. 15. Influence of the diet on rat growth. From Vass et al. [1984].

iron-, copper- and manganese-deficient. The 'yogurt' diet stimulated growth far more significantly than the 'milk' diet, which is due to an increase in the 'feed efficiency'. It was observed that the supplementation of diets with vitamins (a complete vitamin mix corresponding to the recommended intakes) does not affect growth (no significant change as compared to the preceding case).

The iron and copper addition to the initial milk improved rats' growth as compared to unfortified milk. In the same way, rats fed with the 'yogurt supplemented with iron and copper' diet showed a higher growth than the animals on the 'yogurt with no supplementation of these minerals' diet. Yet, as compared to milk supplemented with iron and copper, the superiority of yogurt fortified with iron and copper was shown. On the contrary, a 'complete' mineral fortification reduced all differences between the 'yogurt' and 'milk' diets. It seems that the addition of copper and iron to the diet caused a reduction of the manganese absorption, since the amount of manganese found in the livers of the animals fed with milk and yogurt supplemented with iron and copper was lower than that in the livers of the animals kept on unfortified milk and yogurt diets. Thus, whereas the vitamin supplementation does not seem to play a significant part, the mineral fortification (a mineral complex providing the recommended intakes) cancels all differences between milk and yogurt as regards rats' growth.

In rats, Schmidt et al. [1984] assessed liver regeneration after a partial hepatectomy within a 3-week feeding with milk or yogurt added to a vitamin- and mineral-fortified basic diet. The amount of milk or yogurt contained in the mix was twice as high as that of the basic diet. Rats fed with a yogurt-supplemented diet demonstrated a more significant liver regeneration and a higher growth than rats fed with a milk-supplemented diet. The regenerated liver composition was similar to that of the initial liver.

Relations with the Carcinogenesis Processes

Bogdanov et al. [1978] isolated a glycopeptide fragment from the cell wall of *L. bulgaricus* called blastolysin. This substance demonstrated a specific effect against sarcoma S180, the tumor which was found to be most sensitive to blastolysin. It should be noted that the blastolysin effect was only obtained when treatment (by intravenous injection) began 7–9 days after tumor subcutaneous inoculation. After a single blastolysin intravenous injection, the tumor demonstrated a total necrosis in 30% of mice while in the remaining 70% of animals the tumor continued to grow, although much more slowly than in the control animals. It is interesting to note that tissues with a high proliferative activity showed no changes. Blastolysin inhibited neither erythropoiesis nor leukopoiesis. Moreover, in the animals with tumors, an increase in the leukocyte count was found 24 h after injection of this substance. The fact that blastolysin has no action on tumors in vitro, the leukemoid reaction which it induces, indicates that the activation of the immunological mechanisms seems to play a major part in the antitumor action of blastolysin.

In mice, after intraperitoneal inoculation of Ehrlich tumor cells on day 0, Ayebo et al. [1981] fed mice with yogurt dialysate or retentate, freeze-dried and diluted with water, from day 1 to day 7, while the control animals drank milk. The animals fed with yogurt dialysate demonstrated a 32% reduction of the tumorous cell count and a 23–26% reduction in the DNA synthesis, an effect which was not observed with the yogurt retentate. Therefore, the antitumor compound can be dialyzed.

Besides, the writers collected the yogurt water-soluble fraction during an ether extraction, an aqueous phase they freeze-dried and subsequently diluted with sterile saline water they administered to animals, by intravenous or intraperitoneal injection, on day 1. After the intraperitoneal injection, a reduction of the tumorous cell count as well as the DNA synthesis was observed, yet this reduction was less significant than that caused by the intravenous injection (a 25% reduction of the tumorous cell count/a 32% DNA synthesis reduction). As a conclusion, these authors suggested that the 'antitumor' compound has a low molecular weight, less than 14,000, and is not chemically bound to the cell solid fraction since it can be separated by dialysis.

In another experiment, Ayebo et al. [1982] described the purification of the yogurt dialysate by ion-exchange chromatography and the determination of the in vitro and in vivo antitumor action. Thus, the dialysate was divided into anionic, cationic and neutral fractions. In the in vitro tests, neither the dialysate nor the fractions showed an inhibitory effect. On the contrary, when administered by intravenous injection on day 1, while the Ehrlich tumor cells were inoculated on day 0 and mice were sacrificed on day 8, the dialysate and the anionic fraction exhibited a high tumor-inhibitory effect. Several assumptions can explain the reason why the dialysate and the anionic fraction are provided with an inhibitory effect in vivo which is not demonstrated in vitro: the antitumor compounds might be inactive when they are ingested and then metabolized into an active form, or the inactive form might stimulate the host immunological response against the tumor without exerting a direct action.

Friend et al. [1982] showed, in mice, that the consumption of yogurt diluted 3:1 with water reduces the Ehrlich tumor growth while the consumption of yogurt cells cultivated on an APT broth – Difco All-Purpose Tween broth (glucose/broth)/Difco laboratories, Detroit, Mich. – and resuspended in saline water demonstrates no inhibitory effect.

'Test' injections were carried out from day 1 to day 4 and animals were sacrificed on day 5. The intraperitoneal injection of yogurt cells – cultivated on an APT broth before being resuspended in saline water – exhibited a reduction of the tumorous cell development. On the contrary, with the intraperitoneal injection of the APT broth in which the yogurt ferments multiplication was achieved (broth containing no ferment), demonstrated no reduction, which suggests that the 'antitumor' compound is not exocellular. Part of the yogurt ferments culture, resuspended in saline water, was sonicated and centrifuged, which allowed one to collect the supernatant and the 'insoluble' fraction. When intraperitoneally injected, the 'insoluble' fraction demonstrated a reduction of the tumor development which was not the case with the 'soluble' fraction. The *L. bulgaricus* or *S. thermophilus* ferments, when intraperitoneally injected, exhibited an inhibitory activity. Therefore, the authors concluded that the 'antitumor' compound is not exocellular but related to the cell-insoluble material.

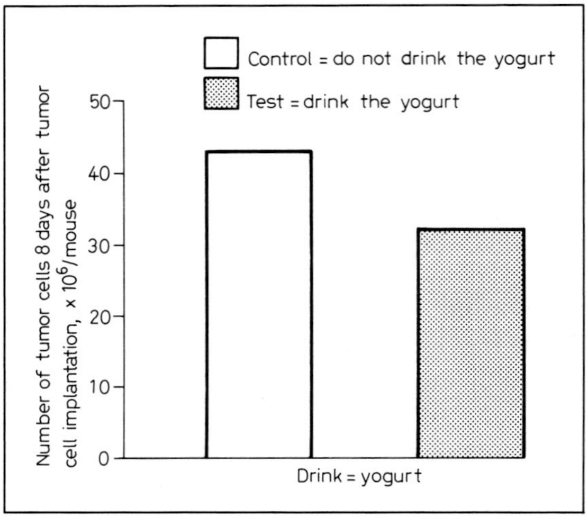

Fig. 16. Effect of feeding yogurt on Ehrlich tumor cell proliferation in mice. From Reddy et al. [1983].

In mice, which were intraperitoneally inoculated with Ehrlich tumor cells on day 0, Reddy et al. [1983] showed that the consumption of yogurt diluted 3:1 with water from day 1 to day 7 exhibits from 24 to 28% inhibition of tumor cell proliferation and from 23 to 31% inhibition of DNA synthesis (fig. 16). Milk and the lactic acid solution exhibited no effect on the tumor cell progression. Yogurt prefeeding for 7 days before inoculation, and feeding for 7 days after inoculation, did not improve the observed tumor reduction. Besides, when feeding with yogurt after inoculation was delayed, the yogurt inhibitory effect was significantly decreased: indeed, when yogurt feeding was only initiated 4 days after inoculation, yogurt had no longer antitumor activity. The yogurt centrifugation showed that the inhibitory effect against the tumor development results from the solid fraction. Yogurt dilution in water demonstrated that the effect is proportional to the amount of yogurt added to the drink. Though yogurt ingestion inhibited the tumor growth in its initial stage, it did not retard death in mice.

In mice, Shahani et al. [1983] investigated the effect on the development of the Ehrlich tumor cells played by the ingestion of colostrum fermented by *L. bulgaricus* or by *L. bulgaricus* and *S. thermophilus* as well as that of milk fermented by *L. bulgaricus,* given as a drink (i.e. diluted in

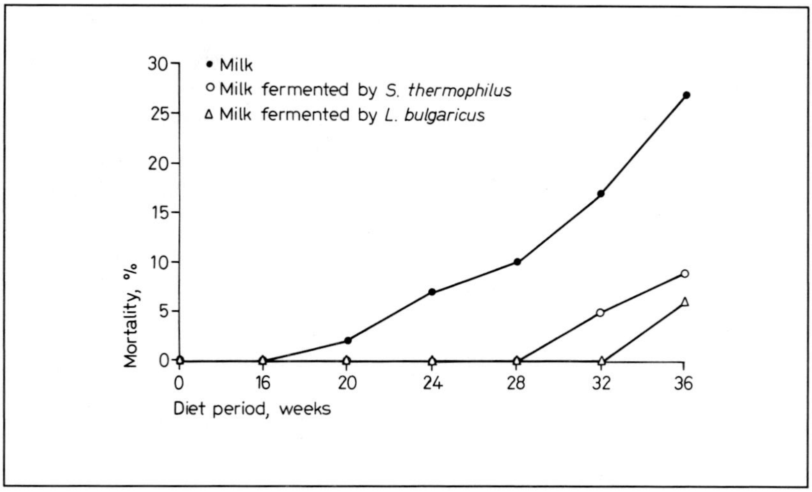

Fig. 17. Mortality of rats after injections of dimethylhydrazine related to the kind of drink consumed. From Shackelford et al. [1983].

some water in a 3:1 fermented milk/water ratio). Tumor cells were implanted on day 0 and the diet was fed ad libitum from day 1 through day 7, while the control animals received non-fermented colostrum. Mice were sacrificed on day 8. As compared to non-fermented colostrum, fermented milk and colostrum reduced the tumor cell counts by 16–40% and DNA synthesis by 20–35%. No significant difference was reported between products fermented by *L. bulgaricus* and those fermented by *L. bulgaricus* and *S. thermophilus.* Furthermore, colostrum provided no additional inhibitory effect as compared to milk.

Besides, Shackelford et al. [1983] studied, in rats, the result of feeding with skim milk, and skim milk fermented by *S. thermophilus* or *L. bulgaricus,* given as drinks, on the effect of dimethylhydrazine (DMH), injected s.c. once a week for 20 weeks, drinks being given 2 weeks before the first injection and continuously through week 36. Control animals were given water, and received saline water injections. At the end of the experiment, the group supplemented with milk fermented by *L. bulgaricus* had a 93% survival rate, whereas animals fed with milk fermented with *S. thermophilus* showed a 90% survival rate, and the milk-fed group demonstrated a 73% survival rate. All control animals survived (fig. 17). No tumor was found in the control group whereas the incidence of colon tumors was not affected by the diet. Rats receiving milk fermented by *S. thermophilus* had a higher incidence of small intestine tumors when compared to rats given milk or milk fermented by *L. bulgaricus.* On the other hand, the number of rats with ear-duct tumors was significantly higher in the milk group as compared to the fermented milks groups. Fermented milks play a protective role against DMH-induced mortality, and affect the location of tumors (carrying them from the ear-duct to the small intestine).

In another type of experiment, Cole et al. [1984] showed that chickens receiving a yogurt-water mix as drink (yogurt accounting for 40% of the mix) demonstrate, as compared to control animals (receiving water), a reduction of the activity of the β-glucuronidase, a fecal enzyme likely to convert procarcinogenic substances into carcinogenic substances.

Modification of the 'Health' Effects by Means of Various Treatments

Freeze-Drying

Effect on the Animals' Growth. On various occasions, we have seen that the freeze-drying of the 'yogurt' and 'milk' diets did not alter the growth stimulation achieved with the yogurt diet as compared to the milk diet, under incomplete mineral supplementation conditions. Freeze-drying conditions are only specified for three of the five works mentioned below. Yogurt freeze-drying resulted in a 97% reduction of the number of live ferments in the experiment carried out by Wong et al. [1983] (a reduction from 5.6×10^8 to 10^7/g) whereas it induced a decrease in the number of live ferments, ranging from 90 to 95% in the studies performed by McDonough et al. [1982, 1985] (a falling from $5–9 \times 10^8$ to $2.5–9 \times 10^7$/g) [Wong et al., 1983, McDonough et al, 1982; Vass et al., 1984; Broussalian and Westhoff, 1983; McDonough et al, 1985].

Heat Treatment

Effect on Lactase Activity. Savaiano et al. [1984] demonstrated that yogurt heating at 63 °C for 30 min results in a changing of the number of live ferments from 3×10^8 to 3.4×10^6/g of product – and in a reduction of lactase activity by 10-fold. In addition, in lactase-deficient subjects, breath hydrogen values were reported to be significantly higher after the ingestion of the heated product than after the ingestion of yogurt. This results suggest that, contrarily to yogurt, the heated product provides no lactase activity to the lactase-deficient subject (fig. 18).

When Besnier et al. [1983] administered during 42 days to germ-free or conventional, just-weaned mice, as drinks, the product resulting from yogurt heating at 100 °C during 15 min, they observed that the total lactase activity of the small intestine wall is significantly reduced in the germ-free animals and slightly decreased in the conventional set of mice as compared to the values registered at the time of weaning. It must be remembered that yogurt consumption results in an increase in the total lactase activity of the small intestine wall in both sets of mice.

Effect on the Pathogenic Bacteria Growth. Experiments carried out in vitro by Yazicioglu and Yilmaz [1966] demonstrated that its heating does not inhibit the yogurt antibacterial effect against some pathogenic bacteria strains. This persistence of the antibacterial effect was confirmed by other writers, especially Pulusani et al. [1979] and ALM [1983].

Effect on Cholesterolemia. Hepner et al. [1979] demonstrated that the supplementation of the regular diet with three 240-ml cups of product resulting from yogurt heating (2% fat) per day for 12 weeks results in a significant reduction of the serum cholesterol level. The same reduction was observed with the yogurt-supplemented diet (fig. 19).

Effect on Immunity. Conge et al. [1980] as well as Vesely et al. [1985] showed that yogurt heating at 65 °C for 1 min in the first experiment, and at 90 °C for 15 min in the second experiment, results in a decrease in the immunity stimulation achieved by yogurt. Besides, yogurt heating (at 90 °C for 15 min) reduced its stimulating effect on the production of γIFN by the human lymphocytes stimulated by concanavalin A [De Simone et al., 1986].

Relations with the Carcinogenesis Processes. Yogurt ferments, cultivated on an APT broth (Difco Laboratories, Detroit, Mich.) then resuspended in saline water, and at last heated for 15 min at 121 °C before being administered to mice by intraperitoneal injection, exhibited no inhibitory effect on Ehrlich tumor cell development, whereas this development was reduced by the intraperitoneal injection of the non-heated saline suspension [Friend et al., 1982]. The authors assumed that there must be an 'antitumor' thermolabile factor, or the presence of live ferments allowing this factor to act. On the contrary, the decrease in the β-glucuronidase activity (observed in the cecal contents) in chickens ingesting yogurt was still reported when yogurt was heated at 80 °C for 20 min [Cole et al., 1984].

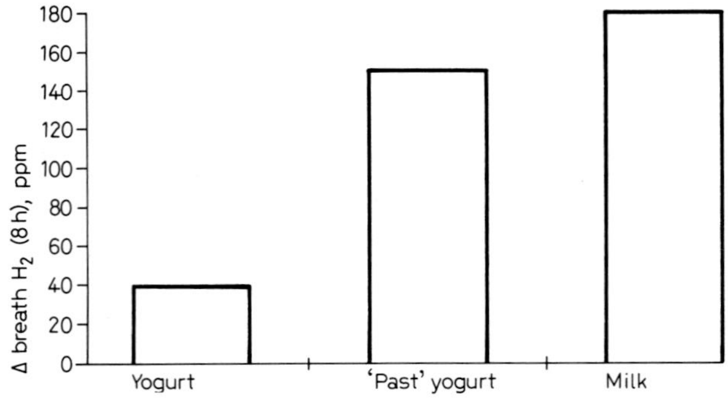

Fig. 18. Change in breath hydrogen after ingestion of several products in lactase-deficient subjects. From Savaiano et al. [1984].

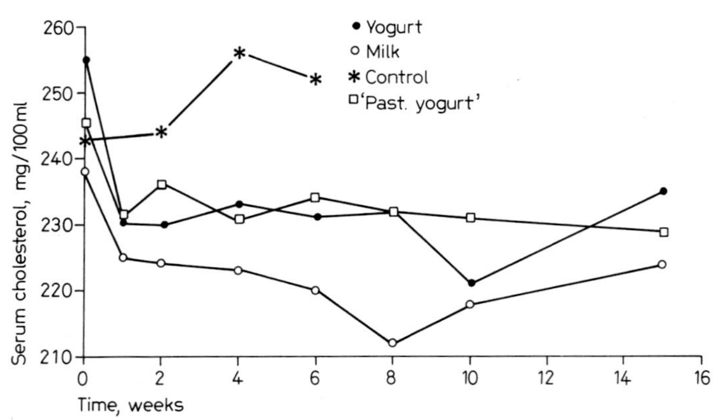

Fig. 19. Effect of milk or yogurt supplementation (12 weeks) on cholesterolemia in man (lipid and cholesterol intakes are the same for the three groups). From Hepner et al. [1979].

Conclusion

As compared to milk, yogurt offers a double nutritional and 'health' interest. Its 'health' properties, such as the providing of a lactase activity, the prophylactic and curative effect on some infections of the alimentary tract, the immunity stimulation ..., etc., are for most of them related to the flora 'live' feature. All over the world, a great number of researchers are interested in yogurt's probiotic properties, and insofar as the food industry provides us with a controlled, reliable product, whose ferments' viability is maintained by the cold chain, and taking account of the achieved works, we can do nothing but encourage its consumption.

References

Abou-Donia, S.A.; Ismail, A.A.; Salama, F.A.; Khader, A.E.; Abou-Zeid, N.A.: The inhibitory effect of some fermented milk flora on the growth of some pathogenic bacteria. Monoufeia J. agric. Res. *3:* 225–236 (1980).

Alm, L.: Effect of fermentation on lactose, glucose and galactose content in milk and suitability of fermented milk products for lactose intolerant individuals. J. Dairy Sci. *65:* 346–352 (1982a).

Alm, L.: Effect of fermentation on *L*(+) and *D*(–) lactic acid in milk. J. Dairy Sci. *65:* 515–520 (1982b).

Alm, L.: Effect of fermentation on milk fat of Swedish fermented milk products. J. Dairy Sci. *65:* 521–530 (1982c).

Alm, L.: Survival rate of Salmonella and Shigella in fermented milk products with and without added human gastric juice: an in vitro study. Prog. Fd Nutr. Sci. *7:* 19–28 (1983).

Ayebo, A.D.; Shahani, K.M.; Dam, R.: Antitumor component(s) of yogurt: fractionation. J. Dairy Sci. *64:* 2318–2323 (1981).

Ayebo, A.D.; Shahani, K.M.; Dam, R.; Friend, B.A.: Ion exchange separation of the antitumor component(s) of yogurt dialyzate. J. Dairy Sci. *65:* 2388–2390 (1982).

Balasubramanya, N.N.; Natarajan, A.M.; Rao, R.V.: Availability of calcium and phosphorus for albino rats from yoghurt. Asian J. Dairy Res. *3:* 131–134 (1984).

Bazzarre, T.L.; Liu Wu, S.; Yuhas, J.A.: Total and HDL-cholesterol concentrations following yogurt and calcium supplementation. Nutr. Rep. int. *28:* 1225–1232 (1983).

Besnier, M.O.; Bourlioux, P.; Fourniat, J.; Ducluzeau, R.; Aumaitre, A.: Influence de l'ingestion de yoghourt sur l'activité lactasique intestinale chez des souris axéniques ou holoxéniques. (Inst. Pasteur) Ann. Microbiol. *134A:* 219–230 (1983).

Bianchi Salvadori, B.; Brughera, F.; Salvadori, P.: Studio sulle variazioni coproculturali nel lattante, in rapporto alla somministrazione di yogurt. Minerva Diet. *7:* 176–180 (1967).

Bianchi Salvadori, B.; Camaschella, P.; Bazzigaluppi, E.: Distribution and adherence of *Lactobacillus bulgaricus* in the gastroenteric tract of germ-free animals. Milchwissenschaft *39:* 387–391 (1984).

Bianchi Salvadori, B.; Gotti, M.; Brughera, F.; Polinelli, U.: Etude sur les variations de la flore lactique et bifide intestinale par rapport à l'administration des cellules lactiques du yaourt. Lait *571/572:* 17–42 (1978).

Blanc, B.: Valeur nutritionelle du yaourt, aliment vivant. Symp. Int. sur les Effets Nutritionnels de la Flore Digestive, Paris 1981.

Boccignone, M.; Brigidi, R.; Sarra, C.: Studi effettuati sulla composizione in trigliceridi ed acidi grassi liberi nello yoghurt preparato da latte vaccino, pecorino e caprino. Annali Fac. Med. Vet. Torino *28:* 223–233 (1984).

Bogdanov, I.G.; Velichkov, V.T.; Gurevich, A.I.; Dalev, P.G.; Kolosov, M.N.; Mal'kova, V.P.; Sorokina, I.B.; Khristova, L.N.: Antitumor action of glycopeptides from the cell wall of *Lactobacillus bulgaricus.* Bull. Exp. Biol. Med. *84:* 1750–1753 (1978).

Boguslawski, W.; Wrobel, J.: An inhibitor of sterol biosynthesis present in cow's milk. Nature, Lond. *247:* 210–211 (1974).

Brand, J.C.; Darnton-Hill, I.; Gracey, M.S.; Spargo, R.M.: Lactose malabsorption in Australian aboriginal children. Am. J. clin. Nutr. *41:* 620–622 (1985).

Breslaw, E.S.; Kleyn, D.H.: In vitro digestibility of protein in yogurt at various stages of processing. J. Food Sci. *38:* 1016–1021 (1973).

Broussalian, J.; Westhoff, D.: Influence of lactose concentration of milk and yogurt on growth rate of rats. J. Dairy Sci. *66:* 438–443 (1983).

Bujanover, Y.; Katz, A.; Peled, Y.; Gilat, T.: Lactose malabsorption in Israeli children. Israel J. med. Sci. *21:* 32–35 (1985).

Burgio, G.R.; Flatz, G.; Barbera, C.; Patane, R.; Boner, A.; Cajozzo, C.; Flatz, S.D.: Prevalence of primary adult lactose malabsorption and awareness of milk intolerance in Italy. Am. J. clin. Nutr. *39:* 100–104 (1984).

Cochet, B.; Jung, A.; Griessen, M.; Bartholdi, P.; Schaller, P.; Donath, A.: Effects of lactose on intestinal calcium absorption in normal and lactase-deficient subjects. Gastroenterology *84:* 935–940 (1983).

Cole, C.B.; Anderson, P.H.; Philips, S.M.; Fuller, R.; Hewitt, D.: The effect of yoghurt on the growth, lactose-utilizing gut organisms and β-glucuronidase activity of caecal contents of a lactose-fed, lactase-deficient animal. Food Microbiol. *1:* 217–222 (1984).

Comité Mixte FAO/OMS d'Experts des Additifs Alimentaires (JECFA): Evaluation toxicologique de certains additifs alimentaires; examens des principes généraux et des normes. 17e rapport: (FAO/OMS, 1974).

Conge, G.; Gouache, P.; Desormeau-Bedot, J.; Loisillier, F.; Lemonnier, D.: Effets comparés d'un régime enrichi en yoghourt vivant ou thermisé sur le système immunitaire de la souris. Reprod. Nutr. Dev. *20:* 929–938 (1980).

Connor, H.; Woods, H.F.; Ledingham, J.G.G.: Comparison of the kinetics and utilisation of *D*(–) and *L*(+) sodium lactate in normal man. Annls Nutr. Metab. *27:* 481–487 (1983).

Cori, C.F.; Cori, G.T.: Glycogen formation in the liver from *D*- and *L*-lactic acid. J. biol. Chem. *81:* 389–403 (1929).

Costet, J.; Delmont, J.: Intolérances au lactose: un diagnostic simple à ne pas négliger. Méd. Digest. Nutr. *39:* 30–32 (1985).

Cuddenec, Y.; Delbruck, H.; Flatz, G.: Distribution of the adult lactase phenotypes – lactose absorber and malabsorber – in a group of 131 army recruits. Gastroentérol. clin. biol. *6:* 776–779 (1982).
Deeth, H.C.; Tamine, A.Y.: Yogurt: nutritive and therapeutic aspects. J. Food Protect. *44:* 78–86 (1981).
De Simone, C.; Bianchi Salvadori, B.; Negri, R.; Ferrazzi, M.; Baldinelli, L.; Vesely, R.: The adjuvant effect of yogurt on production of gamma-interferon by Con A-stimulated human peripheral blood lymphocytes. Nutr. Rep. int. *33:* 419–433 (1986).
De Vries, E.G.E.; Meyer, C.; Strubbe, M.; Mulder, N.H.: Influence of various beverages on urine acid output. Cancer Res. *46:* 430–432 (1986).
De Waard, H.; Stadhouders, J.: Het metabolisme van *D*(–)-melkzuur. Voedingsmiddelentechnologie *16:* 22–23 (1983).
Dewit, O.: Le yaourt a-t-il un intérêt nutritionnel en cas de malabsorption du lactose? Thèse, Paris (1985).
Dillon, J.C.; Macneil, J.; Senghor, G.: Intolerance to powdered milk among Senegalese children showing poor lactose absorption. Can. J. publ. Hlth *73:* 341–344 (1982).
Drury, D.R.; Wick, A.N.: Chemistry and metabolism of *L*(+) and *D*(–) lactic acids. Ann. N.Y. Acad. Sci. *119:* 1061–1069 (1965).
Dubois, G.; Smoragiewicz, W.; Charbonneau, R.; Gagnon, M.: Inhibition de quelques bactéries pathogènes et potentiellement pathogènes par *Streptococcus lactis, Streptococcus thermophilus, Lactobacillus acidophilus* et *Lactobacillus helveticus.* Lait *621/622:* 681–687 (1982).
Dupuis, Y.: Rapport no. 4/laits fermentés et minéralisation. Bull. Fil. (1974).
Ferguson, A.; Macdonald, D.M.; Brydon, W.G.: Prevalence of lactase deficiency in British adults. Gut *25:* 163–167 (1984).
Flatz, G.; Bernsau, I.; Behrens, A.: Lactose absorption and malabsorption in healthy German children: improved phenotypic resolution by simultaneous determination of breath hydrogen and carbon dioxide. Eur. J. Pediat. *138:* 304–306 (1982).
Flatz, G.; Kuhnau, W.; Naftali, D.: Breath hydrogen test for lactose absorption capacity: importance of timing of hydrogen excretion and of high fasting hydrogen concentratin. Am. J. clin. Nutr. *39:* 752–755 (1984).
Friend, B.A.; Farmer, R.E.; Shahani, K.M.: Effect of feeding and intraperitoneal implantation of yoghurt culture cells on Ehrlich ascites tumor. Milchwissenschaft *37:* 708–710 (1982).
Gilat, T.: Lactase deficiency: the world pattern today. Israel J. med. Sci. *15:* 369–373 (1979).
Goodenough, E.R.; Kleyn, D.H.: Influence of viable yogurt microflora on digestion of lactose by the rat. J. Dairy Sci. *59:* 601–606 (1976).
Guix Garcia, J.; Rodrigo Gomez, J.M.; Aparisi Quereda, L.; Serra Desfilis, M.A.; Garcia-Conde Gomez, F.J.: Intolerancia a la lactosa en la población española. Rev. esp. enf. ap. digest. *42:* 367–382 (1974).
Gurr, M.I.: The effect of feeding cultured dairy products on health. Bull. fil. *159:* 18–28 (1983).
Haggerty, R.J.; Luedecke, L.O.; Nagel, C.W.; Massey, L.K.: Effect of selected yogurt cultures on the concentration of orotic acid, uric acid and a hydroxymethylglutaric-like compound in milk after fermentation. J. Food Sci. *49:* 1194–1195 (1984).

Hargrove, R.E.; Alford, J.A.: Growth rate and feed efficiency of rats fed yogurt and other fermented milks. J. Dairy Sci. *61:* 11–19 (1978).

Hepner, G.; Fried, R.; St. Jeor, S.; Fusetti, L.; Morin, R.: Hypocholesterolemic effect of yogurt and milk. Am. J. clin. Nutr. *32:* 19–24 (1979).

Hitchins, A.D.; McDonough, F.E.; Wells, P.; Wong, N.P.: Relationship of dietary carbohydrate and lactic acid to the resistance of yogurt-fed male weanling rats to gastrointestinal salmonellosis. Nutr. Rep. int. *33:* 641–649 (1986).

Hitchins, A.D.; Wells, P.; McDonough, F.E.; Wong, N.P.: Amelioration of the adverse effect of a gastrointestinal challenge with Salmonella enteritidis on weanling rats by a yogurt diet. Am. J. clin. Nutr. *41:* 92–100 (1985a).

Hitchins, A.D.; Wells, P.; McDonough, F.E.; Wong, N.P.: A gastrointestinal and nonsystemic dietary effect of yogurt in the alleviation of rat salmonellosis. Nutr. Rep. int. *31:* 601–608 (1985b).

Jaspers, D.A.; Massey, L.K.; Luedecke, L.O.: Effect of consuming yogurts prepared with three culture strains on human serum lipoproteins. J. Food Sci. *49:* 1178–1181 (1984).

Jenkins, D.J.A.; Wolever, T.M.S.; Taylor, R.H.; Barker, H.; Fielden, H.; Baldwin, J.M.; Bowling, A.C.; Newman, H.C.; Jenkins, A.L.; Goff, D.V.: Glycemic index of foods: a physiological basis for carbohydrate exchange. Am. J. clin. Nutr. *34:* 362–366 (1981).

Jia Ju Zheng; Rosenberg, I.H.: Lactose malabsorption in healthy Chinese adults. Ecol. Food. Nutr. *15:* 1–6 (1984).

Judge, M.A.; Van Eys, J.: Excretion of *D*-lactic acid by humans. J. Nutr. *76:* 310–313 (1962).

Kilara, A.; Shahani, K.M.: Lactase activity of cultured and acidified dairy products. J. Dairy Sci. *59:* 2031–2035 (1976).

Klupsch, H.J.: The content and importance in sour milk products of *L*(+) and *D*(–) lactates. Nth Eur. Dairy J. *6:* 170–175 (1983).

Kolars, J.C.; Levitt, M.D.; Aouji, M.; Savaiano, D.A.: Yogurt – an autodigesting source of lactose. New Engl. J. Med. *310:* 1–3 (1984).

Mann, G.V.: A factor in yogurt which lowers cholesterolemia in man. Atherosclerosis *26:* 335–340 (1977).

McDonough, F.E.; Hitchins, A.D.; Wong, N.P.: Effects of yogurt and freeze-dried yogurt on growth stimulation of rats. J. Food. Sci. *47:* 1463–1465 (1982).

McDonough, F.E.; Wong, N.P.; Wells, P.; Hitchins, A.D.; Bodwell, C.E.: Stimulation of rat growth by yogurt – effect of vitamins and minerals. Nutr. Rep. int. *31:* 1237–1245 (1985).

Mitchell, I. de G.; Kenworthy, R.: Investigations on a metabolite from *Lactobacillus bulgaricus* which neutralizes the effect of enterotoxin from *Escherichia coli* pathogenic for pigs. J. appl. Bact. *41:* 163–174 (1976).

Mourot, J.; Thouvenot, P.; Antoine, J.M.; Debry, G.: Comparison of gastric emptying rate of yogurt and milk in man. 1st Int. Congr. Food and Health, Salsomaggiore Terme, Parma 1985.

Niv, M.; Levy, W.; Greenstein, N.M.: Yogurt in the treatment of infantile diarrhea. Clin. Pediat. *2:* 407–411 (1963).

Odet, G.: Quelques considérations sur la valeur alimentaire des produits laitiers frais. Cah. Nutr. Diét. *8:* 182–186 (1973).

Oh, M.S.; Uribarri, J.; Alveranga, D.; Lazar, I.; Bazilinski, N.; Carroll, H.J.: Metabolic utilization and renal handling of *D*-lactate in men. Metabolism *34:* 621–625 (1985).

Pacini, N.; Ferrari, A.; Canzi, E.; Bianchi-Salvadori, B.: Etude sur la microflore intestinale et sur les transformations biliaires chez des souris alimentées avec du yaourt. Lait *589-590:* 615–624 (1979).

Parente, F.; Sangaletti, O.; Vedova, G. della; Lazzaroni, M.; Petrillo, M.; Porro, G.B.: Measurement of expired hydrogen: an indirect method for diagnosis of lactose malabsorption. Clin. Lab. *7:* 170–180 (1983).

Pointillart, A.; Cayron, B.; Gueguen, L.: Utilisation du calcium et du phosphore et minéralisation osseuse chez le porc consommant du yaourt. Sci. Aliments *6:* 15–30 (1986).

Pulusani, S.R.; Rao, D.R.; Sunki, G.R.: Antimicrobial activity of lactic cultures: partial purification and characterization of antimicrobial compound(s) produced by *Streptococcus thermophilus.* J. Food Sci. *44:* 575–578 (1979).

Rao, D.R.; Reddy, J.C.: Effects of lactic fermentation of milk on milk lipids. J. Food Sci. *49:* 748–750 (1984).

Rao, D.R.; Reddy, B.M.; Sunki, G.R.; Pulusani, S.R.: Influence of antimicrobial compound(s) extracted from milk fermented by *Streptococcus thermophilus* on keeping quality of meat and milk. J. Food Quality *4:* 247–258 (1981).

Rasic, J.; Kurmann, J.A.: in Rasic, Kurmann, Fermented fresh milk products, vol. 1, pp. 69–87, 99–136 (1978).

Rasic, J.; Stojsavljevic, T.; Curcic, R.: A study on the amino acids of yoghurt. II. Amino acids content and biological value of the proteins of different kinds of yoghurt. Milchwissenschaft *26:* 219–224 (1971).

Reddy, G.V.; Friend, B.A.; Shahani, K.M.; Farmer, R.E.: Antitumor activity of yogurt components. J. Food Protect. *46:* 8–11 (1983).

Rossouw, J.E.; Burger, E.; Van der Vyver, P.; Ferreira, J.J.: The effect of skim milk, yoghurt and full cream milk on human serum lipids. Am. J. clin. Nutr. *34:* 351–356 (1981).

Salvadori, P.; Bianchi Salvadori, B.: Studio sulle variazioni coprocolturali nell'uomo in rapporto alla somministrazione di yogurt. Minerva diét. *14:* 8–12 (1973).

Savaiano, D.A.; Abouelanouar, A.; Smith, D.E.; Levitt, M.D.: Lactose malabsorption from yogurt, pasteurized yogurt, sweet acidophilus milk, and cultured milk in lactase-deficient individuals. Am. J. clin. Nutr. *40:* 1219–1223 (1984).

Schmidt, P.; Vass, A.; Szakaly, S.: Effect of fermented milk diets on regeneration of the rat liver. Acta med. hung. *41:* 163–169 (1984).

Shackelford, L.A.; Rao, D.R.; Chawan, C.B.; Pulusani, S.R.: Effect of feeding fermented milk on the incidence of chemically induced colon tumors in rats. Nutr. Cancer *5:* 159–164 (1983).

Shahani, K.M.; Friend, B.A.; Bailey, P.J.: Antitumor activity of fermented colostrum and milk. J. Food. Protect *46:* 385–386 (1983).

Shahani, K.M.; Vakil, J.R.; Kilara, A.: Natural antibiotic activity of *Lactobacillus acidophilus* and *bulgaricus.* Cult. Dairy Prod. J. *27:* 14–17 (1976).

Shapiro, S.: Control of antibiotic induced gastrointestinal symptoms with yogurt. Clin. Med. *7:* 295 (1960).

Simoons, F.J.: The geographic hypothesis and lactose malabsorption. A weighing of the evidence. Dig. Dis. *23:* 963–980 (1978).
Souci, S.W.; Fachmann, W.; Kraut, H.: Food composition and nutrition tables (1981/82) (Wissenschaftliche Verlagsgesellschaft, Stuttgart 1981).
Terre, S.: Caractérisation et production en continu de biométabolites du yaourt. Mémoire INRA, Rennes 1985.
Thakur, C.P.; Jha, A.N.: Influence of milk, yoghurt and calcium on cholesterol-induced atherosclerosis in rabbits. Atherosclerosis *39:* 211–215 (1981).
Thompson, L.U.; Jenkins, D.J.A.; Amer, V.; Reichert, R.; Jenkins, A.; Kamulsky, J.: The effect of fermented and unfermented milks on serum cholesterol. Am. J. clin. Nutr. *36:* 1106–1111 (1982).
Toba, T.; Watanabe, A.; Adachi, S.: Quantitative changes in sugars, especially oligosaccharides, during fermentation and storage of yogurt. J. Dairy Sci. *66:* 17–20 (1983).
Vass, A.; Szakaly, S.; Schmidt, P.: Experimental study of the nutritional biological characters of fermented milks. Acta med. hung. *41:* 157–161 (1984).
Vesely, R.; Negri, R.; Bianchi Salvadori, B.; Lavezzari, D.; De Simone, C.: Influence of a diet additioned with yogurt on the mouse immune system. Riv. Immunol. Immunofarmacol. *5:* 30–35 (1985).
Wagh, M.G.; Ghooi, R.B.; Shetty, R.K.: Lactose intolerance; physiological, clinical and therapeutic considerations. Indian J. Pediat. *51:* 671–681 (1984).
Wong, N.P.; McDonough, F.E.; Hitchins, A.D.: Contribution of *Streptococcus thermophilus* to growth-stimulating effect of yogurt on rats. J. Dairy Sci. *66:* 444–449 (1983).
Yazicioglu, A. von; Yilmaz, N.: Untersuchungen über die Mikroflora von Joghurt und dessen antibakterielle Wirkung. Milchwissenschaft *21:* 87–92 (1966).

P. Bourlioux, PhD, Laboratoire de Microbiologie industrielle,
Centre d'études Pharmaceutiques, F–92290 Châtenay-Malabry (France)

Subject Index